PANDEMIC OF PERSPECTIVES

This volume brings together academics, activists, health professionals, social work practitioners, poets, and artists from different parts of the world to record their visceral experiences and critical reflections of the Covid-19 pandemic. It sheds light on how the pandemic has exposed the inequities in society and is shaping social institutions, affecting human relationships, and creating new norms with each passing day.

It examines how people from diverse societies and fields of work have come to conceptualise and imagine a new world order based on the principles of social and ecological justice, care, and human dignity. It prioritises the realm of imagination, creativity, and affect in understanding social formations and in shaping societies beyond positivist approaches. Documenting the myriad experiences of and responses to the pandemic, the volume foregrounds varied processes of making meaning; understanding impulses, resistances, and coping mechanisms; and building solidarities. Further, it also acts as a tool of memory for future generations, and articulations – artistic, political, socio-cultural, scientific – of hope and perseverance.

Its uniqueness lies in the way it brings together a much-needed interface between science, social sciences, and humanities. A compelling account of our contemporary lives, the volume will be of great interest to scholars of sociology, anthropology, politics, art and aesthetics, psychology, social work, literature, health, and medical sciences.

Rimple Mehta is a Senior Lecturer in Social Work and Communities, School of Social Sciences, Western Sydney University. She has previously worked at the Tata Institute for Social Sciences, Mumbai, and Jadavpur University, Kolkata. She has studied Sociology, Social Work, and Women's Studies. She researches and writes on gender, criminalisation of mobility, trafficking, and incarceration. Her monograph titled *Women, Mobility and Incarceration: Love and Recasting of Self across the Bangladesh-India Border* was published by Routledge in 2018. Her latest co-edited volume titled *Women, Incarcerated: Narratives from India* was published by Orient BlackSwan in 2022. She has researched with women in prisons in Mumbai, Kolkata, the Netherlands and Sydney.

Sandali Thakur is an Assistant Professor in the Centre for Women-centred Social Work, Tata Institute of Social Sciences (TISS), Mumbai. She has taught Women's and Gender Studies/Social Work/Sociology at the Azim Premji University Bengaluru, Rajiv Gandhi Institute of Youth Development Sriperumbudur, Savitribai Phule Pune University, and Tata Institute of Social Sciences Mumbai and Chennai (BALM). Sandali has been part of anti-caste struggles and co-founded Insight Foundation (a New Delhi-based organisation funded by Ford Foundation) to intervene in the area of social exclusion in higher education. She has been an Executive Committee member of the Indian Association for Women's Studies and helped set up the Women's Studies Program at Patna University. In the last few years, she has engaged with research, training and advocacy on violence against women at TISS, Mumbai. Her doctoral thesis explored social relations of caste, class, and gender among 'folk' artists of Madhubani/Mithila. She is currently working towards building an online repository on 'folk'/'tribal'/'indigenous' artists.

Debaroti Chakraborty is an Assistant Professor in the Department of Performing Arts, Presidency University, India. As a researcher-artist and performance thinker, her research interests focus on lived experiences, narratives, oral history and on making cross-cultural and inter-cultural performances. Her doctoral work broadly studies narratives of women in India and Latin America through a comparative perspective in the context of borders. Debaroti has been an instructor at the "Bodies at the Borders" collaborative video-conferencing course between Cornell University, USA, and Jadavpur University. She also teaches Latin American literatures and Comparative Literature as invited lecturer in other Universities. She writes as a performance critic with the *Telegraph*. Her latest co-edited volume titled "Centering Borders in Latin American and South Asian Contexts: Aesthetics and Politics of Cultural Production" has been published with Routledge in 2022.

PANDEMIC OF PERSPECTIVES

Creative Re-imaginings

Edited by
Rimple Mehta, Sandali Thakur
and Debaroti Chakraborty

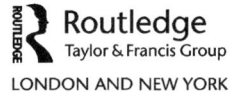

Routledge
Taylor & Francis Group

LONDON AND NEW YORK

First published 2023
by Routledge
4 Park Square, Milton Park, Abingdon, Oxon OX14 4RN

and by Routledge
605 Third Avenue, New York, NY 10158

Routledge is an imprint of the Taylor & Francis Group, an informa business

British Library Cataloguing-in-Publication Data
A catalogue record for this book is available from the British Library

ISBN: 978-1-032-02090-7 (hbk)
ISBN: 978-1-032-34090-6 (pbk)
ISBN: 978-1-003-32052-4 (ebk)

DOI: 10.4324/9781003320524

Typeset in Sabon
by SPi Technologies India Pvt Ltd (Straive)

To Rosie, who always helps me reimagine a better world ~ Jacob Appel

To Amma ~ Mahalakshmi

To my parents, Amit and Amita, and my sister, Sayani, for teaching me how to love unconditionally ~ Soumita Basu

To the thousands of migrant workers who died, lost their jobs and livelihood during the pandemic ~ Aditya Vikram Sengupta

For OG, who reminds me every day that hope is not lost ~ Rusham Sharma

For ASHA Didis (frontline healthcare workers) of Bihar who worked tirelessly during the pandemic to save our lives ~ Harshita Jha

To all the immigrants who bravely face the unfamiliar every day ~ Áshildur Linnet

To the many kinds of care, patience, and support offered by Dr. Nisha Gera, Debashish, Shruti, Silja, Tina didi, Nona, Mukta (and many, many others), who were my constants in a world that was shifting too much and too soon. Thank you! ~ Ridhima Sharma

To Dr. Dakhina Mitra, a fine person and a passionate researcher... for your love of children ~ Chandni Basu

To my parents, Amit and Amita, and my sister, Sayani, for teaching me how to love unconditionally ~ Soumita Basu

To all those who couldn't make it through the pandemic with us, and to all those who worked in various capacities so that the rest of us could; to my parents, Jerry and Swarna; to my sister, Shubathra; and to Raisa who held me through it all ~ Gitanjali Joshua

To all Indigenous and other non-Western Peoples seeking to undo the damage caused by Western 'civilisation' ~ Jim Ife

To those that have survived the pandemic with love and determination, defeating betrayal and lies ~ Nabina Das

To my mother, Alice L. Savage, who reminds me always to cultivate flowers, even in a time of revolution ~ Megan Savage

To Sanjay, our guardian angel ~ Anju Chaudhary

To the survivors of violence and the spirit of the team at Special Cell for Women ~ Trupti Jhaveri Panchal & Aarthi Chandrasekhar

To Bashabi ~ Sandali Thakur

To all those who courageously show up each day to make the world a better place ~ Rimple Mehta

To Sanjay, our guardian angel ~ Anju Chaudhary

To little love from Tot-to ~ Rosalie Purvis

To Anindya, who always helps me have faith in imagination and hope! ~ Debaroti Chakraborty

To all those who struggled to breathe during the pandemic ~ Anup Tripathi

To Sharmila, for keeping hope alive ~ Vaishali Diwakar

CONTENTS

CONTENTS

CONTENTS

CONTENTS

ARTWORKS

ACKNOWLEDGEMENTS

This volume has been possible with the creative vision of each of the contributors. We thank the contributors for joining us in this journey to engage with diverse ideas and forms of expression. We have learnt so much from each of the contributors through their vision for social change.

We thank the enthusiastic and meticulous editorial assistants – Arkadeepra Purkayastha and Anushka Bhattacharya – for being with us in this journey and helping us make this volume a reality. This volume would not have been possible without their hard work and support.

We extend our gratitude to Mary E. John, Anjali Dave, and Bashabi Barua for their engagement with our ideas and suggestions for the volume. We also thank the anonymous peer reviewers for their comments and feedback.

We acknowledge the support and contributions of our present institutions of affiliation – Western Sydney University, Australia; Tata Institute of Social Sciences, India; and Presidency University, India. The research environment, our colleagues, and students in these institutions have provided us the necessary impetus to conceptualise this volume.

This volume has been possible with the support of family and friends who stood by us at a time when every sense of 'reality' around us seemed to collapse. They gave us the necessary encouragement, which emboldened us to embark on this journey of re-imagining.

CONTRIBUTORS

Jacob M. Appel is currently an Associate Professor of Psychiatry and Medical Education at Mount Sinai's Icahn School of Medicine, where he is the Director of Ethics Education in Psychiatry and Assistant Director of the Academy for Medicine and the Humanities. Jacob is also the author of four literary novels, ten short story collections, an essay collection, a cozy mystery, a thriller, a volume of poems, and a compendium of medical dilemmas. Prior to joining the faculty at Mount Sinai, Jacob taught most recently at Brown University in Providence, Rhode Island, and at Yeshiva College, where he was the writer-in-residence. More at www.jacobmappel.com

Chandni Basu is a Guest Lecturer at the Department of Sociology, Rabindra Bharati University, Kolkata. She is also a Visiting Faculty at the Institute of Development Studies Kolkata. She is also affiliated as an Associated Researcher at the Institute of Sociology, University of Freiburg. She has been a Research Associate at the Department of Sociology, University of Frankfurt. Dr. Basu has also worked on a children's project at an asylum seekers camp in Germany. She has variously conducted guest lectures at the Ambedkar University, Delhi; West Bengal National University of Juridical Sciences; University of Strassbourg; University of Leiden; and University of Bonn. Her publications include a chapter in an edited volume *Global Childhoods Beyond the North-South Divide*, 2018. Her research interest includes children and childhood, marginality, knowledge circulation, and the postcolonial.

Soumita Basu is a solution seeker. She is a pioneer in the field of inclusive fashion and runs her own line of Inclusive clothing, Zyenika, where the designs are adapted to people's body types, physical requirements, and challenges. She was motivated to do this from her lived experience from being non-disabled to completely bedridden, and currently with 20 per cent mobility. Soumita started her career as a journalist before taking to a career in action research informing innovations and policies for social development, with particular focus on health, livelihoods, and governance. She holds a Master's in Development Studies from International Institute of Social Sciences (ISS), The Hague, and a postgraduate diploma in Journalism from the Asian College of Journalism.

Chandan Bose is an Assistant Professor of Anthropology and Sociology, Department of Liberal Arts, Indian Institute of Technology, Hyderabad. His research focuses on the meaning of work and livelihood, and ways of knowledge production and sharing among skilled communities. His first monograph *Conversations around Craft* published by Palgrave Macmillan is an ethnographic study of a household of artisans in Telangana, who share their experience of making "crafts" and of being "craftspersons" in contemporary India. At present, Chandan is editing a volume titled *Ways of Studying Craft: Methodological Reflections in Anthropology, Art History and Design* and is currently working with second-generation artisans in urban India to understand how inheritance, technology, and urbanisation help shape visions of a future.

Linda Briskman holds the Margaret Whitlam Chair of Social Work at Western Sydney University in Australia. She conducts research, publishes, and advocates in the areas of Indigenous rights, asylum seeker rights, and challenging Islamophobia. She is a member of the management committee of the Australian Council for Human Rights Education and a co-convenor of Academics for Refugees. Recent books include the co-authored Human Rights and Social Work: Towards rights-based practice (Cambridge University Press 2022), and two co-edited collections, Indigenous Health Ethics: An Appeal to Human Rights (World Scientific 2021) and Social Work in the Shadow of the Law (The Federation Press 2018). Research partnerships are both Australia-wide and international, and Linda is a regular keynote speaker and media commentator on human rights issues.

Jackie Campbell is a Mexican; is a journalist and human rights defender; accompanies women in situations of violence, also peasants in defence of territory; and is against the privatisation of water. She is the creator of the writing workshop for people deprived of their liberty and who are inside prisons called "The Right Eye of Polonius" *(El Ojo Derecho de Polonio)*. With the research "Discrimination in People Affected by Hansen's Disease Institutionalized in Argentina and Their Right to a Full Life in Society" (2019), she obtained a postgraduate degree in Human Rights in Argentina. She is a member of the production team TRIBU2020 that made the documentary "There's No Other Way" (2021).

Debaroti Chakraborty is an Assistant Professor in the Department of Performing Arts, Presidency University, India. As a researcher-artist and performance thinker, her research interests focus on lived experiences, narratives, oral history and on making cross-cultural and inter-cultural performances. Her doctoral work broadly studies narratives of women in

India and Latin America through a comparative perspective in the context of borders. Debaroti has been an instructor at the "Bodies at the Borders" collaborative video-conferencing course between Cornell University, USA, and Jadavpur University. She also teaches Latin American literatures and Comparative Literature as invited lecturer in other Universities. She writes as a performance critic with the *Telegraph*. Her latest co-edited volume titled "Centering Borders in Latin American and South Asian Contexts: Aesthetics and Politics of Cultural Production" has been published with Routledge in 2022.

Aarthi Chandrasekhar is currently Programmes Coordinator at Resource Centre for Interventions on Violence against Women (RCI-VAW), TISS, Mumbai. Her role involves programmes design and strengthening and monitoring of support services for survivors of violence. She provides capacity support to teams and partner organisations across RCI-VAW's projects in India. She has earlier worked with CEHAT engaging with the public health system. She has contributed to working groups reviewing laws and policies pertaining to women and children, guidelines on issues such as custodial deaths, and publications on gender-based violence. A postgraduate in Psychology, her professional expertise and interest lie in feminist praxis with state systems and gender-based violence and solutions.

Anju Chaudhury is a 58-year-old artist who has been running her Art School since 2001 in Dehradun. She completed graduation in Painting and postgraduation in Psychology from R.G. College, Meerut University. Apart from painting, she loves to read Indian Literature. In her free time, she likes experimenting with glass painting. She started her art school 20 years back called Shivangi Art School named after her daughter. Her students hail from all walks of life and age having a common love for Art. She has conducted six solo and combined exhibitions along with her students. These exhibitions were well covered in the media. Her last painting exhibition was inaugurated by Uttarakhand's Governor Krishna Kant in 2017. She works in almost all medium, but oil medium is her favourite. She is a curious lifelong student of art.

Nabina Das is the author of five books. Her poetry collections are *Sanskarnama* (Red River, 2017), *Into the Migrant City* (Writers Workshop, 2013), and *Blue Vessel* (Les Editions du Zaporogue, 2012). Her debut book is a novel titled *Footprints in the Bajra* (Cedar Books, 2010), and her short fiction volume is titled *The House of Twining Roses: Stories of the Mapped and the Unmapped* (LiFi Publications, 2014). Her new poetry collection *Anima and the Narrative Limits* will be appearing in 2022 from Yoda Press. Nabina's poems appear in *Poetry* magazine, *Prairie Schooner*, *Indian Literature* (National Academy of Letters), *The Yellow Nib Anthology* (Queens University, Belfast), etc. Nabina is a 2017

Sahapedia-UNESCO fellow, a 2012 Charles Wallace Creative Writing alumna, and a 2016 Commonwealth Writers features correspondent. Nabina has worked as a Creative Writing teaching faculty in universities and workshops and as a journalist for ten years. A Rutgers-Camden MFA alumna, Nabina is the editor of *Witness: Poetry of Dissent* (Red River Press, 2021) and is the co-editor of *40 under 40, an Anthology of Post-globalisation Poetry* (Poetrywala, 2016). Nabina's first book of translations "Arise out of the Lock: 50 Bangladeshi women Poets in English" is out from Balestier Press, UK.

Vaishali Diwakar teaches Sociology at St. Mira's College for Girls in Pune. Her academic interests are Sociology of film, Gender studies, and Cultural studies. Her publications involve: gender and power in the cinema of V. Shantaram; regional and national identities on the site of cinema; diaspora and Marathi literature; multiplexes and film viewing practices; and social media and teens.

Francesca Esposito is Lecturer at Westminster University of London and Research Fellow at the Institute of Social Sciences (ICS), University of Lisbon. She is also Associate Director of Border Criminologies at the University of Oxford. Her work draws on intersectional feminisms and focuses on border violence, particularly immigration detention, and bottom-up forms of resistance and solidarity. She is a member of the feminist NGO Befree (Rome, Italy), and is engaged in different feminist, antiracist, and abolitionist movements/groups.

Gaia Giuliani is a political philosopher who works as a permanent researcher at the Center for Social Studies, University of Coimbra (Portugal). She hold her PhD at the University of Torino (2005) and since then has worked at the Universities of Bologna, University of Technology Sydney, and Cambridge University, and collaborated as research associate with the University of Padua, Leeds, London (Goldsmiths and Birkbeck College) and Fordham. Her research interests focus on visual constructions of race and aims to deconstruct post-colonial (visual) archives of monstrosity through the analysis of texts coding 'fears of disasters and crisis' and their symbolic and material impact on European and Western self-representations in the context of the post-9/11 terrorist threat, the so-called migrant and refugee crises, and human/environmental catastrophes including the Covid-19 pandemic. Her methodology crosses critical race and whiteness, postcolonial, cultural, and gender studies. Among her books are *Bianco e nero. Storia dell'identità razziale degli italiani* with Dr. Cristina Lombardi-Diop (2013), which won the first prize in the 20th-21st-century category by the American Association for Italian Studies; *Race, Nation, and Gender in Modern Italy* (2019), finalist of the Gadda Prize 2019, and *Monsters, Catastrophes and the Anthropocene: A Postcolonial Critique* (Routledge 2021).

Amitesh Grover is an award-winning inter-disciplinary artist. He moves beyond theatre into visual art, film, installation, and digital art. His works shift away from the artwork or medium and produce open-ended actions, series, processes and projects. His work is anchored in social practice and revolves around themes like absence/presence, staging abandonment, the necessity of mourning, the performance of resistance to keep on living, and how to embody unsayable knowledge. His projects are shown internationally in theatres, galleries, public spaces, and on the internet. He also teaches, writes, and curates for performances.

Jim Ife has held professorial positions in social work and human rights at The University of Western Australia, Curtin University, where he is Emeritus Professor, and Western Sydney University, where he is currently Adjunct Professor. He has been involved in social work education and is active in various community roles since the 1970s, including a period as President of Amnesty International Australia and as Secretary of the Human Rights Commission of the International Federation of Social Workers. He is the author of several books in the areas of community development, human rights and social work, emphasising in particular the relationships between them.

Harshita Jha is currently working with Kudumbashree NRO as a State Project Coordinator for the PRI-CBO Convergence Project in the state of Assam. Her work is mostly focused on poverty reduction through engagement of community-based organisations with Panchayati Raj Institutions. She has done her MA in social work with specialisation in women-centred social work practice from Tata Institute of Social Sciences (TISS), Mumbai. She completed BA in Social Sciences from TISS, Guwahati. Her areas of interest are women and participatory governance and women and social entrepreneurship.

Gitanjali Joshua is a perennial student, who enjoys skipping across disciplines. She is currently exploring an intersection of law, religion, and gender in her doctoral thesis. She loves dinosaurs, the sea, and things that give her a sense of scale. She enjoys visual art and writing fiction and is experimenting with different forms and genres. One of her stories was shortlisted for the Commonwealth Short Story Prize, 2022. She somehow manages to find cats to befriend wherever she goes. You can find some of her work here: https://linktr.ee/GitanjaliJ.

Niro Kandasamy is a Lecturer in History in the School of Humanities at the University of Sydney. She teaches International and Global Studies and researches the historical dimensions of post-migration, international relations, and transnational activism with her geographical focus on Sri Lanka.

Boaz Kukundakwe is a prize winner, inter-disciplinary artist, designer, sculptor, photographer, and educator. Boaz graduated from the school of Fine Arts at Makerere University-Kampala with a Bachelor's degree in Industrial and Fine Arts (2016). He participated in Resilient African Network (RAN) Video and Photo Contest (2016) and won his first prize as the second runner. His mastery in photography led him to participate also in the Uganda Tourism Board (UTB) Photography project of documenting the tourism investments in and around Lake Victoria (2019). He has been commissioned to produce several photos and woodcut prints and other forms of art. He worked as an art teacher at Nsambya Hillside High School (2017–2019). He worked as design director at World Superior Enterprises Limited. From here, he established a company, Art & Beyond, which deals with art on a general scale. His works are unique creations, incorporating amazing characters and stories from Ugandan culture and social life into complex art pieces. Apart from Visual arts, Boaz Kukundakwe is also a singer, songwriter, composer, and performer, who does music with a primary vision of encouraging and instilling hope in people.

Pushpesh Kumar teaches Sociology at the University of Hyderabad. His recent edited work *Sexuality, Abjection and Queer Existence in Contemporary India* is forthcoming with Routledge. He serves on the international advisory board of the Community Development Journal, Oxford University Press, UK.

Áshildur Linnet has a BSc in Human Geography from the University of Iceland and a Master's degree in Human Rights and Peace Education from Universidad Nacional in Costa Rica. She is a migration expert at the Ministry of Social Affairs and Labour. Ms. Linnet worked as a migration expert at the Icelandic Red Cross, as a delegate for the IFRC and as a University teacher in development geography at the University of Iceland. She co-chaired the Platform for European Red Cross Cooperation on Refugees, Asylum seekers and Migrants for four years. Ms. Linnet is one of Iceland's leading experts on migration.

Mahalakshmi has been working in the development sector for seven years and is currently training to be a special educator. She enjoys reading and spending time by the sea. Though she identifies as an amateur, she likes to experiment with different media in her art. In the past few years, she has begun to take it more seriously to express thoughts on gender and identity. She draws inspiration in her style from the Mithila paintings of Bihar, where she spent several years. She now lives in her hometown, Chennai.

Rimple Mehta is a Senior Lecturer in Social Work and Communities, School of Social Sciences, Western Sydney University. She has previously worked at the Tata Institute for Social Sciences, Mumbai, and Jadavpur

University, Kolkata. She researches and writes on gender, criminalisation of mobility, trafficking, and incarceration. Her monograph titled *Women, Mobility and Incarceration: Love and Recasting of Self across the Bangladesh-India Border* was published by Routledge in 2018. Her latest co-edited volume titled *Women, Incarcerated: Narratives from India* was published by Orient BlackSwan in 2022. She has researched with women in prisons in Mumbai, Kolkata, the Netherlands and Sydney.

Debomita Mukherjee is a Research Assistant at the Department of Sociology, University of Hyderabad. She has an MPhil in Sociology, with a focus on the areas of Sexuality and Masculinity. She has co-authored the paper "Subordinated and Marginalised Masculinities and the Covid-19 Pandemic," which has been published in EPW.

Laban Kashaija Musinguzi, PhD, completed his Doctoral Studies at the Amsterdam Institute of Social Sciences Research, University of Amsterdam, Netherlands, in 2016. His PhD explores the intersection between Community Health and Formal Healthcare in poor resource settings. Laban also holds an MPhil from the University of Cambridge, UK, and a Bachelor of Social Work and Social Administration, from Makerere University, Uganda. His research interest is at the intersection of action and applied research in gender-based violence, children studies, general program research, and evaluation. Laban was appointed to chair the Covid-19 Department of Social Work Task Force. Currently, Laban is a Co-Principal Investigator and a Senior Researcher on the following projects: The Situation and Impact of Covid-19 on school-going girls in Uganda funded by FAWEU; Uganda Commercial Sexual Exploitation of Children (CSEC) Prevalence and KAP Study between 2019 and 2022, funded by Global Fund to End Modern Slavery (GFEMS).

Danalakota Vinay Kumar Nakash is a 25-year-old artist based in Hyderabad, India. Trained by his father, National Award winner Danalakota Vaikuntam Nakash, Vinay has been contributing to the traditional practice of Nakash paintings since 2010 when he was 15. Vinay has completed his Bachelor of Fine Arts from Jawaharlal Nehru Architecture and Fine Arts University, Hyderabad. Today an accomplished and independent artist, Vinay has received a number of accolades for this work, among which is the prestigious Kamala Devi Puraskar in 2012, while participating in several national and international exhibitions and workshops.

Trupti Jhaveri Panchal is currently an Assistant Professor and Chairperson of Centre for Women Centred Social Work in School of Social Work at Tata Institute of Social Sciences (TISS) in Mumbai. She is engaged in teaching, research, field action work, and policy advocacy. Currently she leads two projects at TISS, viz. Resource Centre for Interventions on Violence against Women (RCI-VAW) and Special Cell for Women and Children (Maharashtra). In the past 30 years, she has engaged in the area of violence against women and children, especially work with the police and various State governments for expansion/institutionalisation of feminist praxis models and to strengthen the response to survivors through direct intervention. She has co-authored the book *Multi-Agency Response to Violence against Women: Feminist Social Work within the Police System (Vitasta 2019)*. She has Bachelor's and Master's degree in Social Work and has PhD from Tata Institute of Social Sciences.

Binendri Perera is a Lecturer (Probationary) at the Department of Public and International Law of the Faculty of Law, University of Colombo. She is also a Visiting Lecturer at Sri Lanka Law College. She completed her LL.B. at the Faculty of Law of the University of Colombo. She read for her Master's at the Harvard Law School, Cambridge, Massachusetts, where she was a Cogan Scholar (2018/19). Her main research interests are constitutional law, pro-democracy movements, economic, social and cultural rights, and rights of marginalised groups.

Emerson Pessoa is a sociologist/anthropologist and Professor/researcher at University Federal of Rondônia (UNIR), Rolim de Moura (Brazil), in the Department of Countryside Education. His research and activism revolve around critical discussions on bodies, gender, sexuality, and bio-technologies in subjectivation processes. He concluded his Phd in 2020 at the Institute of Social Sciences (ICS) of the University of Lisbon with a thesis entitled: *Encarnando a europeia: biografias corporais, (i)mobili-dades e subjetividades de trabalhadoras do sexo trans e travestis brasilei-ras em Lisboa.*

Rosalie Purvis is a Libra Assistant Professor of Theatre and English at the University of Maine. She holds an MFA in Theatre Directing from Brooklyn College and a PhD in Performing and Media Arts from Cornell. Her research focuses on border studies and inter-cultural performance. Since 2000, she has worked as a theatre artist in New York City, where work has been featured at, among others, the Atlantic Theatre's Second Stage, Dixon Place, La Mama, the Culture Project, Teatro Circulo, 59 East 59, Dance New Amsterdam, 78th Street Theatre Lab, and BAX. Most recently, she joined a Kolkata-based international performing arts collective Chaepani and together they have performed at various international borders.

Stuart Rees, co-founder of the University of Sydney's Centre for Peace & Conflict Studies and Founder of Inaugural Director Sydney Peace Foundation, is Professor Emeritus at the University of Sydney. As an author of numerous books on social justice, health care and international peace negotiations, and of anthologies of poetry, his most recent work is *Cruelty or Humanity*, Bristol: Policy Press (2020). He is a regular contributor to the online platform Pearls and Irritations. In 2005, Professor Rees was awarded the Order of Australia for service to international relations and in 2018 the Jerusalem (Al Quds) Peace Prize.

Alejandra Saavendra is a Mexican illustrator and designer. Since 2008, she has collaborated across different media. In 2009, she joined SacBé Producciones, an organisation that develops audio-visual productions with social and cultural content. She was responsible for the graphics in different web documentary projects such as Frio en el Alma (www.frioenelalma. com) and Geografía del Dolor (www.geografiadeldolor.com) (2014). She was also involved in documentaries about forced disappearance in Mexico; "La Patrona" 2009 and "La Cocina de Las Patronas" (2018). From 2017 to 2019, she was head of the animation department for the documentary feature "Monarca, El Espíritu del Bosque," produced by Grupo Milenio and recently in June 2020 she was in charge of the design and illustration of the project "Migrantes de otros mundos" for Centro Latinoamericano de Investigación Periodística (migrants-otro-mundo.elclip.org).

Megan Savage is a multi-genre writer and educator living in Portland, Oregon. Her fiction has recently appeared in *Hunger Mountain #25: Art Saves*, was featured as the first audio fiction on the More Devotedly podcast, and has been twice nominated for Best New American Voices. Other publications include fiction in *Spork*, lyrical flash nonfiction in *The Gravity of the Thing*, and poetry in *Plainsongs* and *Subtropics*. She holds degrees from Bard College and Indiana University, where she served as Fiction Editor of *Indiana Review*. Currently, she teaches writing at Portland Community College in Portland, OR, where she serves on the Steering Committee for the first-and-only community college writing residency, the Carolyn Moore Writers House.

Aditya Vikram Sengupta is a Film Maker, Artist, and musician based out of India. His films have been premiered at the most prestigious international film festivals like Venice, London, Rotterdam, and Busan. He is currently working on his fourth feature film and spends the rest of his time painting, writing songs, and studying magic.

Ahmed Shamim is an Assistant Professor of Instruction at the University of Texas at Austin. He has taught Bangla in the Department of Asian Studies at UT Austin since 2015. He completed his PhD in Linguistics from the City University of New York. His research interests include Endangered Language Documentation and Description, Phonology, Morphology, Grammar, and Language Policies and Ideologies. He penned two books on Bangla language, literature, and linguistics: *Bangla Kotha* (2013) and *Shobdo Hoy Shobder Ghore* (2018).

Ridhima Sharma completed her MPhil titled "Rethinking the Cow Protection Movement: Gender, Caste and Labor at a Cow-Shelter in a North Indian Town" at the Centre for Women's Studies, Jawaharlal Nehru University, New Delhi. She is about to begin her PhD at the Department for the Study of Religion, University of Toronto, in September 2021. She has taught courses around Feminist Theory and Cultural Studies from 2018 to 2020.

Rusham Sharma is an 18-year-old student, who looks forward to pursuing law as a career ahead. She believes that an introspection of the political environment begins with an active process of learning, unlearning and thriving through networks of interdependence. She is a learning Marxist.

Mary Lourdes Silva is an associate professor of writing at Ithaca College. She received a doctoral degree in Language, Literacy, and Composition Studies from the University of California, Santa Barbara, as well as Masters of Fine Arts in Creative Nonfiction from California State University, Fresno. Her past and current research examine the citation practices of first-year college writing students, pedagogical use of multimodal and multimedia technologies and practices in the classroom, the implementation of institutional ePortfolio assessment, and movement-touch literacy as a modality to teach reflective/reflexive thinking in first-year writing. She studies the culture, literature, and dance of Argentine tango and teaches tango in upstate New York.

Vera Silva completed her Master's in Social and Cultural Anthropology with a dissertation that developed an exploratory study of a feminist anthropology of prisons in Portugal. She is currently a doctoral student at the University of Coimbra, and a member of the Centre for Research in Anthropology (CRIA). Her action-research PhD project is entitled "Configurations of Gender in Women's Prisons: Permanences, Continuities and Variations." Vera has also experience in researching intervention systems on violence against women and children, and on sexual violence. She is an activist in feminist projects and organisations, as well as in projects and networks for the human rights and support of prisoners and their families.

Karen Soldatic is a Professor, School of Social Sciences, and Institute Fellow, Institute for Culture and Society, Western Sydney University. She was awarded a Fogarty Foundation Excellence in Education Fellowship for 2006–2009, a British Academy International Fellowship in 2012, a fellowship at The Centre for Human Rights Education at Curtin University (2011–2012), where she remained an Adjunct Fellow (2012–2020), and an Australian Research Council DECRA Fellowship (2016–2019). Her research on global welfare regimes builds on her 20 years of experience as an international (Cambodia, Sri Lanka, Indonesia), national, and state-based senior policy analyst, researcher, and practitioner. She obtained her PhD (Distinction) in 2010 from the University of Western Australia.

Sandali Thakur is an Assistant Professor in the Centre for Women-centred Social Work, Tata Institute of Social Sciences (TISS), Mumbai. She has taught Women's and Gender Studies/Social Work/Sociology at the Azim Premji University Bengaluru, Rajiv Gandhi Institute of Youth Development Sriperumbudur, Savitribai Phule Pune University, and Tata Institute of Social Sciences Mumbai and Chennai (BALM). Sandali has been part of anti-caste struggles and co-founded Insight Foundation (a New Delhi-based organisation funded by Ford Foundation) to intervene in the area of social exclusion in higher education. She has been an Executive Committee member of the Indian Association for Women's Studies and helped set up the Women's Studies Program at Patna University. In the last few years, she has engaged with research, training and advocacy on violence against women at TISS, Mumbai. Her doctoral thesis explored social relations of caste, class, and gender among 'folk' artists of Madhubani/Mithila. She is currently working towards building an online repository on 'folk'/'tribal'/'indigenous' artists.

Anup Tripathi is an Assistant Professor, Sociology at FLAME University, Pune, India. He has obtained his PhD and Master's degrees from the Tata Institute of Social Sciences, Mumbai. His interest areas are Urban Studies and Housing. His doctoral thesis attempts to conceptualize homelessness in the Indian context. He has worked on the issues of e-governance, urban planning, EIA and SIA in the past.

Sharlotte Tusasiirwe is a Uganda-born, internationally educated social worker. After completing a Bachelor's degree in Social Work in Uganda and a Master's degree in Social Work and Human rights from the University of Gothenburg, Sweden, Sharlotte pursued her PhD at Western Sydney University from 2016 to 2020. Sharlotte is very interested in researching Social Work Education, and her PhD has been focused on how to decolonise social work education and practice to create culturally appropriate and contextually relevant profession. She has researched how African knowledges and Obuntu/Ubuntu philosophies can inform social work. She is interested in theorising how diverse epistemologies from our diverse cultures can be at the centre of social work education and practice. She loves teaching and researching Indigenous knowledges, ageing and age-old wisdom, community-led initiatives, community development and advocacy, and gender, among others.

Sushrija Sakshi Upadhyaya Sushrija Sakshi Upadhyaya is an Associate Consultant in Cyber Security at Ernst & Young's Technology Consulting. She graduated in Political Science from Miranda House, University of Delhi and completed her Master's with specialization in Criminology and Justice at Tata Institute of Social Sciences, Mumbai while working extensively with the prison system. Her postgraduate thesis centred around the Right to Information Act and Activism, wherein she explored the concept of Whistleblowing in the Indian Public Sector. As a data privacy and information security professional, her interest area lies in the constantly evolving cyberspace and its implication on the regulatory landscape. She is also particularly interested in the role that coherent public policy, law, and citizenship practices play in expanding access and opportunities to all.

Anil Vangad hails from a small Warli tribal village in Maharashtra, north of the cosmopolitan city of Mumbai in India. He has been painting for the last 20 years in the traditional art style of the Warlis, experimenting with themes of gods and goddesses as well as contemporary issues of our times. It was the artist's mother who influenced and taught him how to paint. He is not just passionate about painting but also about farming, which is the traditional occupation of the Warlis. Vangad's art works have been exhibited in the United States, Britain, France, Singapore, Hong Kong, and so on. In 2014, his work was introduced to the Santa Fe Folk Art market for the first time. He received the WCC Award of Excellence from UNESCO for his painting in the same year, imprinting Warli art onto the world map.

INTRODUCTION

*Debaroti Chakraborty, Sandali Thakur,
and Rimple Mehta*

It was the early days of the pandemic and the lockdown, when the world was grappling with fear and uncertainty generated by the barrage of information storming from multiple sources, which ranged from speculations to seemingly definitive proclamations. Three of us came together through the digital medium to share our experiences of making sense of all that we were seeing, hearing, and experiencing. We were confronted, on the one hand, with a deep sense of anxiety over our survival and those around us, while on the other, with an aggravating fear of losing human touch. The familiarity of everydayness began to disappear from every walk of life, when we stepped towards making the transition into a new world order. We found that our conversations not only revolved around ways to understand and cope with the new reality that confronted us but the need to critically engage with the rationale of this sudden shift and human responses that stemmed from it. While it is too early to be able to find resolutions, the contexts of what is 'safe' 'universal', 'homogeneous', 'labour', 'essential', 'access', 'discrimination' stimulate crucial debates against the backdrop of the pandemic.

We wanted to create a platform where people from across cultures and professions could articulate their experiences. This volume foregrounds diverse critical and artistic perspectives that may have been triggered by the pandemic but do not remain confined to it. Rather these perspectives, in their parallels and dissonances, make valuable comments on larger structures of contemporary societies which exist irrespective of the current pandemic and also shape human crisis at all levels during the pandemic. Such articulations do not always find representation in media reports, surveys or other official discourses. Our collaboration, therefore, stems from the need to find articulations that would help understand the nature of this transition in diverse contexts of societies, cultures, economic situations, and personal histories. We come from different disciplinary and research backgrounds but what has brought us together and continues to bind us is the concern for the values of social justice, human dignity, and the ethics of care. These values form the ethos of this volume.

DOI: 10.4324/9781003320524-1

The idea for this volume came out of the realisation that Covid-19 has laid bare the unsustainability of the present systems and institutions that undergird those systems and that there is a dire need to imagine alternatives. The other impulse was to document and archive human stories of loss, struggle, reflection, compassion, social action, and resilience, in the face of the pandemic. We wanted to foreground emotional and visceral responses as domains capable of making an alternative history that documents experiences instead of only the statist narrative of mathematical models and projections. This collaboration also generated a valuable meaning-making process in which we worked through several dichotomies such as those of connections and contradictions, compassion and violence, isolation and social mobilisation, in a world that was suddenly marked by unforeseen norms of social behaviour and by the lack of any immediate remedy.

The pandemic has given rise to an avalanche of perspectives that constantly destabilises a monolithic understanding of the world order. Artists have creatively expressed a plethora of experiences – despair stemming from witnessing the pain of communities around them, inability to find 'home' in existing ways of life, hope and hopelessness as they live through the pandemic. Activists have pointed towards the deepening vulnerability of the already marginalised, as existing safety nets and support networks disappear. They have risked their lives and freedoms to unmask hidden agendas of divisive politics beneath the veneer of efficient governance. Medical practitioners have reflected upon their experiences at the frontline, shed light on the inequities that have become more prominent since the outbreak of Covid-19, and explored the field of bioethics in this light (Boyd 2020; Constantine et al. 2020). Feminists have highlighted the double burden borne by women both at home as well as at their workplace (Kabeer et al. 2021; Dewan 2022) and the increase in instances of domestic and intimate partner violence (Mlamb-Ngcuka 2020). The impact of Covid-19 on prisoners as well as those in immigrant detention centres has been highlighted from within criminology as well as other disciplines (Suhomlinova et al. 2022; Caraballo 2020; Tazreiter and Metcalfe 2021). Social workers have articulated the need to prioritise both macro- and micro-level work to facilitate a path to social recovery for individuals and communities (Cross and Benson 2021; McPherson 2020). The glaring divide between the Global North and the Global South is unravelling itself differently at every stage of the pandemic (Mehta and Briskman 2022). There are possibilities of looking at these fields of social observation and practice as existing at intersections rather than as fragmented perspectives. This volume places these multifarious and multidisciplinary articulations within a shared space to throw light on ethico-political paradigms and processes that shape societies during the pandemic and beyond it.

This volume is unique as it cuts across disciplinary and professional boundaries and brings together academics, activists, social work practitioners, novelists, poets, and artists from about 11 countries, exploring themes ranging from bioethics, domestic violence, communication strategies, housing, to Shakespearean tragedy and tango. It brings together a much-needed interface between science, social sciences, and humanities. The volume combines theoretical analysis, reflective essays, along with poetic and artistic expressions – each piece a commentary on a unique and significant aspect of the pandemic. It emphasises the importance of creative social change and the role of art in enabling people find value in their experiences during prolonged periods of isolation, as well as build solidarities. As editors, we envisioned a collection that would be able to valourise visceral experiences, critical thinking, and social activism as necessary and correlated fields of human responses rather than present them within existing sets of academic hierarchies. In addition, the polyphony of voices in the volume also emphasises the need to prioritise layers of human experiences and specificities of contexts in matters of governance, policy building, crisis management, and personal coping mechanisms, which are usually overdetermined by universal and empirical norms.

We embraced an approach towards understanding the impact of this pandemic on society and its institutions and systems, and simultaneously the influence of individual experiences in shaping history. This volume will act not only as a collection of articles, stories, poetry, and artwork that critiques unsustainable socio-economic and political systems but also, as a tool of memory for future generations, and a symbol of hope and perseverance for individuals and communities. In sum, it is meant to archive and document visceral responses while people are reeling under the impact of the pandemic to foreground how affect feeds into processes of making meaning and understanding impulses, resistances, and coping mechanisms. Our underlying conviction is that self-expression soothes, heals, and creates possibilities, by allowing us to connect with ourselves and others.

We brought together, as chapters essays, poetry, and artwork in an attempt to critique and re-imagine ideologies, practices, and institutions through different modes of expression. The chapters have been worked on across different periods of time during the pandemic and lockdowns in 2020 and 2021. Each chapter indicates the month when the contributor began to engage in this process of reflecting, critiquing, and re-imagining. Some contributors have since revised parts of their chapter to incorporate concerns that have emerged in recent times. This introduction itself has been written over a little more than a year – starting from April 2020 to July 2021, and has been re-visited several times. We included multiple forms of expression to open a space for different modes of communication. While some contributors have opted to express themselves in the conventional academic form, others have chosen to present their experiences and ideas in a personal, anecdotal manner, or through poetry and visual art. This has enriched the volume as the visceral nature of responses shaped by subjectivity, personal history, and social location, have been prioritised. We believe that all these different forms of expression have the capacity to create a polyphony, where the

3

process of re-imagining will require each of us from diverse walks of life and different areas of interest to come together and join the polyphony, while also making our individual voices heard. The contributors hail from across the world and have written about their experiences from a wide range of geographical and social locations, presenting intersecting standpoints of age, gender, caste, ability, nationality, race, and ethnicity. Since Covid-19 is a global pandemic, the sentiments, imaginations, and arguments in the volume in a sense speak to each other, crossing spatial and social boundaries.

Through this volume, we question who gets to participate in the re-imagining and make a political claim based on lived experience. Lived experience claims legitimate epistemological significance in the chapters in this volume. The contributors are implicated in the narratives they weave. Their ability to mobilise the self that experiences as well as the self that witnesses and shapes, sharpens their analysis. Their own lived experience, situatedness, resistance as well as conviction render their writings a shrapnel-like character that does not seem to mince words or shy away from inflicting wounds onto the readers in a bid to elicit empathy, compassion, and, of course, action. In this way, different contributors, either through the written word or through artistic expressions, bring into sharp focus the inequalities unveiled by the pandemic, evoking a sense of urgency for re-imagining alternatives.

Responses to Covid-19

Since December 2019, the world has been witnessing unforeseen challenges of Covid-19 pandemic that is taking its toll on human lives, economy, and sense of belonging. Perceptions in the neo-liberal, post-global world are constantly being shaped by politics of the media and the social media in definitive ways (Shaw 2020). If we refer to the past, we will observe that the origin stories around a pandemic usually perceive the outbreak as a threat coming from the outside world characterised by 'the other' like that of the myth of a group of Spanish people who brought smallpox to Mexico (Brooks 1993) or as the result of a deliberate act of deviation by a community like that of the Jews being dirty and causing plague or conjectures among Christian missionaries about the epidemic smallpox being an act of God's punishment (Pringle 2015). In a similar vein, the media was blazing with stories of the emergence of the novel coronavirus due to an accident of leakage from a high-level biosecurity laboratory in Wuhan, a city located in central China. Another origin theory claimed that the virus originated from a wet market in China. These origin theories that circulated in global media raised discontentment to an extent that triggered a culture of banning Chinese goods in many countries. We observed a wave of xenophobia, toxic comments, and jibes hurled at China posited as the 'other'. Amidst such havoc, international and national passage of commodities and people continued for a while, leading to complex forms of othering and heightened fear of contamination.

When the first wave hit, frontline workers risked their lives to provide medical aid to as many as they could, scientists and researchers grappled to make a breakthrough, and media portals flooded with continuous updates about the numbers affected and recent developments in research. As the pandemic wreaked havoc, 'believers of science' and those with the privilege of a home and access to information, isolated themselves, while the rest mostly included either the underprivileged or the 'non-believers of science'. On the one hand, while many were lamenting and coping with the rupture in community life and loss of human touch, in many contexts a toxic culture of stigma, wrought with fear of contamination, was shown towards the ones affected or towards potential carriers (Sotgiu and Dobler 2020).

The pandemic evoked a bouquet of conceptual vocabulary in the initial days – 'social distancing', 'home isolation', 'self-quarantine', 'contagion', 'essential and non-essential' – viewed as the only available mechanisms of fighting against the disease at that moment. Newer kinds of conceptual binaries created newer categories of disposable populations. Self-quarantine, social distancing, home isolation, and all these concepts generated a multiple range of emotions in people across the world. These terms had already shaped the everyday reality of a large number of minority communities, in different contexts, whose lived experiences have been invisible. Undocumented migrants, prisoners, detainees, refugees, asylum seekers, people with mental illness, to name a few, are familiar with the experience of isolation, distancing, and quarantine even prior to the pandemic. The pandemic either meant an increase in the intensity of these experiences or the imposition of a new set of stigmas on groups that are already marginalised. 'Home isolation' was a mockery of the experiences of those rendered homeless because of structural inequalities. The spread of the virus was mapped in a world already marked by existing divisions of privilege.

Essential and Non-essential

The difference between essential and non-essential services and people associated with these services became glaring in the initial phase of the pandemic itself. Sanitation workers, healthcare workers, social workers, on the one hand, and truck drivers, seafarers, and those within the supply chain and logistics domains, on the other, went out to work and risked their lives, so that essential systems and services could continue to run seamlessly. The otherwise stigmatised and invisibilised community of sanitation workers received garlands of gratitude, as the pandemic unmasked their 'relevance' (The Indian Express 2020). However, safety nets, PPE kits, and other kinds of social protection continued to elude them.

People's relationships with food and other essential commodities are shaped by personal and community histories, conditions of living, income, and psychological and social conditioning. The panic of the pandemic exacerbated people's need to stock up basics for emergencies and triggered unusual practices. In the wake of the lockdown, it was reported that people in the United States were hoarding toilet papers (Baertlin and Fares 2020). In India, people were stocking up rice and pulses, while in some places people bought pets and plants (Khosla 2021). This was in sharp contrast with the sight of daily wage earners and labourers, who endlessly queued up for ration (Mitra 2021).

While the pandemic has disentangled for us and created new meanings of what is essential and what is not, it has also created a sinister hierarchy between who is essential and who is not. How did healthcare workers decide whom to treat and whom to refuse treatment, in the face of scarce and fast-diminishing resources? Decisions regarding apportioning of care and withdrawing life-saving equipment from those whose lives are considered to be disposable within the hierarchies of age and 'ability' have thrown up moral-ethical questions that will continue to haunt us. How old or disabled does one have to be in order to get de-selected from the efforts to be saved? Whose life is essential and who is non-essential?

The way in which governmental policies categorised and fixed notions of 'essential' and 'non-essential' also throws open the complex question of the inherent discriminatory attitude towards fields of work, people's position and relationship with society, people's access to education, healthcare, food and shelter and art practices. After the immediate shutting down of theatres and spaces for live arts, the government in some countries like the U.S. and India did not wake to the need of providing alternative modes of arts practice and sustenance for artists. Moreover, the life-affirming value of creative practices is not acknowledged by any of the discourses that seek to quantify the social role of arts to fit the designated categories of 'essential' and 'non-essential'.

It is important to note at this point that these categories which were rolled out as strategies to manage a medical crisis, stem from hierarchical attitudes which pre-existed the pandemic and continue to inform policy-making in various ways even after the severity of the pandemic has now been tackled. For instance, in India, offline classes in schools and colleges were the last to open up while religious gatherings, political gatherings, fairs and festivities had acquired legal permissions for long. Moreover, in 2022, hybrid systems continue to prevail in schools and colleges which are periodically shut down on grounds of other kinds of threats like that of a very hot summer. In the 'third world' context like that of India, a huge percentage of students do not have access to an internet service or a device to attend classes. This loss in the education sector is not accounted for because it easily slips into the category of 'non-essential', now fixed by emergency rulings to manage the pandemic.

'Social Distancing'

The initial days of the pandemic witnessed different kinds of responses to the illness itself as well as to the discourse around it. The term 'social distancing', for instance, which refers to the practice of keeping a safe distance from others continues to be considered as non-negotiable within prevention protocols worldwide, received flak from various quarters (Allen et al. 2020; Long 2020). In a hierarchical society such as India, where the outlawed tradition of untouchability continues to be practised with caste-groups engaged in labour practices considered as 'polluting', the term evokes and legitimises processes of othering. Smita Patil (2021) resurrects the moment of the plague epidemic that had ravaged parts of western India at the end of the 19th century, believed to have travelled to Bombay through the sea route from Honk Kong. The intertwined questions of caste, gender, and custom became central in organising relief for people, as 'upper'-caste men across religions objected to male health workers examining their wives by touching. Food served by people belonging to 'lower' castes was refused by caste Hindus. Due to persisting resistance from select caste/community groups, hospitals aimed at catering to different communities had to be established. In this and several other contexts globally, where there are distinct stratifications, the term 'social distancing' only exacerbates existing social, economic, and political hierarchies. A more neutral term 'physical distancing' was offered as an alternative later in the Covid-19 pandemic, carrying within it the scientific prescription of physical distancing but one that is cognisant of the importance of social connections (Allen et al. 2020).

Social Media

Social media portals remain as living documents containing human impulses of hatred and compassion in these dire situations of survival. The callous attitudes of governments in many countries and the imposition of universal norms of containment without attention to specific contexts led to a huge massacre of lives of migrant workers, daily wage earners, and labourers (Singh et al. 2020). While the atrocities of governing systems and loss of lives have been glossed over by popular media controlled by the state, the public has claimed social media spaces to resist, extend support, form human networks, and connect across borders (Wong et al. 2021). Alongside, it is also noticeable how social media users spontaneously shared personal ways of relating to one's sense of home and to one's creative self in situations of isolation during the initial phase of the pandemic. In the first wave, despite high-brow criticism hurled towards indiscriminate sharing of artistic and culinary explorations in times of human crisis, they continued to flood social media as vignettes of human resilience and longing for validation. The simple yet intimate acts of reaching out to loved ones, sharing artwork and recipes, playing music, writing poems, knitting, doing one's own dance, or sharing one's moment of joy, are extremely precious ways of telling and listening to stories and experiences shaped by these difficult times. However, a heavy curtain fell over such unconstrained sharing of creative impulses over social media, as several countries continued to fight a grim battle with the second and third waves of the viral infection.

India witnessed a harrowing disaster under the second wave of the pandemic, where the public health infrastructure had collapsed. People infected by Covid-19 and their families were frantically searching for medicines, oxygen, and hospital beds; crematoriums were ablaze with endless fire from carcasses while news of the dead was systematically buried (Bhaumik et al. 2021). Amidst this chaos and shock, an unprecedented support was forged over social media by human networks and civil societies working tirelessly towards sourcing funds, information, oxygen, medicine, and care for people (Bahadur 2021). Social media has been a catalyst in this process by providing a quasi-democratic space for sharing information as well as to help garner support and solidarity across borders.

Where Is the Communion?

As protocols of distancing and of containing the virus were rolled out in official statements and press notes, the obscurity and arbitrariness around some of these categories remain unresolved. For instance, in a world where all theatres have been shut down and live performance spaces are forbidden, where is arts practice situated in the grid that maps needs and economy into categories of 'essentials' and 'non-essentials'? Madhu Raghavendra (2021) raised this point through his powerful poem 'Artist':

> I don't mind being the non-essential
> knowing you will come looking
> when things are broken
> and nothing else works.
> Art is non-essential
> Until it is not.

This seemingly inevitable restriction on arts practice and communion renders the occupation of arts practice as a 'non-essential' and may catalyse the formulation of educational policies that de-prioritise arts and humanities. As opposed to natural sciences, the contribution of liberal arts in the context of social development cannot be measured by positivist parameters of growth. Thus, the validity and social need of arts practice have been debated as much as the status of an artist in society. This sudden disruption of arts practice has fuelled discussions on the one hand around the emotional and social need for art and has helped link these discourses with the marginalisation and invisibility of artists across decades. Teaching and learning practices related to the arts and artmaking heavily rely on the realm of experiences, where aspects of the sensorium and communion gain utmost meaning. The present crisis poses a challenge to spaces of collective experiences and thereby to knowledge systems that valourise everyday practices and shared modes of lives. We are faced with a dilemma of how to address the lack of liveness and the disappearance of spaces of communion, as we transition into the world of the digital to perform ways of 'connectivity' and 'normalcy'. The earlier systems of social interaction and community formation face threats of being relegated to the domain of the 'non-essential'. At this hour, we need to revisit the multiple meanings of communion in the context of different cultures, to find ways of restoring the knowledge systems that are embedded in daily practices involving collective and public spaces. In the novel *Things Fall Apart*, Chinua Achebe (2013: 118) writes

> A man who calls his kinsmen to a feast does not do so to save them from starving. They all have food in their own homes. When we gather together in the moonlit village ground it is not because of the moon. Every man can see it in his own compound. We come together because it is good for kinsmen to do so.

Here, Achebe valourises the mundane events of collective experience as practices that forge stronger solidarities in a community and help sustain in the face of infiltration and threats of erasures. This understanding shapes many systems of knowledge formation that, alongside the cognitive, rely on the emotive and artistic ways of making meaning. Educational, economic, corporate, legal, and medical systems spell a set of imperatives that mark virtual platforms with the formal codes and behaviour of workplaces, bereft of human emotions. The virtual platforms of interaction define performance and human interaction through the lens of efficacy, efficiency, and effectiveness as Jon McKenzie (2000) explores in his foundational book *Perform or Else: From Discipline to Performance*.

On the other hand, it is meaningful to re-invent ways of communicating over virtual platforms that can disrupt the culture of invisibility and inaudibility of human presence and make space for creating newer kinds of intimacies as opposed to practices of physical distancing and lack of communion. A remarkable example would be Troy Anthony and Jerome Ellis' made for Zoom performance 'Passing Notes' (2020) that dealt with seven stages of grief and was created to offer a shared space through which strangers could articulate their sense of grief and loss (Schotzko 2020). The title of the performance reflects on the intimate act of passing notes to friends in school with a lot of trust. The virtual intimacies, such as this, can forge a space for sharing vulnerabilities, anxieties, and personal narratives of struggle inside and outside of domestic spaces that do not find voice in the official narratives of the pandemic.

Diverse, Unequal Experiences

The pandemic has defamiliarised our relationship with time, as with much else. The affective states during the suspended time of the lockdown, marked by waiting, delaying, persisting, and maintaining, have characterised the collective experience of time (Baraitser 2017). The disruption/rupture in our taken-for-granted experience of time has had different implications for different people. Women stuck in violent homes, who have waited desperately for the lockdown to end, have felt time coagulate into a viscous fluid, refusing to flow. Migrants waiting/walking to return to their homes have had their journeys punctuated by the absence of a safety net, essential services and the apparition of state brutality. Children wait to go (back) to school. Teachers and learners long to go back to the classroom – away from the veneer of digital accessibility that tend to mask dispassionate, business-like transactions. For many young women pursuing higher education in towns and cities far away from home, the pandemic has meant going back to the fraught space of the home, where they find themselves straddling the very different worlds of online education on the one hand and gendered experience of restrictions and domestic responsibilities on the other. Similarly, for queer individuals, moving from campuses that allow for questioning norms and fashioning identities back into the space of the home has perhaps meant an existential reversal in their temporal world. Educational campuses are supposed to be spaces marked by the freedom to explore the self and the world, forge friendships, intimacies, and bonds based on democratic values, where, in the words of bell hooks (2018), there is no love without justice – for many, perhaps an entirely new way of thinking about and organising relationships. At the same time, non-normative bodies located variously on the spectrum of social abilities look at the opening up of the world with apprehension, as the new normal does not necessarily promise a transformed one. While many metropolitan cities had almost erased the struggles of the homeless, the migrant workers, and the urban poor, the pandemic also left many people from middle-class families jobless (Inani 2021). These people, who have suddenly lost sustenance, are often not covered by support groups since they were previously contained by a sense of economic and moral stability of the so-called middle class.

The pandemic is not a leveller as was initially proclaimed. It has further deepened the hierarchies of power across gender, class, caste, race, sexuality, ability, age, ethnicity, nationality, and other axes of stratification (Bowleg 2020; Zarkov 2020). Economic vulnerability of the masses has become glaringly visible, and the response of governments has ranged from being protectionist to being apathetic/callous towards the desperate measures people took to deal with lockdowns and the concomitant loss of livelihood and shelter (Sengupta and Jha 2020). Will the institutions of the new world continue to be inhabited by people and cultures that uphold exclusionary, discriminatory norms and practices? If access and mobility continue to elude and productivity persists as the marker of human worth, doesn't staying captive in the liminal time-space of the lockdown offer a more emancipatory existence? What are the ways in which we need to re-think deprivation, accessibility, mobility, health, and well-being?

Care and Labour

Pedagogues and thinkers have expressed strong views about the creation of a new hyphenated space the private-domestic across virtual platforms, that foregrounds newer subjectivities, vulnerabilities, and negotiations informed by a sudden shift of all aspects of our life to the digital (Schotzko 2020). The work-from-home situation has also deepened gender inequities, shaped by different registers of class, that surface in the hyphenated private-domestic space in latent ways. Helen Lewis's (2020) *Atlantic* article, 'The Coronavirus is a Disaster for Feminism', discusses the gender inequities that unfold through corporate and academic structures, particularly in precarious situations when domestic labour cannot be easily or safely shared or outsourced. Lewis (2020) shares instances of women, in heterosexual relationships, who have been forced or co-opted to take a break from their professional careers to respond to constant domestic needs or in favour of their partners' jobs who happen to be a frontline worker.

Women's role of care and nurture has become more entrenched during the pandemic, often at the expense of their own careers. This has been particularly difficult for women who are seen to be the primary caregivers in many cultural contexts. In several families across the world, expectation from women to take care of domestic chores and home-schoolers increased during the lockdown, to the detriment of efforts towards a sustainable reorganisation of gendered household labour. Several women precariously balanced performing both wage work and unpaid care work within the space of the household.

Many women shared on social media about how their professional, creative, or academic pursuits have taken a backseat because they have been unable to balance humongous responsibilities at home and the compulsion to be present in the virtual workspace on almost a 24x7 basis. Women academics are known to take on an additional burden both at home as well as at their space of work. They have borne the brunt of the pandemic while having to take care of their infants and home-schoolers and teaching their students online (O'Keefe and Courtois 2020; Docka-Filipek and Stone 2021). The decrease in the number of submissions in academic journals made by women academics during the pandemic is a tell-tale sign of society's primary expectation of them: care work (Viglione 2020).

In the Indian context, there has been a steep decline in women's workforce participation amidst rising unemployment rates in general (Dewan 2022). The probability of getting back work lost to the pandemic is much less in the case of women, creating conditions of chronic dependencies (Deshpande 2020). Domestic workers, a largely women-dominated workforce, whose cheap labour allows families to flourish, have been laid off and recruited again depending on the extent of the fear of infection perceived by their employers. Their precarity has increased, given the uncertainty around wages as they are not paid when they are not called for work or are unable to get to work due to fear around their own health. The pandemic has unpacked these unresolved inequities by compelling a quick transition in patterns of living, working, and relating to private and public spaces. It reveals the divides that already existed but were shielded behind manifold registers of privilege.

The discourse around social reproduction that had become relegated to the background has resurfaced in recent times and has been rightly receiving much attention after the pandemic struck (Stevano et al. 2021). The question of care has been resurrected in the context of the pandemic as one of the most fundamental elements of regeneration and reproduction of life, yet that has been one of the most invisibilised and overlooked dimensions of social life. The pandemic has excavated the structures of care and dependency that lay hidden. The dependence of humans on other humans, non-humans, and the environment has manifested itself in multiple ways during the lockdown.

Pandemic of Perspectives

The pandemic has intervened and ruptured existing weaves of our social fabric. It has either introduced newer hierarchies or has deepened existing divides into gaping holes that might need years of critical reform work to be sutured. As discussed, a series of neologisms have been put in place as codes for understanding and interacting in this unfamiliar social world shaped by the pandemic. Most of these binaries – essential/non-essential, accessibility/inaccessibility, disposable/non-disposable, physical distancing/ social distancing, productivity/non-productivity, vaccinated/unvaccinated and others – serve to map and manage the crisis but fail to address the specific contexts and experiences of people. In this section, we discuss, through the different chapters in this volume, experiential aspects of the pandemic beyond statistics and neologisms.

Touch

The narrative of touch is undergoing an unprecedented transformation since the transmission of the Covid-19 infection is based on human contact. People have also been lamenting the loss of touch as a vital sensory experience that informs consciousness, memory, and sense of familiarity. Robin Dunbar, Emeritus Professor of Psychology at the Oxford University, said, 'Physical contact is a part of the mechanism we use to set up our relationships, friendships and family memberships' (Stokel-Walker 2020). He brought a physiological aspect into perspective by pointing out that the stroking of hairy skin triggers the release of the endorphin system in our brain, which translates into a feeling of warmth. Thus, the loss of human touch has evoked deep ruptures in the psyche, often intensified by experiences of isolation.

How does one experience touch and yet communicate or transcend the fear related to spaces/objects of community use, 'unknown' bodies, 'sick' bodies? The protocols of distancing have prompted privileged sections of societies to move into home isolation, while large masses of the population, living in slums, on the streets or in other cramped situations, are perceived to be potential carriers of the virus and thus cordoned off as castaways (Banerjee and Bhattacharya 2020). Since the initial phase of the pandemic, a growing inhumaneness has been displayed towards 'sick' bodies, labouring bodies, or migrant bodies.

Shamim's poem and Saavendra's artwork, in this volume, evoke the bodies that are cast away, forgotten by the protocols of distancing. Saavendra's piece represents naked bodies of refugee women who hold hands and dance in a circle. Much like the witches of Shakespeare's Macbeth, the frenzied dance of the refugee women embodies resistance and a moment of solidarity that foreshadows a preparation. Shamim's poem evokes a sense of numbness that stems from the fear of touching human bodies. Shamim laments how this talks to repressed hostilities and a barrenness of human emotions. The pandemic has unravelled deep contradictions in one's inner life as one copes with an increasing despair of losing touch and at the same time with an evolving relationship with a sense of 'home' textured by objects, emptiness, people, and rituals of living.

Das and Savage's poems speak to each other from starkly different cultural contexts in terms of their unique ways of understanding an intimate relationship through habits of the everyday couched in nuanced meanings of 'touch'. Lourdes Silva's chapter *My Tango Life Cancelled* poignantly explores the visceral as well as affective quality of touch in her life of being a Tango dancer. She shares the deeper imprints created by touch and the lack of it in her life during the pandemic. Finally, after 56 days, when she dances Tango with her practice partner, she discovered a renewed meaning of this dance form, revealed through the sensory and emotive experience of touch. This chapter strongly resonates with Eleanor Morgan's article 'Lost Touch: How a Year without Hugs Affects Our Mental Health', in which Morgan expresses how the visceral experience of touch translates into a component of memory, of smell, of groundedness and catalyses the process of recuperation from difficult physical or mental states (Morgan 2021). Sensory experience of touch is a way of relating to the world around and thus as a mode of making meaning.

Social behaviour and patterns of building relationships are couched differently in different cultures and contexts. Most of these behavioural gestures are associated with touch, like that of the double air kiss in France, the tight embrace in Italy, the robust handshake in the Netherlands or the physically more distant gesture of *namaste* (the palms meet each other by way of showing respect) in India. In the wake of the pandemic, physical contact was unexpectedly curtailed. People negotiated with what could be appropriate ways of social interaction such that we can abide by the safety protocols and yet not harm people whom we socially meet and care for. While practices of wearing masks, lockdowns, and restrictions on mobility and business enterprises were imposed on the public domain, the limits of ensuring safety were now pushed to the realm of the personal, which are often informed by affordability and subjectivity. Re-writing the narrative of touch involves revisiting the ideas and practices of distancing and those of touch and allowing newer social modes to evolve.

Home and the World

The experience and consciousness of 'home' represent a multitude of meanings. It incorporates the material, emotional, and existential dimensions of lives. The experience of home has changed drastically during the pandemic. Staying home/observing home isolation has been considered a way to care for fellow humans. But who is able to or can afford to stay at home? Those who do not have their own space to self-quarantine were evicted from the public space they had come to claim, even if precariously. Homelessness was met with a renewed sense of disgust, as it evoked the fear of contagion.

The idea of 'home' has been explored by a few chapters in different ways in the volume. Tripathi's chapter, for instance, raises an important question of decent housing as a basic right for all and an end to structural inequalities that have historically dominated housing access in India. Chaudhury and Mahalakshmi's artworks draw our attention to the gendered idea of the home. The contemplative woman in Chaudhury's artwork seems to bear witness to a multitude of emotions while reminiscing her past during the pandemic – bitter, sweet, bittersweet. In Mahalakshmi's artwork, on the other hand, the woman is seen located in the midst of the home-quagmire; her pandemic-induced incarceration within the boundaries of her home being not a radical departure from but a continuation of her pre-pandemic predicament. The tenacity with which patriarchal, heteronormative institutions such as family and marriage exist well into the present, perhaps by morphing to snugly fit into neo-liberal, capitalist, and right-wing socio-economic systems, has made women's journeys out of the labyrinth even more elusive. In many cultural contexts, for women, home is where the 'self' is entwined within a web of relationships that structure their lives in myriad ways (Gilligan 1995). But women also question their own place within it and in the larger world.

For women confined within their homes with violent partners, staying at home/observing home isolation meant a severe compromise of their safety, survival, and well-being. In all these instances, the promise of 'home' as a safe space remains elusive. Campbell frames the violent murders of women by their partners in Mexico as 'normal' and 'banal' that go unnoticed till activists like her draw public attention towards the issue, at the risk of back-lash and threat to their own safety. Women ask why their everyday lives should be organised by violence and why home should be a space where they are crucified every day and must resurrect themselves every day. Why do care and justice elude women with such persistence? Beyond the space of the home, the structural violence experienced by migrant women in India during the lockdown, carrying children and meagre belongings, walking hundreds of miles to reach home, in the process giving birth, menstruating, and dying, forecloses the possibility for them of articulating any aspiration for or claim towards the ethics of care and justice (Hans et al. 2021).

Briskman provides another perspective to the meanings of home during Covid-19 by making a reference to the experiences of migrant and refugee communities in the social housing complexes in Melbourne. She alludes to the politics of language and how appropriate information did not reach the refugees in these housing complexes as interpreters were not mobi-lised by the state with the same sense of urgency as would have been effective to curb the spread of the virus in those communities. Her analy-sis of bordering practices highlights how state borders keep shrinking into smaller and smaller bubbles, leaving a number of disadvantaged communities in isolation. A sense of 'homelessness' prevails for refugee and migrant communities within Australia and globally as they grapple to have their voices heard and their presence visibilised in destination countries.

Governance

The post-2008 policy of austerity in the Global North and a continuous rollback of welfare in the Global South have generated unprecedented levels of precarity, amidst predatory capital accumulation. Withdrawal of basic provisioning for people whose labour sustains human life has left them at the mercy of individual employers, community networks, and 'fate'. Repeated acts of abandonment by the state occur alongside targeted violence on them, harming vulnerable people during the time of crisis when care is most needed. Sengupta's artwork depicts faceless migrants huddled together challenging the state and civil society to come out of its stupor and respond to the lived realities we have either denied or invisibilised. Nakash's artwork and Bose's commentary of the same urge us to revisit systems of governance and view them from the knowledge standpoint of the 'common' person.

Upadhyaya alerts us to the threats that the existing modes of governance pose through increased surveillance of its citizens. She evokes the work of Yuval Noah Harari (2020), who has argued that the kind of surveillance strategies governments in several countries have devised and implemented in the name of fighting the pandemic would have met with huge dissent, had they been mobilised under any other circumstances. It is as if the compulsions of Covid-19 management have not left any room for dissent. She urges citizens to 'keep an eye' on the strategies of the state and thereby equalise state-citizen power relations. Well-informed citizens can seek accountability from the state in this post-truth world, where facts are manufactured via the Ideological State Apparatuses (Althusser 1971).

The top-down, statist ideas about governance have been challenged by a few chapters in this volume. Jha sees strengthening of local self-governance through substantive devolution of power in the form of allocation of resources as non-negotiable in responding to a crisis like the Covid-19 pandemic. Based on field research, she argues that states in India that have strong local governance structures and processes have been able to respond to the pandemic much more effectively than their counterparts. She emphasises on the need for governments to invest more in the infrastructures of care. Panchal and Chandrasekar's chapter foregrounds ways in which a collaboration between a School of Social Work within a higher education institute in India and the police system was effectively mobilised to reach out to women affected by domestic violence during the pandemic. State power was harnessed in the interest of women by deftly employing the skills and perspectives of working with people. The chapter argues that social workers be considered essential workers, as they act as a crucial bridge between the government and people and facilitate access to services for the latter.

Some of these approaches of engaging with the state come into sharp contrast in the multiple ways governments across the world have repressed their people for attempting to seek accountability. From the Black Lives Matter movement in the United States to the nation-wide protests against the exclusionary Citizenship Amendment Act in India, from the opposition to the enactment of laws that are feared will change market equations against farmers in India, to the myriad forms of public outcry in several nations challenging policies of their governments, the past few years have witnessed powerful mobilisation of dissent against the excesses of repressive regimes (The Hindu 2019).[1] After the pandemic struck, some of these articulations moved to the digital space, some were repressed by states citing 'social distancing' protocols, while the others continued to be performed on the streets for a bit longer till they fell prey to states' cleansing drives. Pandemic policies also gave rise to protests in multiple countries. Popularised by the video OTT service Netflix's one of the most-watched shows during the pandemic *Money Heist*, the Italian song 'Bella Ciao', (Katz 2020) among others, resonated as an anthem of resistance in many of these protest movements (Pleyers 2020).

Religion and Godlessness

The pandemic has given new meaning to places of worship. Just before the pandemic, India experienced a raging debate on whether menstruating women should be allowed on the premises of the Sabrimala temple. While there were strong arguments on both sides, what stood out in the debates was the concern over the sanctity of the physical space of the temple, which was at the risk of being 'polluted' by the bodies of the menstruating women (Kumari 2019). Religious spaces are marked by hierarchies of purity and pollution. The pandemic has compelled believers to let go of the stronghold of the hierarchies of religious spaces as well as that of spaces of religious communion. The pandemic forced people to witness and experience sermons by religious heads from their personal space, while sermons were also recorded in isolation (Graff 2020).

Grover, in his chapter in this volume, explores how situations triggered by the pandemic puncture the tools of ruling of the modern state machinery by rendering it godless and by placing human resilience at the centre. He poignantly observes that all places of worship have been shut down; people have lost faith in the mediators of religion while scientists, doctors, nurses, and artists are taking care of lives. This historical juncture stands testimony to the utter collapse of the flawed ethical and moral principles that framed the political arrangement of many secular states. Paradoxically, Kumar and Mukherjee's paper focuses on how the Covid-19 pandemic has exposed the brutal methods through which the modern state in India devises 'legitimate' methods to politically arrange bodies and minds and renders many lives disposable within the logic of the secular state. What could be the new limits of reason in a world where structures that connected the personal with the political have crumbled?

Creative Communications

Effective communication of strategies to prevent the spread of the virus has been seen as the key to the efforts made by institutions, both at the global and regional levels. The WHO guidelines and advisories were interpreted and communicated to the populations in different countries. The universal modes of communication and the content of the communication further marginalised and invisibilised the experiences of disadvantaged groups of people. In many contexts, the challenge in countries around the world has been to translate the messages in a mode and language that is accessible to different communities. Tusasiirwe, Musinguzi, and Kukundakwe in this volume discuss the ways in which artists adopted Indigenous strategies to effectively communicate the message of safety against the virus to the communities in Uganda. They emphasise on the need to integrate Indigenous practices along with creative modes of communication to reach out to the most marginalised and disadvantaged groups of people. Linnet contextualises the experience of Iceland as an island nation and the ways in which they worked effectively to contain the virus. However, in their efforts at effective communication they realised that they had not been able to reach out to the immigrants, as they had failed to translate and contextualise the information for them in the first instance. Her experience of working in the Red Cross and bringing about changes at the institutional level to cater to and communicate with diverse groups of people will be an important resource for those seeking to devise effective means of communication in their contexts.

Joshua recreates the everyday life of the pandemic through artistic representations that are both mundane and political. The seeming banality of the images pierces through the viewers to present the layers of complexity unveiled by Covid-19. Vangad's artwork creatively traces the source of the pandemic in the shift from the slow, pastoral life of yore to the fast-paced expansion of the present time. He brings together varied themes of development, climate change, rural–urban inequities in a way that communicates layers of meaning to those witnessing this artwork. His artwork alludes that a crisis of this scale can only be addressed by slow, sustainable ways of existing. Chapters such as those of Joshua; Vangad; Tusasiirwe, Musinguzi, and Kukundakwe; and Linnet display the power of audio-visual modes of communication in language and aesthetic forms, which may be accessible to a diverse range of people and transcend the limitations of universalised modes of communication.

Questioning the 'Normal' and the Normative

The premium that humans have placed on productivity, defined in the narrowest sense of the term, has created and sustained the figure of the 'normal' human whose existence in the world is predicated upon performing a series of scripted acts intended to regulate and control. Any deviation from the script is met with violence at worst, and derision and ridicule, at best. There is little room for diversity, difference, and spontaneity. The script is, as it were, cast in stone. And at the heart of the human condition is this struggle to measure up to and align with that script.

Several chapters in the volume strike hard, albeit in different ways, at some of the foundational beliefs and values that human civilisation hinges on – for instance, the impulse to engage in the process of othering. It seems as though the full import of one's self can be experienced and asserted only by invalidating, even demonising the 'other'. Soumita Basu, Kandasamy Perera, Soldatic, and Rusham Sharma explore this question in the context of the accepted norms of efficiency and productivity. Rusham Sharma's poignant self-reflection points to the compulsive need to be productive to define oneself and the despair that comes with being 'inactive' or 'unproductive'. She, unabashedly, brings to the fore her subjective experience as a teenager situated within the structures of school education, which is undergoing a paradigmatic shift shaped by remote methods of teaching and learning. Kandasamy et al present findings of their research on disabled people in Sri Lanka and raise significant questions around ethics and public policies. Soumita Basu argues that those who fail to measure up to the normative ideals of bodily capacity and productivity far outnumber those who seem to conform, thereby questioning received ideas about 'majority' and 'minority'. She notes that it took a pandemic to institutionalise an idea such as 'work from home' when the disabled community has always demanded it. Paradoxically, the parameters of availability that situations of 'work from home', shaped by the pandemic demand, ultimately de-centre the needs of the disabled community.

Education

The pandemic has galvanised seismic shifts in the functioning of education systems. One may notice a prominent change in the form of pedagogy that prioritises remote practices of teaching and learning to keep pace with the 'normal' rhythm of academic processes like evaluation, semesters, admission to higher institutions, and others. However, there remains a lacuna in the content of pedagogic practices that continue to offer the same modules but often in a more compromised way due to a sudden shift to virtual modes of teaching. Educators world over have had to adapt to and design new pedagogical methods to reach out to their students. The challenges faced within the primary, secondary, and tertiary education sectors are vastly different. As discussed, the shift of primary education to the space of the home has had ripple effects on working parents, especially women, who have had to split time between supervising their children's online classes while also catering to work commitments.

The resistance towards online education among certain sections during the pandemic triggered conversations around the digital divide created as a result of disparate access to the internet. These concerns expanded to include the ability to acquire gadgets that would suit such a system; whether the environment of all homes was conducive to further remote learning; the physical discomfort (both long-term and short-term) that was caused by staring into screens for hours; and the quality of education that was imparted and acquired through such a medium.

Besides the challenges to learning, the discriminatory practices of hiring contract staff in academic institutions were also glaringly visible during the pandemic. Those on contract, whether professional or academic staff, were the first to be seen as 'dispensable' or their positions made redundant. The pandemic was seen as an opportunity to display the inability of the academia to sustain the employee strength that it previously had. Riddhima Sharma and Diwakar's chapters highlight the challenges confronted by the faculty and students in institutes of higher education. They allude to the inherent problems of a neo-liberal logic used within the University system, which is based on 'merit and choice'. Such a premise does not take into consideration differences and structural disadvantages experienced by different groups of students. Diwakar analyses the experiences of students through Bourdieu's lens to bring forth the challenges faced by students in access to education because of the difference in cultural and social capital. The pandemic has, to an enormous extent, reversed the gains made through decades of policy and practice of reaching education to one and all. It has created additional barriers for accessing education for a vast majority from disadvantaged and marginalised groups.

Of Trauma and Loss

For many who work in the health sector, the Covid-19 pandemic has been an entry point into understanding personal narratives of trauma or loss as well as the fissures that inform social morality and value systems at large. Appel, who has been working as an emergency room physician in New York City since the early days of the pandemic, reflects, in this volume, on how vulnerability to the lethal virus was informed by a stark economic and racial disparity. Privileged white people, who could afford, fled from the city or shut themselves in their luxurious apartments while mostly the lower-income African-American and Latino communities, the non-white people, continued to work, fight, or succumb to keep the city functional. Appel draws upon instances from earlier catastrophes to emphasise that social justice and access to healthcare systems have been controlled by wealth and power. He contemplatively situates the individual within a larger paradigm of the social order to comment that our subjective sense of ethics and priorities will contribute towards shaping the new world order, after we transcend the horrors of the Covid-19 pandemic. Purvis' chapter 'Narrating the Moment of Transmission' stems from her subjective experience of listening to people's narratives of anxiety related to illness and explores how a deeper understanding of these narratives might help foster a space of care and compassion in society. She reflects on her work as an artist with people living with HIV and Hepatitis to recollect how they constructed narratives around the moment of transmission of the disease. She observes that all the narratives she came across during the pandemic followed a similar pattern in the way they were steeped in varied emotions of guilt, fear, anxiety, and repentance about the moment of transmission. At a deeper level, these emotions were related to their inner lives and situations of trauma that they might already be dealing with. The way Purvis draws a poignant connection with her personal experience through motherhood reveals how an incident of deep loss leaves imprints that psychologically and physiologically surface across a length of time in moments of unexpected encounters. This chapter, though very different from Appel's, also speaks of how, in retrospect, the pandemic may provide us with a window to recognise the gaps and find ways to re-think human emotions and values in the context of a collective.

Creative Re-imaginings

The pandemic is a moment in the long histories of violence and marginalisation. It has just made it more visible and created a sense of urgency among many who would have otherwise continued to live a life of denial or ignorance. We wonder why a radical moment is required to make us stop and reflect. What has changed as we move from one wave of the pandemic to the next? Has there been a reprioritisation? Has there been a rupture in the thought-process and action? Is there a way to transcend fear, anger, trauma, and grief as we re-invent subjective coping mechanisms? Is it transformative?

Chandni Basu's imagination of a child-friendly city as a bird-friendly place embodies a social and ecological utopia, where architectural innovation synergises with human compassion to re-imagine spaces of flourish for all sentient beings. Esposito et al, in their creative cross-cultural collaboration, acknowledge how the impact of the Covid-19 pandemic needs to be understood distinctively in specific cultural contexts. Their political project, as discussed in a chapter in this volume, seeks to re-imagine a world shaped by empathetic connections that would be forged on the basis of self-care, care for others, and earth care. Chapters such as those of Ife prod us to acknowledge tragedy and re-imagine in Kafkaist ways: *reverently*, *reflectively*, and *lovingly*. In a similar vein, Rees' chapter asks important questions of language and its uses. He points out that the language of poets and musicians helps us realise some of the values of socialism and dismiss the fears by demystifying it.

Looking Back, Looking Ahead

As we complete this introduction in July 2021, the pandemic is shaping social institutions, affecting human relationships, and creating new norms with each passing day. Malcolm Bradbury and James McFarlane (1976) aptly introduce Modernism by stating,

> Overwhelming dislocations, those cataclysmic upheavals of culture, those fundamental convulsions of the creative human spirit that seem to topple even the most solid and substantial of our beliefs and assumptions, leave great areas of the past in ruins, question an entire civilization or culture and stimulate frenzied rebuilding.
>
> (19–20)

Analogous to such an exploration of Modernism, the volume brings together experiences of isolation and the multitude of emotions generated in situations of lockdown that have provided the context to question our widely-held beliefs. They conceptualise a new world order based on the values and principles of human dignity as well as social and ecological justice. A world where love, care, compassion, and empathy may be a possible logic to define our relationships with the human and non-human world. A more nuanced understanding is required of this period in history, which is marked by uncertainty, and calls for the need to envision a new reality.

We argue that the so-called shifts in different kinds of social phenomena that we have been perceiving after the pandemic broke out cannot be attributed to Covid-19 alone. Be it the issue of increased burden of housework on women; the spike in domestic and family violence against women, children, and queer persons; the collapse of health and other governance systems; the precarity of existence confronted by the disadvantaged; the inhuman treatment meted out to migrant labourers; the racism and religious hatred towards specific communities; the perverse marginalisation and exclusion of disabled, queer, lower caste-marked, racialised bodies from public policies; or animals reclaiming habitat that had been lost to the unstoppable avarice of the human kind – these phenomena were already part of the pre-pandemic world. The pandemic therefore proves to be what all moments of crisis are – a mirror that forces us to look at our festering self. On a more optimistic note, it provides a window of opportunity that demands us to envisage, strategise, and operationalise radical transformation. Re-imagining the world order will require a re-organisation of social relations, where systemic and everyday violence gives way to justice and care.

The visceral responses, creative re-imaginings, and artistic explorations that stem from grim realities of the pandemic reflect stories of human resilience and a deep-seated desire to search for hope in dark times. These works, which often remain unacknowledged in the mainstream archives of history, provide aesthetic, philosophical, and political insights that help suture the devastated pieces and bolster the frail reconstructionist visions of future. It is important to acknowledge this moment of a sudden pause and to try to address with acuity and sensitivity, the fundamental questions that this catastrophe has stimulated. The stories of human struggle and solidarity that have also emerged in this crisis provide insights to re-think about newer modes of social engagement rather than of alienation, of imagining communities amidst cataclysmic ruptures, and of rebuilding ideas of social justice and equal opportunity. Nicholas Berger (2020), in his online article 'The Forgotten Art of Assembly', recognises the human need to be sensitive to this moment of pause that might help us find an internal process to share grief and to foster a renewed approach towards arts. He writes:

> We must lean into this pain. We must feel the grief. We must mourn. Mourn the loss of work, the loss of jobs, the loss of money, the loss of life. Mourn the temporary loss of an art form that demands assembly. Lean into the grief. Lean in. Lean in. Lean in. We must remind ourselves that mourning is a human act, not a digital one. It is only in this acknowledgment that we will survive. The internet isn't going to save us, we are.

The pandemic has made us face the idea of death and destruction as an inevitable philosophical truth, as embedded in many ritualistic practices, as well as a real condition which compels preparedness, acceptance, and reconstruction. The pandemic may have stimulated denial as an emotional mechanism to resist the shock of an unimaginable number of death, but at the same time it has re-invoked an engagement with philosophical discourses around death which is related to discourses of a 'post-truth' world. Literature, oral stories, artwork, like an anchor, help re-imagine rituals of mourning, of love, of touch, and of care, of loss and of life-affirming practices in acts of the everyday, in times when the existing social order collapses.

Elena Bernabé (2020) from Indigenous Peoples Cultures speaks of an internal passage of waiting during which one might re-invent newer ways of relating to the world. It harnesses knowledge from a body of rites of life, of ritualistic acts of doing to re-interpret the meaning of quarantine. While the narrative of the virus propels a fear of death and the loss of a sense of community, this piece drums up a vocabulary around quarantine that is deeply rooted to life, the ethics, and practices of community existence.

Grandma, how can I live this quarantine?

"My daughter, quarantine is a special, mysterious and sacred period. In my days, new born children could only leave the house for the first time after their 40th day of life. It is a period of waiting and preparing for a new life. It is the period that produces a great change."

And how do you prepare for this change?

"With simple, genuine and loving actions. Every morning comb your long hair with dedication and untie all the knots, even the most hidden ones that you have always neglected. It is time to put all the knots in the comb. Then dedicate yourself to untangling even your beloved ones skeins. With patience and you will try to find the end of the skein, the exact starting point of the thread. Already with these simple but powerful actions you will create order outside and inside of you. Undoing physical knots with your hands you will begin to touch your internal knots."

And after undoing the knots, what can I do, grandma?

"Remove all parts of you that are no longer fertile. In many funeral rites of ancient peoples it is believed that the deceased leaves the body entirely on the 40th day after his death. In these 40 days, my daughter, cut your hair, eliminate clothes that you have not worn for a long time or that you no longer want use, open the windows of your home well to let the stale air out, cultivate new thoughts by abandoning the old, dedicated to creating new habits, new customs, new traditions."

Grandmother, I'm afraid that after this isolation nothing will change. Man quickly forgets…

"How others will react to this quarantine is none of your business. Make a commitment to change and not forget. Make sure this storm shakes you up so much that it completely revolutionizes your life."

Note

1 For a broader view of the movements in different parts of the world, see: https://carnegieendowment.org/publications/interactive/protest-tracker

References

Achebe, Chinua. (2013). *Things Fall Apart*. UK: Penguin. Print.

Allen, H., Ling, B. and Burton, W. (2020). 'Stop using the term social distancing – start talking about physical distancing, social connection', *Health Affairs*, April 27 [online]. Available at: https://www.healthaffairs.org/do/10.1377/forefront.20200424.213070/full/ [Accessed 12 August 2021].

Althusser, Louis. (1971). *Lenin and Philosophy and Other Essays*. New York: Monthly Review Press.

Baertlin, L. and Fares, M. (2020). 'Panic buying of toilet paper hits U.S. stores again with new pandemic restrictions', *Reuters*, November 21 [online]. Available at: https://www.reuters.com/article/us-health-coronavirus-toiletpaper-idUSKBN2802W3 [Accessed 12 August 2021].

Bahadur, Aditya. (2021). 'How India's civil society rose up in the face of Covid-19', *Indian Institute for Environment and Development*. Available at: https://www.iied.org/how-indias-civil-society-rose-face-covid-19 [Accessed 16 March 2022].

Banerjee, D. and Bhattacharya, P. (2020). The hidden vulnerability of homelessness in the Covid-19 pandemic: Perspectives from India. *International Journal of Social Psychiatry* 2021, 67(1), 3–6. Available at: https://journals.sagepub.com/doi/pdf/10.1177/0020764020922890 [Accessed 17 March 2022].

Bandyopadhyay, R., Banerjee, P. and Samaddar, R. (2021). *India's Migrant Workers and the Pandemic*. UK: Routledge.

Baraitser, Lisa. (2017). *Enduring Time*. USA: Bloomsbury.

bell hooks. (2018). *All About Love: New Visions*. USA: William Morrow Paperbacks.

Berger, N. (2020). 'The forgotten art of assembly', *Nicholas Berger*, April 4 [online]. Available at: https://medium.com/@nicholasberger/the-forgotten-art-of-assembly-a94e164edf0f [Accessed 12 August 2020].

Bernabé, E. (2020). 'Abuela, ¿como se afronta el dolor?' *Crónicas de la Tierra sin Mal*. Available at: https://cronicasinmal.blogspot.com/2020/08/el-dolor-como-afrontarlo.html?spref=fb&m=1

Bhaumik, S. et al. (2021). 'Low-value medical care in the pandemic – Is this what the doctor ordered', *The Lancelet Global Health*. Available at: https://www.thelancet.com/journals/langlo/article/PIIS2214-109X2100252-7/fulltext [Accessed 16 March 2022].

Bowleg, L. (2020). We're not all in this together: On COVID-19, intersectionality, and structural inequality. *American Journal of Public Health* 1971, 110(7), 917.

Boyd, K. (2020). Ethics in a time of coronavirus. *Journal of Medical Ethics*, 46(5), 285–286.

Bradbury, M. and McFarlane, J. (1976). *Modernism: A Guide to European Literature 1890–1930*. Harmondsworth, New York: Penguin.

Caraballo, K. (2020). Immigration, law, and (in)justice: Coronavirus and its impact on immigration. *International Criminal Justice Review*, 30(4), 448–457.

Brooks, Francis J. (1993). Revisiting the conquest of Mexico: Smallpox, sources and population. *Journal of Interdisciplinary History* (Summer 1993), XXIV(I), 1–29.

Cross, F.L. and Benson, O.G. (2021). The coronavirus pandemic and immigrant communities: A crisis that demands more of the social work profession. *Affilia*, 36(1), 113–119.

Docka-Filipek, D. and Stone, L.B. (2021). Twice a "housewife": On academic precarity, "hysterical" women, faculty mental health, and service as gendered care work for the "university family" in pandemic times. *Gender, Work, and Organization*, 28(6), 2158–2179.

Deshpande, A. (2020). The COVID-19 Pandemic and Gendered Division of Paid and Unpaid Work: Evidence from India, IZA Discussion Papers, No. 13815, Institute of Labour Economics (IZA), Bonn.

Dewan, R. (2022). India. 'Pandemic, Patriarchy and Precarity: Labour, Livelihood & Mobility Rights'. DAWN Discussion Papers No. 35. DAWN. Suva (Fiji).

Graff, Garrett M. (2020). 'Here in spirit: An oral history of faith and the pandemic'. Available at: https://www.wired.com/story/here-in-spirit-oral-history-of-faith-amid-pandemic/ [Accessed 17 March 2022].

Gilligan, C. (1995). Hearing the difference: Theorizing connection. *Hypatia*, 10(2), 120–27. Available at: http://www.jstor.org/stable/3810283.

Hans, A., Kannabiran, K., Mohanty, M. and Pushpendra, (2021). *Migration, Workers, and Fundamental Freedoms: Pandemic Vulnerabilities and States of Exception in India* (1st ed.). India: Routledge. Available at: https://doi.org/10.4324/9781003145509

Harari, Y. (2020). 'Yuval Noah Harari: The world after coronavirus: Free to read', *Financial Times*, 20 March [online]. Available at: https://www.ft.com/content/19d90308-6858-11ea-a3c9-1fe6fedcca75 [Accessed 21 June 2020].

Inani, Rohit. (2021). 'Job lost, income cut: How Covid-19 financially dented India's middle class'. Available at: https://www.business-standard.com/article/economy-policy/how-a-year-of-coronavirus-financially-dented-india-s-middle-class-121083000181_1.html [Accessed 17 March 2021].

Kabeer, N., Razavi, S. and van der Meulen Rodgers, Y. (2021). Feminist economic perspectives on the COVID-19 pandemic. *Feminist Economics*, 27(1–2), 1–29.

Katz, B. (2020). 'Why Netflix's 'Money Heist' is the most in-demand show in the world', *Observer*. Available at: https://observer.com/2020/04/netflix-money-heist-la-casa-de-papel-most-watched/ [Accessed 13 August 2021].

Khosla, V. (2021). 'Pet industry thrives during pandemic; prices of exotic dogs go up', *The Economic Times*, June 13 [online]. Available at: https://economictimes.indiatimes.com/news/india/how-much-is-that-doggy-in-the-window-woof-woof/articleshow/83464822.cms?from=mdr [Accessed 12 August 2021].

Kumari, Rashmi. (2019). 'Menstruating women and celibate Gods: A discourse analysis of women's entry into Sabarimala temple in Kerela, India'. *Third World Thematics: A TWQ Journal*, 4(4–5), 288–305. Available at: https://www.tandfonline.com/doi/abs/10.1080/23802014.2019.1682946?journalCode=rtwt20. [Accessed 17 March 2022].

Lewis, Helen. (2020). 'The coronavirus is a disaster for feminism', *Atlantic*, March 19. Available at: https://www.theatlantic.com/international/archive/2020/03/feminism-womens-rights-coronavirus-covid19/608302/ [Accessed 10 January 2021].

Long, N. (2020). From social distancing to social containment. *Medicine Anthropology Theory*, 7(2), 247–260.

McKenzie, Jon. (2000). *Perform or Else: From Discipline to Performance.* New York: Routledge.

McPherson, J. (2020). 'Now is the time for a rights-based approach to social work practice'. *Journal of Human Rights and Social Work*, 5(2), 61–63.

Mehta, R. and Briskman, L. (2022). 'Covid and social work responses from India and Australia: Strategic and meaningful solidarities for global justice', in *The Coronavirus Crisis and Challenges to Social Development*, eds. Maria do Carmo dos Santos Gonçalves, Rebecca Gutwald, Tanja Kleibl, Ronald Lutz, Ndangwa Noyoo and Janestic Twikirize, Cham: Springer, pp. 3–15.

Mitra, Debraj. (2021). 'Queue for food grows longer, shows depth of distress', *The Telegraph*, June 4 [online]. Available at: https://www.telegraphindia.com/west-bengal/calcutta/covid-19-queue-for-food-grows-longer-shows-depth-of-distress/cid/1817693 [Accessed 12 August 2021].

Mlamb-Ngcuka, P. (2020). 'Violence against women and girls: The shadow pandemic'. Available at: https://www.unwomen.org/en/news/stories/2020/4/statement-ed-phumzile-violence-against-women-during-pandemic [Accessed 5 February 2021].

Morgan, E. (2021). 'Lost touch: How a year without hugs affects our mental health', *The Guardian*, January 24 [online]. Available at: https://www.theguardian.com/lifeandstyle/2021/jan/24/lost-touch-how-a-year-without-hugs-affects-our-mental-health [Accessed 12 August 2021].

O'Keefe, T. and Courtois, A. (2020). 'Who does the 'Housework of the University' during a pandemic? The impact of COVID-19 on precarious women working in universities', *Gender & Society Blog*. Available at: https://gendersociety.wordpress.com/2020/06/30/who-does-the-housework-of-the-university-during-a-pandemic-the-impact-of-covid-19-on-precarious-women-working-in-universities/

Patil, Smita M. (2021). Gender equity and Covid-19: Dalit standpoints. *Economic and Political weekly*, 56(11), March 13 [online]. Available at: https://www.epw.in/engage/article/gender-equity-and-covid-19-dalit-standpoints [Accessed 12 August 2021].

Pleyers, G. (2020). The pandemic is a battlefield. Social movements in the COVID-19 lockdown. *Journal of Civil Society*, 16(4), 295–312.

Pringle, H. (2015). 'How Europeans brought sickness to the New World', *ScienceMag*, June 4 [online]. Available at: https://www.sciencemag.org/news/2015/06/how-europeans-brought-sickness-new-world [Accessed 12 August 2021].

Raghavendra, Madhu. (2021). *Being non-essential.* Red River.

Sengupta, S. and Jha, M.K. (2020). Social policy, COVID-19 and impoverished migrants: Challenges and prospects in locked down India. *The International Journal of Community and Social Development*, 2(2), 152–172. doi: 10.1177/2516602620933715.

Singh, S.K., Patel, V., Chaudhary, A. and Mishra, N. (2020). Reverse Migration of Labourers amidst COVID-19. *Economic and Political Weekly*, 55, 32–33.

Schotzko, T.N.C. (2020). A year (in five months) of living dangerously: Hidden intimacies in Zoom exigencies. *International Journal of Performance Arts and Digital Media*, 16(3), 269–289, December 14 [online]. doi: 10.1080/14794713. 2020.1827206 [Accessed 12 August 2021].

Shaw, D.M. (2020). Invisible enemies: Coronavirus and other hidden threats. *Journal of Bioethical Inquiry*, 17(4), 531–534.

Sotgiu, G. and Dobler, C.C. (2020). Social stigma in the time of coronavirus disease 2019. *The European Respiratory Journal*, 56(2), 2002461.

Stokel-Walker, C. (2020). 'How personal contact will change post-Covid-19', *BBC*, April 30 [online]. Available at: https://www.bbc.com/future/article /20200429-will-personal-contact-change-due-to-coronavirus [Accessed 12 August 2021].

Suhomlinova, O., Ayres, T.C., Tonkin, M.J., O'Reilly, M., Wertans, E. and O'Shea, S.C. (2022). Locked up while locked down: Prisoners' experiences of the COVID-19 pandemic. *The British Journal of Criminology*, 62(2), 279–298.

Stevano, S., Mezzadri, A., Lombardozzi, L. and Bargawi, H. (2021). Hidden abodes in plain sight: The social reproduction of households and labor in the COVID-19 pandemic. *Feminist Economics*, 27(1–2), 271–287.

Tazreiter, C. and Metcalfe, S. (2021). New vulnerabilities for migrants and refugees in state responses to the global pandemic, COVID-19. *Social Sciences*, 10. Available at: http://dx.doi.org/10.3390/socsci10090342

The Hindu. (2019). 'The decade's major movements that became strong voices of resistance', *The Hindu*, December 29 [online]. Available at: https://www.thehindu. com/society/the-decade-of-protest/article30412780.ece/photo/3/ [Accessed 12 August 2021].

The Indian Express. (2020). 'Sanitation workers in Ambala welcomed with garlands and applause', April 10 [online]. Available at: https://indianexpress.com/article/ trending/trending-in-india/ambala-haryana-sanitation-workers-coronavirus-6356611/ [Accessed 12 August 2021].

Wong, A., Ho, S., Olusanya, O., Antonini, M.V. and Lyness, D. (2021). The use of social media and online communications in times of pandemic Covid-19. *Journal of the Intensive Care Society*, 22(3), 255–260. Available at: https://journals.sagepub. com/doi/pdf/10.1177/1751143720966280 [Accessed 16 March 2022].

Viglione, G. (2020). 'Are women publishing less during the pandemic? Here's what the data say', May 20 [online]. Available at: https://www.nature.com/articles/ d41586-020-01294-9 [Accessed 12 August 2021].

Zarkov, D. (2020). On economy, health and politics of the Covid19 pandemic. *European Journal of Women's Studies*, 27, 213–217.

TOUCH

1

MY TANGO LIFE CANCELLED

8 March – 3 May 2020

Mary Lourdes Silva

Day 1: My Tango Life Cancelled

One by one, milongas, practicas, festivals, tango classes, and seminars were cancelled worldwide. My Facebook notifications screen looked similar to an airline terminal monitor during a snowstorm, one cancellation after the next. Sadly, I had to do the same and postpone indefinitely our weekly milonga, which had successfully debuted only three weeks prior. Soon after all the cancellations, *tangueros* worldwide scrambled online to find solace and camaraderie within pop-up Facebook groups, such as *I'm not dancing tango so I did this instead*. Restricted by local and nationwide ordinances to embrace, lock palms, and allow tendrils of infected sweat to fall onto our cheeks and chests, tangueros retreated from the material and temporal conditions of tango to the virtual infinite spaces of the Internet. It was not long before the corners of the Internet filled with clever memes about Covid-19 plus cats, dogs, Zoom sessions, or anti-social distancing. In some corners, tangueros made space for virtual milongas.

A milonga is an Argentine tango dance event, where couples, friends, and strangers arrive at a location, typically a dance studio, hotel, community centre, bar, restaurant, or house to listen to the classics from the golden age of tango during the 1930s and 1940s. We invite a partner to dance this improvisational form that solely relies on touch as its primary mode of communication. Ironically, the invitation begins without touch, with the *cabeceo*, an opportune, sometimes anxious, gaze across a crowded room for the perfect dancer to fill their arms during a tanda, a collection of three to four tangos by a single orchestra. If the dancer consents, they return the gaze with a gentle nod. If it is a male, typically, he walks past the elbows, shoulders, and hips of the crowd to stand in front of her and extend his arm. At first touch, they can now speak in silence.

In tango, we dance with strangers from all over the world at local milongas, tango marathons, and festivals. Most often, we forget the names of our

DOI: 10.4324/9781003320524-3

favourite dancers, even physical traits like weight and height; however, we never forget the way our favourite dancers embrace us; it is their fingerprint and their DNA that wraps our bodies like a double helix bracelet. Dancers will travel hundreds or thousands of miles to reconnect with a beloved dancer just to *feel* once again – feel without hesitation, feel without judgement, feel without fear.

Day 10: I Haven't Touched Anyone

Living alone in a remote rural community had its benefits. I could not inadvertently leave a plume of respiratory droplets for a loved one to inhale. I could not race by neighbours on a busy city sidewalk and suck in their Covid-19 exhaust while we waited for the light to turn green. I could leave an Amazon box on my front porch and wait three days for the virus to mysteriously evaporate like a puff of cartoon smoke. Most importantly, I could avoid touch.

Living in a remote rural community was familiar territory. My entire childhood up until the summer my mother died was on a dairy farm. In the brittle cold mornings of winter, the suckle of a newborn calf warmed my hands after it finished a bottle of warm milk. We were surrounded by dogs who leapt onto our laps without manners and nipped our ankles when we rushed to the 6 am school bus. The boys worked year-round outside, and the girls kept house unless our parents were short-handed outside. I left this world behind for city life to finish my bachelor's degree. Any city-dweller of a multi-million occupancy city like New York or Buenos Aires would call Fresno or Santa Barbara *towns*, where I finished three different education programs. But for this dairy girl, I lived the city life: surrounded by hundreds at any given second but never quite close enough to care about most of them. I never thought I would return to rural living when I landed my first salary job. Between the tango and frequent trips to tango cities, rural living was the time needed to finish my academic work until it was time to surround myself once again with the warm embrace of strangers.

No time in recent history has the world had to confront an invisible enemy in which the one thing that can save us is physical separation – no hugs, no kisses, no holding hands. Touch is the one sense that all humans share in common, the one sense that we cannot ever turn off. Touch is our connection to the world – it is how infants imprint onto their mother's bosom; it is how toddlers learn spatial awareness and develop their motor skills and cognitive functions; it is how adolescents test their boundaries; it is how teens and young adults discover independence and each other's bodies; it is how parents nurture and protect their offspring; it is how my father grasped his wife's hand one last time before dropping his head to the side of the hospital pillow; it is how soft the white petals felt on his coffin, in the shade of a six-foot grave.

Day 21: My Skin Stings without Touch, Like Hands Submerged into a Winter River

What distinguishes tango from other improvisational dances (e.g., modern, jazz, and ballet) is the significance of touch. Touch is the only sensation that is always active. Cultural historian Constance Classen, author of *The Book of Touch*, writes how our culture has become more "eye-minded" and has grown to fear touch or has become disdainful of touch. Touch in tango reminds us that our body is the primary modem of communication. Gunther Kress and Theo van Leeuwen, authors of *Multimodal Discourse: The Modes and Media of Contemporary Communication*, explain that we experience the world differently when we engage with the material world through the body. Without touch, knowledge is merely an abstraction, a quadratic formula of symbols and signifiers without any tangible resolution or purpose. In tango, without touch, we are still, motionless, left standing alone with the music calling us.

After three weeks without touch, I recall my last practice session with one of my practice partners. I lead as well as follow. Although more women in tango are learning to lead around the world, a great majority of dancers adhere to traditional gender roles of leading and following; however, the queer tango movement of the early 2000s allowed more queer women and non-queer women to perform both the lead and follow roles to better express their interpretation of the music. At milongas in the United States, Canada, and Argentina (the birthplace of tango), if a woman is leading another woman, you would mainly see the couple dancing in an open embrace where their chests maintain a hand prayer's distance between the two, whereas a male–female couple may press breast on chest to feel the warm blood pulsing between their embrace. At a festival in San Diego, a woman once told me, "I never know where to put my breasts when I dance with a female leader." I told her to keep them where she last left them. In American and Latina culture, women are more likely to hold hands with girlfriends, hug, caress, and welcome an old friend with a kiss, but in tango, touch is the passageway to our most fragile self. Once we arrive, there is no way of knowing what we will feel – a shard of a once-healed heartbreak, the intoxicating rush of love hormones, and a glimpse of a shadowed memory. And in our culture, women feel safer to experience those surprising moments with a male dancer, breast to chest, moving to the pulse of the music as one body.

Once again, it's safe to blame the media for another gender social construct. From 1976 to 1983, Argentina's dictatorial government prohibited public gatherings like milongas. Once the country returned to being a democracy, tango dancers travelled to Paris, where it became fashionable once again to dance tango after a generation of Elvis and The Beatles. In the decades to follow, magazines published images of women in the throes of passion in a man's embrace, and successful movies like *The Tango Lesson*

(1997) popularised the tango trope of the teacher–student love story, which almost always featured a story between a cisgender male and female.

On 7 March, I met with my practice partner at her house. After about two hours of tango fundamentals, basic walking, and rehearsing a simple sequence from my Buenos Aires library of tango videos, I asked her, "Do you want to know what it feels like to embrace dancers in Buenos Aires?" Male tango dancers from Buenos Aires are known around the world for their firm affectionate embrace and movement. One woman commented, "It's like riding a velvet truck." On a humid summer day in Buenos Aires, his sweat is my sweat; his blood circulates my blood; his body is mine and mine is his.

My partner replied, "Yes, of course!" eager to learn some bottled imported secret from Argentina. I embraced her, heart to heart, my right arm wrapped all the way around her back. Without any tension or strain, I left no room between our embrace for any doubts. I asked her to take a deep breath with me and let go of her embrace: "let go of what it's supposed to look like; let go of what it's supposed to feel like; let go of letting go. Just be with me."

We danced to "El Adiòs" by Ángel Vargas. With each breath, each phrase, each pivot, I could feel our embrace coil, soften, and expand while Angel Vargas wailed in his suffering about some lost lover. Phrase after phrase, while staying on axis, I could feel her body settle more and more into my chest like a sleeping toddler. For the first time, I could feel her entire spine coil; I felt the gravity of her right thigh in a back *ocho*, the pencil point of her foot as she connected to the ground. Our embrace was like a motherboard and I could feel absolutely everything in her body. There were no secrets between us. Nothing to hide.

When the song finally ended, we stood there – silent-coiled and breathing. I could not let go. She did not let go. Before I could make sense of what happened in those three minutes, I began to sob, but this time, she held me like a mother soothing a fallen toddler in her arms. The next Vargas song began to play on my playlist. She modified the embrace, and this time, I followed while she led. Phrase after phrase, as the tears dried, I slept in her arms – coiled and breathless.

Day 30: The Great Fortune of a Pre-Covid-19 Death

If my father had been alive during Covid-19, I would have been more worried about his health like the rest of America. I was fortunate that the virus had not made its way across our shores during Christmas. In October, while living in Buenos Aires for the year, I learned that he had weeks to live due to his congestive heart failure. I waited to finish out the rest of my trip in Argentina, knowing for the past nine years he had been slowly dying from congestive heart failure. I flew into California on the 24th like an empty-handed Santa Claus, eager to celebrate his last Christmas with the entire family.

I walked into the living room. He sat on his electronic recliner chair, jaw limp like a snapped branch on a tree trunk. Each breath exhausted him. He said very little during my visit, although I had been gone for a year. He was never the kind of father who inquired about his kids' lives. He was a proud immigrant who had laboured and sweated for 55 years to provide a life for six kids and our mother, who died 23 years prior, to cancer, and later his second wife. Our father never felt the need to have a close relationship with any of his kids. During his lifetime, fathers raised their kids from a distance with their hands planted deep in the earth working the ground for economic prosperity. It's typically mothers who raise their hand to discipline and embrace. And when our mother passed away, we always felt the love of our father from a distance, signed checks for our education, a co-signer on multiple loans, or a clipped article about my graduate student award found in the dairy office after the funeral. On that final Christmas day, he kept to tradition and loved us from afar, sitting on his recliner chair while his kids and grandkids sat around the kitchen and TV, laughing and sharing stories after ten-plus years of a family divided and once again reunited, for the moment.

On Jan 11th, it was time for me to leave. I had to drive 3000 miles to New York to start the spring semester. It would not be long before the world feared touch. I walked over to his recliner chair, touched his long-sleeved flannel shirt to brace myself, and leaned down to leave one kiss on his warm cheek. My father was never affectionate. After the age of six or seven, our parents never kissed us. Actually, hugging was quite rare as well. My only memories of hugging my mother were when she would introduce me to strangers, and I would cling to her wide hips to avoid talking to anyone. In the early 20th century, psychologists and doctors would warn parents against hugging and kissing their children to avoid spoiling them and raising morally inferior children. I hardly doubt that my uneducated immigrant parents paid much attention to the conventional wisdom of psychologists; however, it was very much a part of their culture to avoid coddling children. In our household, touch was associated with pain – the prickly sting of a spanking, the careful tug of a rusty nail embedded in our barefoot, the pinch pull of a baby tooth, and a mother's palm pressed against our cheeks as the warm olive-oil-soaked cotton ball soothed an aching ear. Without pain, how else would we know that our parents loved us?

When I kissed his cheek, I somehow knew it would be the last time. In fact, it was the first time in my life that I kissed him, a tradition that I imported from Buenos Aires. It happened so naturally as if that had always been our tradition. It was at that moment when he looked at me in a way that he had never looked at me before, so naturally, as if it had always been our tradition to love each other. At that moment, I held back my tears. Two weeks later, he was dead. At the funeral, I chose not to touch his corpse. It was my story. I wanted it to end with the ghost of our first kiss.

Day 56: Tango Is a Pain Worth Longing For

On 1 March, just before the United States closed its doors for Covid-19, I discovered that my father wrote me out of the will in 2005 because I had a loving 13-year relationship that ended in 2014 with my ex-partner, who is now one of my dearest friends. My racist father could not stand to see his daughter with a divorced Mexican barely getting by with his artwork to support his three kids. Even from the grave, my father made sure that "that man would not get a single penny." During our relationship, we were both poor but did our best to make each other happy. We never even asked for a single penny from my father who left behind a legacy, the great American story of rags to riches. My siblings will always remember him as the Great Provider, working the earth to support his family. For me, he made sure that he should be remembered as the Great Punisher instead, who often punished us with brute force or the threat of cutting off funds. He could now punish comfortably from the grave, using money once again to further divide our family. The pain of rejection and abandonment was far too much for me to bear, yet, then Covid-19 happened. And touch was taken from me, ripped right from my hands. The sting of its absence and the longing for its return, surprisingly, brought me some temporary relief. Wanting what the world wanted so badly allowed me to join them in that pain, and temporarily forget a far greater pain, a life's worth of scars, a quilted masterpiece, all ripped apart at once.

On day 56, it was time. The cool dollop of Purell soothed my anxious hands. Her eyes creased above her mask, a gesture that signalled that she was ready. I walked towards her in the middle of my living room, lifted my left arm, and invited her palm to form a seal with mine – my first skin-to-skin contact after two months of quarantine. Her palm was warm and sticky from the imitation Purell that she bought during the onset of the crisis. My right arm reached around her back, hesitant to embrace her closely. We danced, a hand's prayer distance apart, counter-clockwise around my small New York apartment.

For two hours, I imagined a micro storm of viruses swirling between our bodies and the only layer of protection between us was a millimetre-thick layer of cotton over our nose and mouth. I tried to connect to my dance partner and connect to the steady tempo of Di Sarli, trying desperately to ignore the fears of Covid-19 that intruded on our dance like an impatient tanguero waiting for his turn. I wanted to trust science. After two months of quarantine, daily sanitisation of our apartments, wearing masks, and living alone, the likelihood of us being symptomatic was infinitesimal. But the threat of infection, that hollow space between our bodies remained, pushing me further away from the embrace. However, at one point, I made her laugh. Behind a mask, laughter has physical volume. Like a balloon, it quickly stretches the microfibers of the cotton mask, deflates on inhalation, and leaves behind a spray of tiny droplets, like blood splatter at a crime scene. My face was less than a gun's length from hers. *Am I safe? Is she safe?*

After an hour of dancing, she called it. Gratitude for touch filled me with joy. I forgot about the masks and sticky residue of hand sanitiser on our palms. Without hesitation, I hugged her, sealed our hearts together, wrapped both arms around her, felt our cheekbones connect, and sighed. This time, inhaling, expanding our embrace until it burst at the seams.

For over a month, we danced with masks and hand sanitiser, each time, the embrace feeling more at ease, softening at the creases. Although we could embrace once again, something was missing. I should have felt satisfied. With over 135,000 Covid-19 deaths by early July, and hundreds of thousands of Americans living alone without the means to touch or embrace another person during this time, what more could I ask for?

Tango is more than touch. It is the longing for something untouchable; it isn't only the red lipstick stains on white-collar shirts and sticky wooden floors; it's the month-long agitation for the departure date to Buenos Aires; it isn't only the crowded floors and sweat-soaked blazers; it's the anticipation for a D'Arienzo tanda and the agony of heels splitting toenails after 40 blessed hours of dancing; it isn't only the stale potato chips, sleep deprivation, and the pulsing ache at the bottom of our feet; it's the dull heartache of anticipation for our favourite dancer to finally choose us. Tango is the unavoidable dance between pain and love that still stings after a winter's kiss between a father and daughter. We allegedly long for touch, but in reality, we long for the pain of longing, a welcomed distraction from a far more permanent pain that punishes us from the grave.

Day 189: Broken Vows

I place my palm onto her bare chest and feel each breath race to some imaginary finish line. Without the ventilator, her muddied lungs work three times harder. For six months, due to Covid-19 restrictions at nursing homes, our family was prohibited to see, to visit, and to touch our physically and mentally disabled sister. Since the age of 43, Philomena lived at the facility because our father could no longer lift her after shattering his pelvis, sleep-walking down a flight of stairs. For six months, Philomena lived without touch. She was fed. She was bathed. But the nurses didn't know that she smiled whenever we held her crippled hand while listening to music or that swiping right on baby photos made her giddy with joy. If Americans had just worn masks, my sister would not be in some ICU dying. I would not feel her chirping heart beneath the palm of my hand and witness the indigo hue of death fill her lips. My tango life cancelled no longer mattered.

In a post-Covid-19 world, we will touch again. Tango dancers will rejoice in their reunion, strangers will embrace and take pause, and we will vow never to take touch for granted again. And like life, so too such vows will pass.

2

POEMS

Nabina Das

Come Eat My Lotus Heart

Beloved, I want you to be my lotus-heart
Step across; come see my lotus-heart.

Germination has deserted this firmament.
So only you can come free my lotus-heart.

The bazaar no longer has our footprints --
Don't now make me flee my lotus-heart.

TV sets blare inside homes. Can they hear
What birds speak in glee: "My lotus-heart!"

How to again kiss? We cannot even touch!
Did I lose, Navi, in this melee, my lotus-heart?

(First published in *tinfoildresses* Spring 2021)

Limits

It began with examining specks
lying over the floor. As if gems.
Our nail waste, tangled hair, dead skin.
Dead bits of ourselves showcased.
Like spent dragonfly wings. Life
in its limitlessness kissed by death.
But a kiss is like kintsugi. It repairs.
Also, it doesn't believe in limits. Mostly
remaining off limits in its morphology.
But it began with gauging each square
foot of the space we tend to step on.
How much of this air? How much vacuum?
What inches accord us our coordinates,
were the questions. As against each
footprint we left on the wet surfaces
of our dreams, life became microscopic.

DOI: 10.4324/9781003320524-4

Measure the limits of life in coffee cups
the poet said! You did too. When alone
we tried saying loving words from
another era in history. You showed me
how to hold a butcher's knife right. Left
me with my own throbbing heart.
It began with dicing time, love, life, as
they died. As sparks in flight. All night.
    (First published in *The Environmental Situation Room* by The Kala
                      Chaupal Trust, April 2020)

'For Calling the Spirit Back from Wandering the Earth in Its Human Feet'

(Title quoted from a poem by Joy Harjo)

Nights have a special place
in our awakening. It's from
the night that we came. Wandering.

Who's the Believer then? Shall we pray
in the dark watches of the night
when daylight shows only misery:
the practice of tahajjud, in the darkest night.

The day is all lime-sprinkled. Laundry
Soaking like our hearts in fear. Disinfectants
Wrapping us as we seek barakaat.

Shab-e-Baraat, Shab-e-Baraat --
the Night of Forgiveness flowers
faster than flames.

Send us dua, night birds sing.
Send us the extracts from
your Lailat-ul Dua, the sap of your deeds,
say day flies stuck on human spoils.

Amid EMI flats and concrete rises
Burnt smell of broken hearths
Footfalls driven out of homes.
See how our past catches up with us.

Make this the night of records,
for every night. The day of gathering
bounties each day. Call the spirits back.

Today, my eyes like Christ's eyes
cannot find enough moist earth
to rest the wounds of my people.
                    (First published in *tinfoildresses* Spring 2021)

3

REFUGEE WOMEN FROM DIFFERENT CONTINENTS DANCE IN A CIRCLE

Alejandra Saavendra

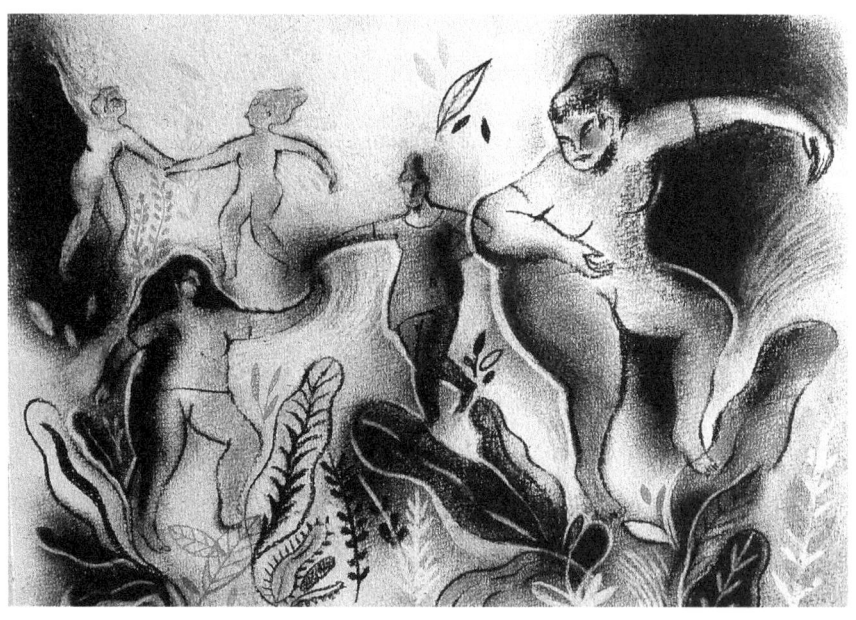

Artwork 3.1 Refugee Women from Different Continents Dance in a Circle.

DOI: 10.4324/9781003320524-5

4

POEMS

Megan Savage

My Mother, a Return Peace Corps Volunteer, Comments on the March 2020 Global Evacuation of Peace Corps Volunteers

I remember when you came home, from the Peace Corps. You spoke English rather haltingly.

> – Nancy Norman Aldridge

I remember you telling me that it was a rule of thumb that it took half as long to adjust as you had been away

> – Gillian Bagwell

Sending heartfelt compassion
and sympathy
to the over 7,000 Peace Corps volunteers
suddenly being evacuated
from 61 countries
and returned to the U.S.
jobless,
with positions terminated.

Re-entry to the U.S.
is the most difficult cultural adjustment/
transition of all,
even if you are a Peace Corps volunteer
in "normal" times
(as I was)
and your return is planned for.

It is MUCH harder to return
to a country you thought
you knew,

DOI: 10.4324/9781003320524-6

after months
or years,
than to make the cultural adjustment
to living in the new,
"foreign,"
"different"
country
the Peace Corps has trained you
to live in.

My Mother, a Sociologist with Breast Cancer, Tells a Story on May Day, 2020

I was in grad school at Michigan State
the year that Kent State happened.
The students who were demonstrating against the Vietnam War
got shot, the national guard came and shot at them,
and you know,
there was death.

So grad students all over the country,
not only grad students
but a lot of people,
went on strike,
which we did at Michigan State,
which is a whole nother story.

Anyway, I was in the grad student room
one time in May that year.
I think it was May 5,
I might be wrong,
that Kent State happened.

One of my female friends came in
with a bunch of flowers
that she had picked
because it was May
and she was all excited
about spring
and everything.

And then a male friend,
both of them were grad students
in the same Sociology department

with me, he was from Libya,
and he came in and he took
one look at her flowers and he said,
No Flowers Until After the Revolution.

I always felt like
you can't stop life.
You have to be able
to do the two things
at one time.

My Mother Masters the Art of the French Omelette

She uses a fork and the same type of pan
and number of eggs,
that the *New Yorker* writer suggests.
And she does the thing in the pan
so the runny part goes to the edge.

Of course, she doesn't flip it like he describes,
"slipping the spatula under the lip
of the omelette," and squeezing in an unorthodox
third flip, for a layered result — instead she slides
a metal plate over the pan
(the green one from the camping set)
and flips the omelette like so.

She is sure she learned to make omelettes
from some cookbook or other, not at home.

You remember what my mother always said, right?
She didn't want us to spend lots of time learning to cook;
she wanted us to learn to read,
and then we could use cookbooks.
(I always think my sister was thinking of that
when she gave me that paperback Fanny Farmer
as a wedding present).

Actually, her mother taught her a lot of cooking,
but other than dinner salads she assembled nightly
while her mother cooked the rest,
it was fun stuff. Cookies, pies, cakes, biscuits,
bread, taffy, popcorn, and so forth.

My mother's mother, one of twelve,
grew up on a farm in Dodge City, Kansas,
during the Great Depression, worked
as a soda jerk to save the money to put herself
through nursing school, became
the head of the contagious disease ward
at Cook County, Chicago's largest
public hospital, before antibiotics, before
hand washing was common practice,
before raising five children
(the ones who lived)
and before releasing her children's father
to World War II, to tending wounded soldiers on the front
in Sardinia and North Africa.

Cookies, pies, cakes, biscuits,
bread, taffy, popcorn, and so forth, peanut butter fudge.

Later still, became a docent at the Field Museum
of Natural History, where she taught herself
hieroglyphics,
and gave Katherine Hepburn a private tour
(a highlight of her life).

Use tongs, I tell my arthritic mother.
It will make it easier to maneuver
the vegetables. *Cooking tongs?* she asks.
My mother called those "forceps."

My Mother's Breast Cancer Surgeon Asks with Interest about Her Record of TB Treatment

i.   My mother would just as soon
     leave her shirt off. She is a doctor's daughter and
     the performance of modesty
     is uncomfortable in this context.
     In this context, her breast is a body part.

     The surgeon has seen her medical chart, and
     asks about her record of surgeries,
     as he palpitates her breast.
     Collects an oral history and makes small talk
     as he feels for the lump in the tissue and lymph nodes.

Born and raised in Denver, Dr. Imatani
is a third-generation Japanese American. His summers
spent helping family with their pickle company
made him appreciate the value of hard work,
leading him to his career in medicine.

I take notes as he circles. He says "tubal ligation"
and I catch my breath, but don't ask what I might
want to. I was interested to see isoniazide
on your chart, the surgeon says, in an avuncular way.
Tell me about that.

It was a long time ago. The paper under
my mother rustles as she moves. After
I came back from the Peace Corps,
in Turkey, she says.

ii.   I had a friend there,
wife of a shopkeeper,
a mother. A traditional woman.

Towards the end of my time,
she was sick, coughing.

But she did not want to go see
a (male)
doctor.

Finally she went and was examined
somehow
by being seen in a mirror,

so I was told;
it turned out to be tuberculosis.

Around then we were ending
our two years and leaving.

We were processed a final time
by the US Public Health Service doctor
assigned to us.

We were checked every 3 months
as I recall
so when they saw a positive

on my TB test they knew
when it happened,
and I knew
where I was exposed.

They said it was early stage TB
and prescribed a year of medication
(isoniazide) and to get annual chest X-rays.

After I returned to the US
I learned my friend had died.

When I came back
I was a grad student at Michigan State.
I went to the health service
to let the doctor know I was on isoniazide
but he seemed like he never heard of it.

Anyway my annual chest X-rays
were clear.

Eventually medical recommendations
were to avoid so much radiation
(research changes)
so since everything had been clear
for a few years
I stopped.

iii. The nurses don't understand
her humor. She jokes with them
at every visit, and they always look confused.
Portlanders are so literal, we say.

Can I have a Snoopy bandaid? She asks
the nurse with the Mickey Mouse scrubs.
Oh, yes, the nurse says, I'll get you one.
And my mother gives me a look.

Later, she tells the nurse, Candy,
who is struggling to connect a tube to the port
inserted surgically in my mother's chest,
I know what the doctors
are doing. Candy smiles,
a benign and reassuring smile.

They put something in the chemo
To make my hair fall out, my mother says.
It's their plan, so we will have to worry
about wigs or hats or scarves.
About how we look and
how to clean the hair from our pillows.
It's all one big scheme on their parts,
to make sure we
have something to focus on
besides the cancer.

In a Time of Distance

My cousin is afraid to journal
because writing breaks her open.

My mother's hijab, fifty years old and
recovered from a drawer,
smells musty but won't slide
across her balding head
like silk scarves do.

And anyway, why cover the head
When home alone?
Not modesty, only
to catch the fine fallen hairs
that make a mess on her pillow.

Present the self a ceremony.
Listen.

These are the facts of the third week in March:
The blossoms covered by unseasonable snow.
The friend in hospice as quarantine starts.
Sensitive skin of my ribs, sheets that cause pain.
The absence in the chemo ward waiting room.
No one to see St. Helens appear from under the clouds.

Listen.

This poem doesn't have a sad
Or a happy
ending.
It does what it needs to do,
It poems.

5

KARTIK'S LAST WORDS

Ahmed Shamim

ইতি কার্তিক
-

স্পর্শকাতর মানুষগুলো
ছোঁয়াচে রোগে মৃত্যুর ভয়ে নৃশংস খুনি হলে
অবাক হয়ো না চন্দনা,
বাকস্ফূর্তি রেখো, কথা বোলো:
শৃঙ্খলের দুর্বল আংটাগুলো খুলে ফেলে
শক্ত শেকলে
নিজেদের আটকে বাঁচার চতুর চেষ্টায়
দর্শন পাল্টে
উৎকট নিরাসক্তিতে নতুন জীবন পাওয়া
মানুষগুলোকে বোলো,
আমাদের কী ছিল:
স্পর্শের কাঙাল শরীর
আর শারীরিক সম্পর্ক।

If these distant people,
in fear of dying from contagious diseases
turn into ruthless murderers,
don't find your tongue tied in terror, Chandana, talk!
Tell these shrewd citizens of the upcoming world,
the neo-humans, the philosophically void
progeny of virulent apathy, who
by weeding out the weak links of their shackles
are getting ready to tightly chain themselves to live,
what we had:
a world of touch-loving bodies,
a world of physical intimacy.

DOI: 10.4324/9781003320524-7

HOME AND THE WORLD

6

PLETHORA OF EMOTIONS ENGULF THE EVERYDAY LIFE

Anju Chaudhury

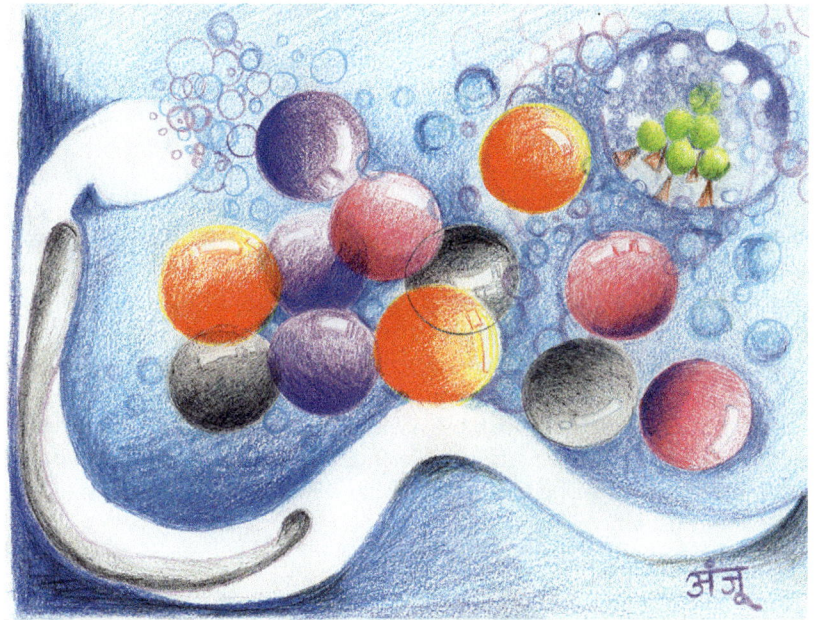

Artwork 6.1 Plethora of Emotions Engulf the Everyday Life.

The lockdown forced us to reflect on our inner world. Abstraction has always given me a window to express myself. This artwork is a reflection of the solitary time and thoughts engulfing the individual. The forced confinement at home brought to the fore a range of complex emotions – difficult memories and happy moments. Thoughts are like bubbles that are connected to each other. Some memories are clearer and more prominent than the rest.

DOI: 10.4324/9781003320524-9

7

POST-COVID-19 URBANSCAPE

Re-imagining Housing as Infrastructures of Care
May 2021

Anup Tripathi

Introduction

Covid-19 pandemic presented all of us with a challenge. The challenge of maintaining social distancing and following lockdown and containment measures as well as obtaining treatment through home isolation in cases with mild symptoms by mostly remaining in the confines of our homes. So far, the most potent response to the Covid-19 pandemic is physical or social distancing, which has emerged as the most effective containment measure. However, it is simply not possible to follow social distancing norms in the densely populated informal settlements in Indian cities. It is estimated that social distancing norms will become more commonplace in future (Stiepan 2020; Mishagina et al. 2021; Yuko 2021) as human populations become more susceptible to zoonotic infections and spread of pandemics (Christou 2011; Dodds 2019; Awaidy and Al Hashami 2020; Harypursat and Chen 2020).

Housing, according to the World Health Organization's Social Determinants of Health, along with infrastructure, socio-economic conditions, and social exclusion, is a key determinant of population health. It has been widely recognised for years that housing is a public health issue (Barker 2020). People living in poor-quality, cramped, and unsuitable accommodation are more likely to suffer from a wide range of illnesses, such as cancer, respiratory, and cardiovascular diseases. India has the largest inadequately housed population in the world with around 35 per cent of urban dwellers living in slums (The World Bank 2021). Indian cities are inhabitant sites of various kinds of informal, precariat housing arrangements. 'Precariat Housing' is any kind of dwelling arrangement that is not formal and regularised (Tripathi 2017, 2018). Most of the urban poor engaged in various kinds of economic activities house themselves in such precariat housing arrangements.

DOI: 10.4324/9781003320524-10

The 'idea of home' encapsulates two characteristics – a physical structure for living and an embodiment of emotions. A well-constructed physical structure of living not only protects from elements but also checks against communicable diseases. Thus, from the point of view of health, a properly constructed house with adequate sanitation facilities is essential. The current Covid-19 pandemic situation forces us to reflect on the embodied, relational, and affective cartographies of the space in our inhabiting practices in the urban. Housing (both individual houses and the broader housing system) supports or hinders the capacity of households to care in different degrees (Power and Mee 2019). However, a broader articulation between care and housing remains substantially under conceptualised (Ibid.). In this article, I am making a case for considering housing as an infrastructure of care and how universal housing as well as several other general interventions in housing can be used to augment the healthcare infrastructure to fight against zoonotic infections in the future.

Social Distancing and Staying at Home

Housing is a key site through which Covid-19 is experienced (Garber 2020, as cited in Rogers and Power 2020). Social distancing and social isolation are important public health measures that depend on people having access to safe and secure housing (Rogers and Power 2020). To break the chain of transmission, the medical fraternity has prescribed following the social distancing protocols. Many governments the world over, including the Government of India, enforced lockdown as a containment measure. Due to the lockdown and as per the advice of the WHO and medical community, two different but interrelated responses emerged. One was to stay at home and not to go outside unless absolutely necessary popularised through the hashtag and slogan #stayathomesavelives ('Stay at Home, Save Lives') (MyGov Cell 2020). The second was sanctified through the emergent practices of work from home (W-F-H) for white-collar professionals and remote or online learning for students and educators. Both of these responses have a couple of implicit assumptions in them. First, it assumes that everyone has a house (rented or owned), where they can stay put without having to worry about maintaining a physical distance. Second, it assumes that the houses are big enough to accord personal space to all the family members regardless of the family size. Third, the houses have the necessary infrastructure and space to convert into and act as infirmary, hospice, quarantine, home office, classroom, as well as recreational and social spaces.

Many of these assumptions were put into practice through government guidelines and regulations as soon as the pandemic started spreading in India in 2020. As hospitals became flooded with Covid-positive patients, the government recommended home isolation for patients showing mild symptoms and gave them 'Corona Kits' that contain different types of allopathic, Ayurvedic, and Unani medicines. Later on, in the first half of 2021 when the country was ravaged by a devastating 'second wave' of infections, a number of doctors who were providing teleconsultations recommended not only medicine prescriptions but also oxygen cylinders and oxygen concentrators and, in some cases, even home ICUs for patients undergoing treatment at home. In some sense, care practices that could be performed at home were envisioned through such a guideline. Additionally, stringent lockdowns and work-from-home options were exercised in the hope that they would help in breaking the chain of transmission and containing the spread of infection.

However, given the reality of housing in the country, especially in the urban areas, the idea that one can break the chain of transmission without social distancing has fallen flat on its face. According to a news report, in Dharavi (Mumbai), which is the largest slum in the country, eight to ten people live together in poky 100 sq. ft. dwellings, and about 80 per cent of the residents in this slum use community toilets (Biswas 2020). The narrow lanes of the slum are dotted with homes and factories coexisting in single buildings. Most people residing over here are informal daily-wage workers who do not cook at home and buy their food from outside. Apart from slum areas, many informal workers also reside and rest in interstitial city spaces like hume pipes, railway platforms, shop awnings, and vehicles like autos, taxis, and buses. Similar informal housing conditions prevail in various other metropolitan and medium and small towns of the country, where it is impossible to practise social distancing within the confines of one's home. According to Khan and Abraham (2020), almost a third of the rural population and half of the urban population in India live in houses where the per capita space available is less than a single room, which effectively means that isolating a person with the risk of infection is extremely difficult (Khan and Abraham 2020). This implies that home quarantine/self-isolation measures would be difficult to implement among 60 per cent of the population in the event of the spread of infection (Ibid.).

At the same time, the availability of running water in houses is a necessity to ensure frequent handwashing with soap. Khan and Abraham (2020) cite the NSSO data, which reveals that 40 per cent of urban households and 75 per cent of rural households in India do not have access to tap water in the house or within their residential premises (Khan and Abraham 2020). Additionally, about 8 per cent of the Indian population uses public sanitation facilities and a quarter of the population has no access to any sanitation facility, making it difficult to follow good hygiene (Ibid.). Maintaining social distancing, following hygiene, and complying with self-isolation guidelines is extremely difficult for a majority of the population due to existing housing and sanitation facilities. While some people are likely to prioritise a level of physical distance and isolation in their residential searches, it is critical to note that many individuals in the country are unable to do so in densely populated areas due to caste and religion-based residential segregation and concentrated poverty. In this regard, pandemics such as Covid-19 become another layer that further isolates and disadvantages low-resource neighbourhoods (Jones and Grigsby-Toussaint 2020).

Pandemic and the Resurfacing of Housing Crisis

Covid-19 has amplified spatial inequalities (Jones and Grigsby-Toussaint 2020). As per a study in the UK, there is a link between Covid-19 deaths and the housing crisis (Barker 2020). The study suggests that areas with more overcrowded housing have been worst hit by coronavirus. Additionally, there is a higher incidence of deaths due to Covid-19 among the homeless and people living in temporary accommodations. Covid-19 deaths are also positively correlated with social housing shortages. Poor-quality housing and overcrowding are almost certainly contributing to poor mental health during the lockdown (Ibid.). Thus, there is evidence that failure to get to grips with the housing crisis has helped make society vulnerable to coronavirus.

Globally, we are in the throes of a housing crisis, which is characterised by a chronic shortage of affordable housing for the vulnerable in society, and in many cases, for the working and middle classes as well (World Economic Forum 2019; United Nations General Assembly 2020). The lockdowns imposed in several countries have led to economic stagnation as well as revealed the absence of safe housing needed to survive during the pandemic (Farha 2020). The UN has shed light on an 'international housing crisis' (Farha 2018; Rolnik 2013), from volatility of housing systems, to evictions, overcrowding, unaffordability, substandard conditions, homelessness, and displacement (Fields and Hodkinson 2018). For people experiencing homelessness or for those who sleep rough, the idea that you can retreat to a private dwelling is, in many cases, simply not an option. This can lead to a whole host of connected issues, ranging from a greater risk of exposure to Covid-19 to a greater risk of coming into contact with the authorities when the public spaces of our cities are placed in lockdown (Rogers and Power 2020). Inadequate housing conditions for millions of marginalised people have contributed to excessive, and largely preventable, levels of death and suffering. The economic crisis caused by the pandemic is further entrenching these inequalities.

India has been witnessing all these housing-related issues. Due to the surge in the number of Covid-19 cases in the second wave of Covid-19 in India, the healthcare staff, families, NGOs, volunteers, government employees, etc., have once again come under severe strain while catering to the needs of the patients. Due to the shortage of beds in the hospitals (James 2021), many patients had to be treated in their homes. In India, there is an estimated shortage of around 18 million houses, with 99 per cent of this in the economically weaker sections of society (Gopalan and Venkataraman 2015). As a result, most of the urban population in the country resides in informal housing arrangements of various kinds, ranging from declared slums to non-declared slums, squatters, housing in interstitial city spaces, pavement dwellings, precarious dwellings, homelessness, etc. Most such informal housing is built by the people and not the market and the state. These informal settlements are marked by explicit blockage to service delivery and legal contestation resulting in their informality.

Let us consider the case of Delhi – the megacity serving as the capital of India for the past 110 years. According to Gautam Bhan, despite the currency of terms like 'encroachment' and widespread 'land grab' in the popular imagination, slums are occupying a minute portion of city land – less than 0.6 per cent of total land area, and 3.4 per cent of residential land in the 2021 Delhi Master Plan (Bhan 2020). This tiny percentage supports no less than 11–15 per cent but possibly up to 30 per cent of the city's population, mostly settled for decades. As against this figure, in 2017, for parking, Delhi's 3.1 million cars used 13.25 square kilometres of land or 5 per cent of all residential area. Thus, cars in Delhi have more space than the informal housing space of the working classes! Similar examples illustrating the apathy of the state and market actors to provide affordable housing to the poorer sections of the society can be found in almost all the urban areas of the country. To make things worse, the state actors have actively exacerbated the housing crisis in the middle of the pandemic. In September 2020, the Supreme Court of India ordered the eviction of 48,000 slum clusters located within safety zones along railway tracks in Delhi within three months (The Hindu 2020). Later, the Supreme Court stayed an order passed by the Karnataka High Court (Plumber 2021) by which it had directed the state government to reconstruct at its own cost the huts/shanties of migrant workers in Bengaluru, which were burnt down near the Kacharakanahalli slum in Bengaluru East, by unknown 'miscreants', when the occupants had left for their native places after the announcement of the lockdown (Plumber 2020).

Indian cities are marked by the problem of inadequate housing. However, the housing crisis has been aggravated by the pandemic as informal housing arrangements fall short of the standard prescription of fighting the pandemic – i.e. stay at home, maintain social distancing and practise home isolation in case of infection. Chronic lack of healthcare infrastructure, sanitation and water facilities for the urban poor and their settlements especially at a time when practising good hygiene is foremost only adds insult to the injury. Thus, the pandemic resurfaces a housing crisis not tackled systematically across sectors and has now become a long overdue duty for the state, market, and civil society to resolve. To resolve the housing crisis prevalent in the country, certain interventions as being demanded by civil society practitioners, housing rights activists, and academicians are required in this sector. Additionally, envisaging housing as an infrastructure of care is warranted with regard to the pandemic situation of the present and future.

Interventions Required in Housing

According to Leilani Farha, former United Nations Special Rapporteur on the right to adequate housing, 'housing is the frontline defence in the fight against COVID-19' (Reckford 2020). In the cities of the world, two population groups are particularly at higher risks – those living in emergency shelters, informal settlements, or those who are homeless and those facing job loss and economic hardship, which could result in mortgage and rental arrears and evictions (Ibid.). The right to adequate housing is, at its core, the right to a place to live in dignity and security. It is interdependent with other human rights, particularly the right to equality and non-discrimination and the right to life (Farha 2017). According to another report transmitted by the Secretary-General at the 75th UN General Assembly, access to adequate housing has become even more critical during the pandemic (Rajagopal 2020). The report quotes Balakrishnan Rajagopal, the Special Rapporteur on adequate housing, as: 'In the context of COVID-19, having no home, lacking space for physical distancing in overcrowded living areas or having inadequate access to water and sanitation has become a death sentence, handed out predominantly against poor and marginalized communities' (Ibid.). According to Raquel Rolnik, the right to adequate housing has to be understood as a 'gateway to other rights'; it is a condition that has to be fulfilled to ensure the exercise of belonging in all its aspects (Rolnik 2014). Thus, to tackle the housing crisis, several interventions are warranted by the state and market actors.

The World Economic Forum has recommended several measures to tackle the housing crisis post the Covid-19 pandemic. Some of the important recommendations are (a) focusing on healthy housing equipped with adequate water, sanitation, and hygiene facilities; (b) meeting the critical housing targets in the UN's Sustainable Development Goals (SDG); (c) employing specific housing finance strategies to help low-income families; (d) raising awareness of housing as a significant contributor to national economies; and (e) providing relief for families at risk of being evicted or of losing their homes (Reckford 2020). All these recommendations are helpful in the Indian context and must be applied as such.

Recognising auto-construction (Holston 1991; Caldeira 2017) in housing is another intervention that is warranted in the country as it acknowledges peoples' agency and labour in city building. Autoconstruction is a radicalising process in which people build their own houses in urban areas under precarious material and legal circumstances (Holston 1991). Housing oneself in a city outside legal settlements including regularised slums requires tremendous fortitude and enterprise in an individual, family, or group of individuals. The different kinds of inadequate dwelling arrangements on pavements, shop awnings, unauthorised slums or 'homeless settlements', parks, pavements, platforms, etc., indicate that the people residing in them look at housing as an opportunity to lead a stable or better life.

The everyday life of such people shows that there are various kinds of material dimensions to housing like identity, citizenship entitlements, healthcare and sanitation, incomes and expenditures, finances and savings, availability of food and livelihood, social networks and relationships, etc., which are socially produced and reproduced (Tripathi 2017). Through their struggles, grit, and determination, people living in such inadequate housing arrangements add on different dimensions to housing, thereby making it a composite idea required for a decent living rather than a mere physical structure for living. By actively housing themselves outside the formal housing system, these people seek to consolidate their 'gains'. Hence, auto-construction should not be merely looked at from the point of formal property rights but as a strategy of inhabitation and active housing by the poor. Housing policies intent on market-led provisions limit the possibility of auto-construction and incremental housing. They also limit the toehold of the migrants in the city and exclude them from the land markets. Thus, the territorialisation of the poor happens through the identification of informality or illegality in the self-built unplanned and unserviced settlements. Although the occupation in such areas is against the norms and laws, it serves a functional value in providing housing alternatives to a poorly paid working force (Rolnik 2014). It is pertinent that informal housing arrangements like slums should not be considered as encroachments for personal gain. On the contrary, they mark the state and market failure to provide affordable and legal housing. In fact, slums are the only affordable housing stock built at scale by any actor in the city. It is the starting of a solution to urban inequality rather than a problem to be solved (Bhan 2020). Most importantly, recognition of auto-constructed housing by the state and non-state actors helps the urban poor and migrant workers in claiming public services and safeguarding territorial claims.

Informal settlements are not just a collection of houses but housing. The difference between the two is how workers survive in cities despite low wages. A house can be resettled, perhaps, but housing cannot simply be transplanted (Bhan 2020). Housing requires not just a *pucca* (permanent accommodation) structure but the possibility of employment and affordable mobility. It is linked to admission for children in local schools, employers' homes that domestic workers can walk or cycle to, public institutions wherein trust has been built between the authorities and the locals, arrangements for child-care with known neighbours, and streets that vendors and rickshaw drivers have mastered as markets. This is why the urban poor exercise a great deal of caution in choosing the space for 'housing' themselves. Location is an essential element of the right to adequate housing, as it is the most straightforward link between housing, inhabitation, and citizenship. Therefore, any recognition of auto-construction in housing should also delineate the logic exercised by the urban poor and migrant workers for housing themselves in a particular location.

Recognising auto-constructed housing is just one part of the overall solution. The second part is upscaling and upgrading the existing housing infrastructure. Although their informality is a challenge, it is central to thinking about urbanism in the Global South in general and India in particular. A normative framework of 'decent habitation' along the lines of the Decent Work framework as developed by the International Labour Organization (ILO) may be deployed for the same (International Labour Organization, n.d.). Any housing arrangement that is not decent or proper for habitation and living – be it slums, homeless clusters, or inadequate housing arrangements of various kinds must be upgraded to decent housing through state action. Stringent laws must be passed in the legislatures, which seek to end indecent habitation and upgrade existing housing arrangements through in-situ upgradation, apart from enlarging the role of the state in welfare. There is an enormous range of housing in India and hence it constitutes a big arena for state action in terms of improving the quality and quantity of housing stocks in the country. Rather than privileging formal property settlements as the dominant mode of housing, different forms of property rights should be acknowledged and recognised. Disconnecting service delivery from tenures and acupuncturing and retrofitting services in the complex and dense informal settlements as interim measures should become part of the essential housing strategy in a country like India. This is not to suggest that new housing stocks should not be built for the urban poor. However, the predominant approach should be that of upgradation. We require upgrading as opposed to redevelopment as the predominant approach since it does not completely transform the built environment, thereby ensuring that livelihoods and living patterns of the people are not disrupted to a great extent. Redevelopment is often not able to uphold the lives in the same way as *in-situ* upgradation, as evident from the examples of Latin America and Thailand. Regularising settlements on an 'as is where is' basis is the fastest, cheapest, safest, and most effective way to secure tenure and respect a lifetime of investment (Bhan 2020).

Ensuring affordable rental housing in Indian cities is another policy goal that merits the attention of policymakers and administrators. Historically, housing policies in India have been ownership centric. Therefore, it is important to explore rental housing solutions. To that end, the Affordable Rental Housing Complexes (ARHCs)[1] as a sub-scheme of the Pradhan Mantri Awas Yojana (PMAY – Urban)[2] for the migrants and the urban poor is a welcome step. The scheme envisages (a) utilising existing government-funded vacant houses to convert into ARHCs through a public-private partnership or by public agencies and (b) construction, operation and maintenance of ARHCs by public/private entities on their own vacant land (Ministry of Housing and Urban Affairs 2020). It is important to realise that poor working classes in the cities lead multi-local lives and not just migrant lives in the urban areas. Proximity to the workplace is an important consideration while deciding on a housing option. Therefore, the link between housing and livelihood for the migrant workers must be understood before devising any kind of social or rental housing options for them. At the same time, building multiple forms of rental housing is important, especially employer responsibility rental housing. The employers hiring low-wage contractual migrant workers should share the responsibility of providing decent rental housing options to their workforce so that these workers living on meagre wages do not have to squatter or reside in precariat housing. The government could also think of converting vacant public housing into rental housing options for migrant workers. The current economic situation in the wake of the Covid-19 pandemic demands an emergency program of comprehensive relief for renters and homeowners, whether they are working or not. The goal should be to secure people's right to remain in their homes for the duration of this crisis period and until the economy begins to recover.

Perhaps, the most important general intervention that is required is to work towards affordable social housing for the needy. It can be achieved through a policy push that calls for a 'Housing for All' approach seeking universal social housing while at the same time, discarding markets as the most rational and efficient allocator of public goods. In the times of the neo-liberal policy paradigm, it is even more essential that we recreate and fight for the idea of 'public' and reclaim housing as a public good. While conceptualising and implementing public housing, we must rescue it from welfare discourse and see the inadequately housed people as active agents in shaping their destinies. Not only is it important to remain conscious of the structural factors that serve to shape their agency, but it is also pertinent to incorporate their voices and recognise their agency while building social housing for them. To that effect, new institutional mechanisms for delivering public housing may be envisaged.

Lastly, we must seek intervention in institutional setups like prisons and shelter homes, etc. The close-packed accommodation at government incarceration facilities put the populations in these facilities at high risk of infection and need to be reduced to a minimum, while those convicted of nonviolent crimes should be released from prison. To ensure everyone can safely shelter in place and practice social distancing, we need to address ongoing problems of overcrowding in shelters as well as homelessness in our cities. There is a need to set up more homeless shelters and various other types of shelter homes that could serve not only as housing facilities but also as enablers for the destitute, vulnerable, and socially excluded people, rather than being places of confinement. Such shelter homes can be conceived as service homes for providing various types of services and citizenship entitlements to persons in need of care and protection. The services may include providing identity documentation, legal aid, psychiatric care, counselling, healthcare, adult education, vocational training and job placements, livelihood, *Anganwadi* or ICDS-related services, recreation, repatriation, daycare centres, etc. It is imperative that the state being the ultimate protector and caretaker of all its residents provides care, support, and protection to them.

Thus, in response to the joint economic and health crises of today, there is an opportunity to develop and implement inclusive housing strategies that stimulate the economy and improve community health outcomes. A robust body of research has established that housing is an economic sector with strong multiplier effects on both employment and consumption, particularly in countries with well-developed credit markets (Pugh 1994; Mayer and Somerville 2000; Adelino et al. 2015; Mian and Sufi 2015 as cited in Acolin, Hoek-Smit and Green 2020). The housing finance institutions in India need to provide affordable interest rates particularly to people working in the informal sector. At the same time, the public and the private real estate sectors must work towards reducing the cost of housing and making it affordable for the economically weaker sections. While these actions may seem challenging, they actually represent the minimum effort necessary to get us through the present crisis. They are not the ultimate solution to this nation's housing crisis. Unfortunately, for that, we need much more.

Envisaging Housing as Infrastructure of Care

Covid-19 has made a compelling case for re-imagining housing as an infrastructure of care apart from being a physical space of living and embodiment of emotions. Domestic houses are increasingly being understood as hubs of care practices and relations (Power and Mee 2019). During the second wave, as hospitals in India struggled to provide beds for the Covid patients, the medical fraternity started prescribing home isolation for asymptomatic patients as well as for patients with mild symptoms, which reflected in the subsequent government directives mandating the same. It saved many individuals and families from incurring out-of-pocket health expenditure as costs for the hospitalisation of Covid-19 patients have increased exponentially. These patients could now be tended to by their family members and neighbours with on and off visits by the healthcare professionals, as and when necessary. During the second wave of Covid-19 in India, as hospitals became overwhelmed with demands for oxygen beds and ICU beds, many people procured critical care products like oxygen cylinders, oxygen concentrators, BIPAP, etc., and even set up home ICUs for patients in home isolation. Thus, the space of the home gets established, firstly, as a central location for care work, and secondly, as a space and locus of meaning that informs the performance of care (Power and Mee 2019).

Dwelling in a home entails processes of accommodation with the housing structure, as residents adapt their home to suit their needs and alter their practices to suit their accommodation (Miller 2002 as cited in Power and Mee 2019). However, such arrangements also necessitate a house large enough to practise isolation as well as provide critical care with at least one additional bedroom that can be spared for the patient. Additionally, even for practising home quarantine, a similar requirement needs to be met.

Apart from an additional room, availability of water and adequate sanitation facilities is also warranted under such a situation. Unfortunately, for a large population in urban India, adequate housing arrangements and water and sanitation facilities are still a far cry. Nevertheless, home quarantine and isolation as standardised ways of fighting Covid-19 infection highlight the necessity of housing as an important hub of care practices and relationships apart from hospitals and health centres. Their efficacy should prompt us to realise their importance as care infrastructure. Foregrounding care as a relational practice recognises that care is central to human existence and vital to the maintenance of life. That is why we need a framework as well as a policy push that seeks to forge connections between care and housing through centring care within an analysis of the house-as-home (Power and Mee 2019).

As a former Covid-19 patient with moderate to severe symptoms who underwent home isolation for recovery, I must state that I greatly benefitted from the care provided to me by my family members and doctors who provided teleconsultation to me. Covid-19 infection sometimes causes serious weakness in the body, and it is very difficult to manage things on your own. The care that one's neighbours or family members can provide like giving food, procuring medicines, health supplements, etc., as well as checking on breathing status, body ache, body temperature, SPO2 levels, etc., is critical to treatment, recovery, and recuperation. My personal experience tells me that apart from the role of medication, non-institutional care is extremely crucial for the treatment of Covid-19 patients. There are many families and individuals who cannot get such care as either they are alone in the house or all the members in the family have the infection. In such cases, the role of relatives, neighbours and friends in extending care to them becomes critical to their treatment and recovery. Ensuring housing situations that can facilitate such a type of sociality and non-institutional care arrangements is critical to the re-imagining of the post-Covid-19 urbanscape.

The sociality and communal way of living in various kinds of housing arrangements have come in handy in testing times like the current pandemic. According to Jean Luc Nancy (2020), Covid-19 reminds us 'of our togetherness, interdependence, and solidarity' and therefore heightens our capacity for solidarity (Quarshie 2020) and care (The Care Collective 2020) during and possibly beyond the pandemic (Rogers and Power 2020). This is manifested in the way various voluntary organisations and individual volunteers, as well as neighbourhood organisations, have been helping Covid-affected people. However, there are concerns about Covid-19's impact on the global economy and the flow-on impacts on solidarity and care networks (Davies 2020; De Angelis 2020, as cited in Rogers and Power 2020). It should make us only cautiously optimistic about our capacity for care and solidarity (Iveson 2020), and many of us can already feel our solidarity and care networks straining under the pressure of Covid-19 at home.

Infrastructures are proposed as a gathering force and political interme-diary of considerable significance in shaping the rights of the poor to the city and their capacity to claim those rights (Amin 2014). They are not just pre-figured objects or necessarily public, capital goods, but as dynamic patterns that are the foundation of social organisation (Star 1999 as cited in Power and Mee 2019). Envisaging housing as an infra-structure of care should take into account the changing societal backdrop along with state inaction on the issue of housing. Housing designs, spaces, and materials iteratively shape the performance of care. At the same time, more than a container within which people live and practice care, hous-ing actively shapes inhabitance (Dowling and Power 2012; Miller 2002, as cited in Power and Mee 2019). As society is becoming more and more modern and individualistic, the traditional caregiving arrangements are falling apart which earlier used to take care of the poor and needy albeit in the charity mode as well as people with special needs like older adults, children, and women.

Once housing is cognised as an infrastructure of care, there is also a need to understand how such infrastructures are being constructed. Infrastructures – visible and invisible, grand and prosaic – are implicated in the human experience of the city and in shaping social identities (Tonkis 2013 as cited in Amin 2014). It is the familial ties and social relationships on the streets and homeless clusters, housing colonies, and neighbourhood associations as well as community and professional networks with physi-cal spaces to interact that help in the formation as well as strengthening of infrastructure of care. Housing as an infrastructure of care can be con-ceived as a strategy of the people who form active communities. Thus, infrastructures – visible and invisible – are deeply implicated not only in the making and unmaking of individual lives but also in the experience of community, solidarity, and struggle for recognition (Amin 2014). At the same time, considering housing as an infrastructure turns on efforts to revalue social housing as a public asset (Power and Mee 2019) that can greatly augment our healthcare infrastructure.

Conclusion

The variegated nature of the housing sector in India demands diverse policy interventions – focus on supporting and enabling incremental growth, envi-ronmental improvements, and affordable rental housing, rather than a uni-dimensional approach that promotes new house construction (Indorewala 2017). In the post-Covid-19 urbanscape, a housing justice wish list would include a number of interventions in housing. It would include recognition of decent housing as a basic right of all Indians; focus on healthy housing equipped with adequate water, sanitation, and hygiene facilities; widespread availability of public and social housing, effective rent control; the abolition of homelessness; and providing relief for families at risk of being evicted or of losing their homes. It would insist on an immediate end to the caste, gender, religious, ethnic, and class inequalities that have historically dominated housing access in India. Recognising auto-construction in housing is another intervention that is warranted in the country as it acknowledges peoples' agency and labour in city building. At the same time, it is pertinent to upscale and upgrade the housing infrastructure in the country in a big way to make our cities more secure, habitable, and sustainable. It can be achieved through a policy push that calls for a 'Housing for All' approach to seeking universal social housing for the needy. We need to recognise the role of universal housing as the pivot of social care for all sections of society and its transformative potential for the cities of the future. Apart from the large-scale social housing projects, Indian cities also require affordable and decent rental housing provisions for the migrant workers, and shelter homes for the socially excluded and vulnerable sections of the society like the destitute, abandoned, elderly, and mentally ill, homeless population groups. Finally, a specific intervention that is warranted is to recognise that housing systems organise the possibilities of care at the household and social scale and to implement policies to that effect without compromising on the quality and scale of existing institutional care infrastructure. Envisaging housing as a non-institutional infrastructure of care is pivotal to foster care practices and supplement healthcare infrastructure in the post-Covid-19 city. It would not only make us better prepared to deal with any zoonotic infections in future but also make our housing systems more inclusive, healthy, and robust.

Notes

1 http://arhc.mohua.gov.in/
2 https://pmay-urban.gov.in/

References

Acolin, A., Hoek-Smit, M., and Green, R. (2020). 'Cornerstone of recovery: How housing can help emerging market economies rebound from COVID-19', *Habitat for Humanity's Terwilliger Centre for Innovation in Shelter* [online]. Available at: https://www.habitat-tt.org/wp-content/uploads/2020/11/Cornerstone-of-Recovery_Oct2020-Habitat-and-Terwilliger-Centre.pdf [Accessed 25 March 2021].

Amin, A. (2014). 'Lively infrastructure', *Theory, Culture & Society*, 31(7/8), 137–161 [online]. Available at: https://doi.org/10.1177/0263276414548490 [Accessed 5 June 2020].

Awaidy, S. A., and Al Hashami, H. (2020). 'Zoonotic diseases in Oman: Successes, challenges, and future directions', *Vector-Borne and Zoonotic Diseases*, 20(1), 1–9 [online]. Available at: https://doi.org/10.1089/vbz.2019.2458 [Accessed 30 May 2021].

Barker, N. (2020). 'The housing pandemic: Four graphs showing the link between COVID-19 deaths and the housing crisis', *Inside Housing*, 29 May [Online] Available at: https://www.insidehousing.co.uk/insight/the-housing-pandemic-four-graphs-showing-the-link-between-covid-19-deaths-and-the-housing-crisis-66562 [Accessed 29 May 2020].

Bhan, G. (2020). 'Affordable housing is the solution to urban inequality, exclusion', *Hindustan Times*, 30 September. Available at: https://www.hindustantimes.com/opinion/affordable-housing-is-the-solution-to-urban-inequality-exclusion/story-2lxI9nIzrMekwC1s9nX3KI.html [Accessed 1 October 2020].

Biswas, S. (2020). 'How Asia's biggest slum contained the coronavirus', *BBC News*, 23 June. [Online] Available at: https://www.bbc.com/news/world-asia-india-53133843 [Accessed 1 July 2020].

Caldeira, T. P. R. (2017). 'Peripheral urbanization: Autoconstruction, transversal logics, and politics in cities of the global south', *Environment and Planning D: Society and Space*, 35(1), 3–20, SAGE Journals [online]. Available at: https://doi.org/10.1177/0263775816658479 [Accessed 10 January 2018].

Christou, L. (2011). 'The global burden of bacterial and viral zoonotic infections', *Clinical Microbiology and Infection*, 17(3), 326–330 [online]. Available at: https://doi.org/10.1111/j.1469-0691.2010.03441.x [Accessed 1 July 2020].

Dodds, W. (2019). 'Disease Now and Potential Future Pandemics', In: *The World 's Worst Problems* (pp. 31–44). Springer, Cham [online]. Available at: https://doi.org/10.1007/978-3-030-30410-2_4 [Accessed 7 May 2021].

Farha, L. (2017). 'Report of the Special Rapporteur on Adequate Housing as a component of the Right to an Adequate Standard of Living and on the Right to Non-discrimination in this Context' (A/HRC/34/51), *United Nations General Assembly*. Available at: https://digitallibrary.un.org/record/861179?ln=en [Accessed 1 June 2020].

Farha, L. (2018). 'Access to justice for the right to housing', *United Nations Human Rights Office of the High Commissioner*, 25 July [online]. Available at: https://www.ohchr.org/EN/Issues/Housing/Pages/AccessToJustice.aspx [Accessed 25 June 2020].

Farha, L. (2020). 'How can billions of people 'stay home' to beat Covid-19 without a safe place to live?' *Guardian*, last updated 29 April at 8.33 BST [online]. Available at: https://www.theguardian.com/society/2020/apr/29/how-can-billions-of-people-stay-home-to-beat-covid-19-without-a-safe-place-to-live [Accessed 31 May 2020].

Fields, Desiree J., and Hodkinson, Stuart N. (2018). 'Housing policy in crisis: An international perspective', *Housing Policy Debate*, 28(1), 1–5 [online]. Available at: https://doi.org/10.1080/10511482.2018.1395988 [Accessed 15 June 2020].

Gopalan, K., and Venkataraman, M. (2015). 'Affordable housing: Policy and practice in India', *IIMB Management Review*, 27(2), 129–140. Available at: https://doi.org/10.1016/j.iimb.2015.03.003 [Accessed 15 June 2020]

Harypursat, V., and Chen, Y. K. (2020). 'Six weeks into the 2019 coronavirus disease outbreak: It is time to consider strategies to impede the emergence of new zoonotic infections', *Chinese Medical Journal*, 133(9), 1118–1120 [online]. Available at: https://doi.org/10.1097/cm9.0000000000000760 [Accessed 1 July 2020].

Holston, J. (1991). 'Autoconstruction in working-class Brazil', *Cultural Anthropology*, 6(4), 447–465 [online]. Available at: http://www.jstor.org/stable/656164 [Accessed 6 January 2021].

Indorewala, H. (2017). 'Structure of housing deficiency in India and policy response at the national level: A Review', Mumbai: KRVIA. Available at: https://mdl.donau-uni.ac.at/binucom/pluginfile.php/405/mod_page/content/31/P7_WP2.5_Case_Study_1_National_Policy_KRVIA.pdf [Accessed July 2021].

International Labour Organization. (n.d.). *Decent Work*. Available at: International labour Organization Website: https://www.ilo.org/global/topics/decent-work/lang--en/index.htm [Accessed 15 August 2016].

Iveson, K. (2020). 'Kurt Iveson: Listening to the city in a global pandemic', *City Road Podcast*. Available at: https://soundcloud.com/user-283789701/kurt-iveson-listening-to-the-city-in-a-global-pandemic [Accessed 11 April 2020].

James, N. (2021). 'Young doctors 'overwhelmed' as beds, oxygen shortage leaves patients gasping', *The Hindu Business Line*, 20 April [online]. Available at: https://www.thehindubusinessline.com/news/amid-crippling-shortages-of-hospital-beds-and-oxygen-healthcare-workers-are-struggling-to-save-lives/article34365229.ece [Accessed 25 April 2021].

Jones, Antwan, and Grigsby-Toussaint, Diana S. (2020). 'Housing stability and the residential context of the COVID-19 pandemic', *Cities & Health* [online]. Available at: https://doi.org/10.1080/23748834.2020.1785164 [Accessed 23 August 2020].

Khan, Mohd. Imran, and Abraham, Anu (2020). 'No 'Room' for social distancing: A look at India's housing and sanitation conditions', *Economic and Political Weekly*, 55(16), 18 April.

Ministry of Housing and Urban Affairs. (2020). 'Affordable Rental Housing Complexes (ARHCs) for urban migrants/poor'. Available at: http://arhc.mohua.gov.in/ [Accessed 15 May 2021].

Mishagina, N., Laszlo, S., and Strumpf, E. (2021). 'The importance of new social norms in a COVID-19 outbreak,' *Policy Options*, 31 March [online]. Available at: https://policyoptions.irpp.org/magazines/march-2020/the-importance-of-new-social-norms-in-a-covid-19-outbreak/ [Accessed 7 May 2021].

MyGov Cell. (2020). 'Stay at home, save lives pledge', *Unified Online Pledge Platform of MyGov* [online]. Available at: https://pledge.mygov.in/stayathome/ [Accessed 19 January 2021].

Nancy, J.-L. (2020). Communvirus. Verso. Available at: https://www.versobooks.com/blogs/4626-communovirus [30 March 2021].

Plumber, M. (2020). 'State duty bound to protect right to shelter': Karnataka High Court directs Govt to reconstruct migrants' huts burnt down during lockdown', *Live Law*, 4 December [online]. Available at: https://www.livelaw.in/news-updates/right-shelter-migrants-huts-burnt-karnataka-high-court-166826?infinitescroll=1 [Accessed 23 June 2021].

Plumber, M. (2021). 'Supreme Court Stays Karnataka HC order directing state to reconstruct migrants' huts destroyed during lockdown', *Live Law*, 4 February [online]. Available at: https://www.livelaw.in/top-stories/supreme-court-reconstruction-kachakaranahalli-huts-karnataka-high-court-169408#:~:text=The%20Supreme%20Court%20on%20 February, by%20unknown%20 miscreants%2C%20when%20the [Accessed 10 June 2021].

Power, Emma R., and Mee, Kathleen J. (2019). 'Housing: An infrastructure of care', *Housing Studies*, 35(3) [online]. Available at: https://doi.org/10.1080/02673037.2019.1612038 [Accessed 1 June 2020].

Quarshie, A. (2020). Solidarity in time of crisis. Verso. Available at: https://www.versobooks.com/blogs/4619-solidarity-in-times-of-crisis [31 March 2021].

Rajagopal, B. (2020). 'Report of the special rapporteur on adequate housing as a component of the right to an adequate standard of living and on the right to non-discrimination in this context' (A/75/148). *United Nations General Assembly.* Available at: https://undocs.org/A/75/148 [Accessed 1 June 2020].

Reckford, J. T. M. (2020). '5 ways to tackle the housing crisis after COVID-19. Pioneers of change summit', *World Economic Forum*, Geneva. [online]. Available at: https://www.weforum.org/agenda/2020/11/5-ways-to-tackle-the-housing-crisis-after-covid-19/ [Accessed 5 January 2021].

Rogers, Dallas, and Power, Emma (2020). 'Housing policy and the COVID-19 pandemic: The importance of housing research during this health emergency', *International Journal of Housing Policy*, 20(2), 177–183 [online]. Available at: https://doi.org/10.1080/19491247.2020.1756599 [Accessed 10 December 2020].

Rolnik, R. (2013). 'Late Neoliberalism: The financialization of homeownership and housing rights', *International Journal of Urban and Regional Research*, 37(3), 1058–1066 [online]. Available at: https://doi.org/10.1111/1468-2427.12062 [Accessed 3 June 2021].

Rolnik, R. (2014). 'Place, inhabitance and citizenship: The right to housing and the right to the city in the contemporary urban world', *International Journal of Housing Policy*, 14(3), 293–300 [online]. Available at: https://doi.org/10.1080/14 616718.2014.936178 [Accessed 15 June 2021].

Stiepan, D. D. (2020). 'COVID-19: Will social distancing be the new normal? A Mayo Clinic expert discusses what the future might look like', *News Network*, 17 April [online]. Available at: https://newsnetwork.mayoclinic.org/discussion/covid-19-will-social-distancing-be-the-new-normal-a-mayo-clinic-expert-discusses-what-the-future-might-look-like/ [Accessed 15 May 2021].

The Care Collective. (2020). COVID-19 pandemic: A crisis of care. Verso. Available at: https://www.versobooks.com/blogs/4617-covid-19-pandemic-a-crisis-of-care [30 March 2021].

The Hindu. (2020). 'Supreme Court orders removal of slums along railway tracks in Delhi', *The Hindu*, 3 September [online]. Available at: https://www.thehindu.com/news/cities/Delhi/supreme-court-orders-removal-of-slums-along-railway-tracks-in-delhi/article32510738.ece [Accessed 5 September 2020].

The World Bank. (2021). 'Population living in slums (% of urban population) – India', *The World Bank* [online]. Available at: https://data.worldbank.org/indicator/EN.POP.SLUM.UR.ZS?view=chart&locations=IN [Accessed 15 May 2021].

Tripathi, A. (2017). 'Cognizing Homelessness: A gaze into the lived experiences of the homeless people in Mumbai (unpublished)', *Tata Institute of Social Sciences, Mumbai.*

Tripathi, A. (2018). 'Homing in on the 'Homeless' in India: A proposed schema', *FLAME University Newsroom*, 13 November [online]. Available at: https://www.flame.edu.in/newsroom/homing-in-on-the-homeless-in-india-a-proposed-schema [Accessed 5 May 2021].

United Nations General Assembly. (2020). 'Guidelines for the Implementation of the Right to Adequate Housing. Report of the Special Rapporteur on adequate housing as a component of the right to an adequate standard of living, and on the right to non-discrimination in this context' (A/HRC/43/43). *Human Rights Council, Forty-third Session* [online]. Available at: https://undocs.org/en/A/HRC/43/43 [Accessed 30 May 2020].

World Economic Forum. (2019). 'Making affordable housing a reality in cities. Insight report', *World Economic Forum*, Geneva [online]. Available at: http://www3.weforum.org/docs/WEF_Making_Affordable_Housing_A_Reality_In_Cities_report.pdf [Accessed 6 May 2020].

Yuko, E. (2021). '14 everyday habits that could (and should) change forever after coronavirus', *Reader's Digest*, 23 March [online]. Available at: https://www.rd.com/list/everyday-habits-that-could-change-forever-after-coronavirus/ [Accessed 9 May 2021].

8

QUARANTINED FOR LIFE

Mahalakshmi

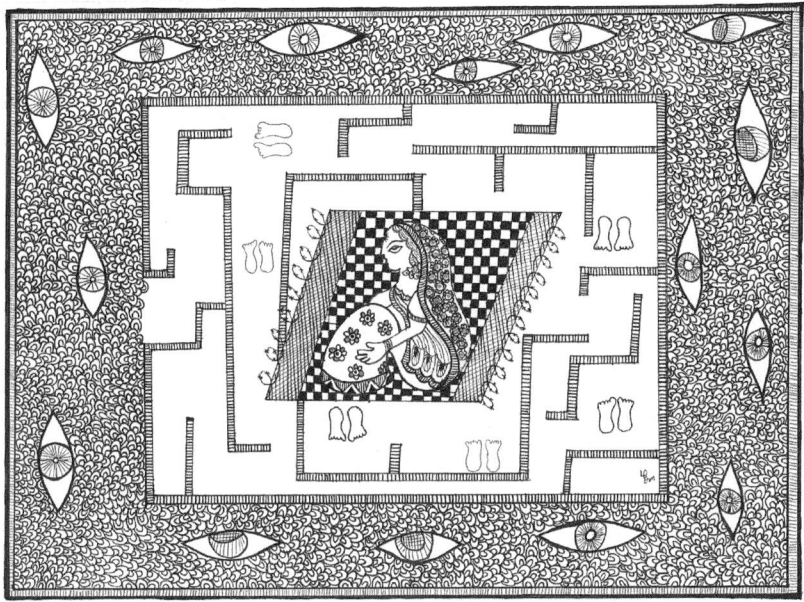

Artwork 8.1 Quarantined for Life.

The lockdown due to Covid-19 brought back vivid memories of my mother. I lost her to cancer in 2018. She spent most of her life indoors, cooking and taking care of the family. Many women in Indian society spend their entire lives in a sort of quarantine at home. Even though I am educated, while working and being at home I struggle with my own identities, my choices, and my idea of independence. I try to stay firm and push my boundaries, solve the puzzles in life, and try to mark my footprints. Sometimes, I feel helpless and tired, since I know I am not completely free from the eyes of society watching me incessantly. The fight is always on and will continue, but I carry hope because I know the fight is worth it.

DOI: 10.4324/9781003320524-11

9

CALLING ON AUSTRALIANS OF CONSCIENCE

Reflections from March to July 2020

Linda Briskman

Introduction

It is July 2020 as I write from my home in Melbourne, designated by the Global Liveability Index as one of the world's most liveable cities. We are entering week two of a six-week second lockdown, just as we were slowly waking up from the uncertainty of an extended first. The social and cultural fabric of the city seems on the cusp of extinction. Fear is engendered by official statements of prosecution for breaches of restrictions, a rising death toll, and a long-term financial abyss. We are confronted by promenading police, overhead drones, and deployment of more than 1,000 military personnel, tasked with ensuring compliance with directives. With constantly changing scenarios, no one knows what is next. There is a sense of collective depression. The subjects of public health and economic health dominate, with social wellbeing less considered, although mental health professionals have noted the impact of lockdown, and domestic violence advocates have spoken of a spike in incidents. What can people of conscience do, as we bear witness to this perplexing time?

This is an essay in two parts, derived from observation, speculation, critical reading of the media, and lament for the world of 2020. I write as a global citizen, recognising that although health, social, and economic impacts are grim in Australia, they cannot compare to what is occurring elsewhere in both the Global North and the Global South. My musings are inwardly focused on my own country while recognising the global hold of the virus and the disproportionate impact on those structurally marginalised. In the context of this essay, I adopt the term 'Australians of Conscience' as denoting those who subscribe to social justice tenets for all and who decry the influence of neo-liberal discourses and practices that deny rights to disadvantaged sections of the Australian community.

I narrate a story of two Melbournes, revealing a dichotomy between the 'haves', of which I am a member, and the 'have nots', living not too

DOI: 10.4324/9781003320524-12

far away. Those whose opportunities in life have given them a Covid-19 head start and those who are disempowered by place of birth, missed opportunities and discrimination. In the first section, I recount my personal pandemic experiences and broad observations of the impact, including alarm at the upsurge of control and surveillance. I then turn, in part two, to people locked down in government housing provision, known as social housing, who are united by a lack of choice, low incomes, wicked policies – hidden away by apathy writ large. My overarching inquiry is to envisage the role of people of conscience in recognising and bridging divides.

Participant Observation: Reflections on Life in Lockdown

With the imposition of social distancing, Covid-19 has created new meanings of home and community. A form of house arrest. When my household transformed from a haven to a workspace, boundary-setting collapsed. Work pressures outweighed home pleasures through relentless tasks previously relegated to an emotionless office. My friends' circle disappeared into the world of virtual realities, with enforced disabling of cafés, cinemas, and book clubs. Newspapers thudding at my doorstep each morning were limited to Covid-19 reportage. The earlier vitality of the neighbourhood was now replaced by an eerie silence.

Non-apathetic people of conscience recognised their privilege to maintain an income, to feel relatively safe from virus encroachment, and to continue connections, even if less than optimal – reflecting burgeoning of social empathy. This welcome acknowledgement soon shifted to relief at being abrogated from the responsibility of privilege, once the crisis boosted government income support for new and long-term unemployed, temporary housing for the homeless and provision for the hungry, the latter largely implemented by the non-government sector. The voices of those cheated of life chances were rarely heard and reported, and were spoken *about* and not *with* by more prosperous sections of the society, including professionals and the media. Prominent commentator Julie Szego (2020) asks us to imagine what it would be like if others were routinely speaking for you and your views were rarely sought. For those who experience persistent seclusion and insecurity, the power of the pandemic was familiar. Flaws were exposed in the Australian image of the 'Lucky Country'.

Coronavirus advances stealthily. It begins at a leisurely pace and then explodes, catching us unaware and ill-prepared. It haunts us with uncertainty and produces fear. New terminology enters the vocabulary – super spreaders, aggressive suppression. Those who care are lessened in their ability to do so, with health professionals and hospital workers among the infected or exposed. Numbers in intensive care units increase. Unlike in the beginning, they are not all elderly. Trust in political and health leadership waxes and wanes along with numbers.

Lockdown One took place from mid-March until early June. Despite severe restrictions on gatherings of many types, it created innovative novelty for some. Rates of infection were relatively low and working from home and supervising children's online learning had some advantages for the well-resourced. The more affluent with kitchen gadgets and internet-enabling devices took pleasure in sharing lockdown recipes (sourdough bread was a favourite), exercising through online individual and group programs, and providing advice on ways to keep children occupied when playgrounds closed. Some found creative ways to celebrate birthdays and connect children with grandparents by digital or drive-by means.

From 1 June, there were moments of opportunity after Lockdown One ended. I was born a day too early as my 31st May birthday meant that I could only embark with my children and theirs on a socially distanced walk from café to café for permitted takeout. Release from Lockdown One represented a 'new normal'. It is self-indulgent to say, but I had craved the return to cafes with friends, family, and newspapers. But it was different. Numbers were restricted, tables set well apart, hand sanitisers were omnipresent, and patrons were required to provide names and phone numbers. Booking a taxi was met with an ominous message of 'regularly sanitised cabs'. Some cafes and restaurants were wary of opening, with number restriction reducing viability and predictions that a second lockdown was imminent. This prophecy came true when Melbourne announced Lockdown Two on 9 July after a consistent rise in Covid cases, just as staff were being re-employed and food orders filled. Some businesses may never recover, and we were officially told to brace ourselves for a recession in the future.

Victorians found themselves banned from other states, something not experienced since the Spanish Flu of the early 20th century when there was a metaphorical ring of steel between Victoria and New South Wales. Borrowing from the UK experience, humorists describe the new bordering as V-exit and drew a map that excluded Victoria, a state of more than 6 million. I could not enter Sydney, which was my working home for the previous three years.

As I sat out the pandemic in Melbourne, I was a constant consumer of news as soon as I woke up until the night ended and sometimes in-between, when dreams of Covid were sleep-denying. I watched the daily count, always in triple digits, with hospital admissions rising and deaths occurring. When it came to other news, Donald Trump's shenanigans, for example, I became fatigued but here I was absorbed. A song rang through my head as I shuffled around the floor in a meagre attempt to keep fit, *Dancing with Myself* by Billy Idol. And, I became unrecognisable with my face mask when venturing into public for the few permitted activities, such as exercising or stockpiling supplies.

Although my life was not the same, I am one of the lucky ones with a job, warm house, caring partner, children I can connect with virtually and good friends. But I too felt vulnerable, as I was told for the very first time that I am in a risky age group. As a person of conscience, I reflect on my own interests as trifling. I note that the pandemic is life-changing for people who have only known a buoyant economy with low unemployment. A fortunate few, who obtained work after losing their jobs, found themselves in occupations they would never have imagined, such as in sanitising teams. I ponder what the future holds for those experiencing protracted unemployment. Their hopes that someone somewhere will give them a chance are increasingly being dashed.

The future for my academic peers is uncertain. Universities are reducing staff and each and every person I know inwardly asks: '[W]ill it be me'? Am I too new, do I have enough publications and grants, will my courses be eliminated or, in my case, am I past my use-by date? The impact on students in the future is not known, as it's likely that in the interest of cost savings, virtual teaching may become increasingly dominant. International students-in-waiting are locked out by hermetically sealed borders.

There have been glimmers of hope, with the government bolstering social security payments, providing measures for businesses to stay afloat, paying attention to housing the homeless and offering time-limited free childcare by way of example. This is surprising for a federal conservative government driven by 'the market' and largely opposed to government intervention. Hopes that this would herald the dawn of a fairer era faded, with retraction of measures mooted, while at the same time increasing expenditure on military hardware because of a vaguely expressed and unconfirmed international threat said to arise from the pandemic. And it was revealed that the government spent almost 3.5 million dollars, hiring 35 private management consultants for less than four months to coordinate its Covid-19 response (Baxendale 2020).

I watched a blame game in place with systemic mistakes twisted into assertions of human error. These include the release, without checking, of passengers on a luxury cruise ship arriving in Sydney, resulting in positive diagnoses and deaths. In a quarantine hotel in Melbourne, another cluster arose when a staff member from a private, profit-driven security company contracted the virus from those confined, which subsequently multiplied in his community.

I observed ministers of the government accusing people of refusing Covid tests. Despite the talk-up, it is unlikely that the numbers were overwhelming, and there was a failure to consider causal factors such as inability to understand instructions in English, fear of authority and anxiety about not being able to maintain livelihoods, if testing positive.

I watched racism rise. At first, it was confined to the Chinese, with reports of people being targeted because the origins of the virus were from China. Islamophobia in Australia and elsewhere is vicious and rapacious. With reports of clusters from Eid celebrations after Ramadan and in an Islamic school, there is a likelihood that Islamophobia will fester, resulting in Muslim organisations springing to the defence of how Muslim communities have responded to transmission and offering organisational support.

At every turn, politics comes into play despite the unconvincing mantra of governments that 'we are all in this together' or 'do the right thing', resulting in message fatigue. Prime Minister Scott Morrison, in a clumsy attempt at national empathy with the Melbourne surge, declared, "we are all Victorians now because we're all Australians." But we are not. Victoria became the pariah state and although Australians are used to unconscionable bordering for asylum seekers, we are not used to heavily policed state border controls, with a combination of home detention and state extinction. Arguably, the country is becoming increasingly authoritarian and we are all under the eye of authorities. Australia prides itself on being an open and free society, although some groups could never realise their civil rights. Now everyone is subject to erosion of liberty.

The first alert for civil libertarians was the Covid-19 Safe App, to be downloaded on mobile phones. Several concerns arose, including the security of data despite government guarantees, and we know that governments are not known for keeping promises. With information to be stored by Amazon US, qualms emerged that the data might be used for other purposes. Apart from the costs associated with the app itself, a massive advertising campaign was undertaken to get people to sign up. I did not. And subsequently, the app has been shown to be technically flawed and of little benefit, while manual and genomic tracing is more effective. The government fudges criticism.

In local neighbourhoods, it was disturbing to see police roaming where they never did before. For people who breached the somewhat ambiguous rules, massive fines were imposed. Although names were not revealed, public shaming occurred with authorities telling media intimate breach details. Warnings were minimised; hefty fines maximised.

Vigilantes arose in civil society. One culprit is public radio, which encourages listeners to talk back on what they see and then joins in admonishment. In an attempt to inspire joy in a now gloomy society, a listener called in about a neighbourhood street where people developed an idea to nourish the soul. Christmas lights in windows. Another caller rang in. She rebuked people driving past and accused them of breaching the rules for permitted activities, stating that she'd report. Another chastised those buying pots and pans as a non-essential activity. Others, no doubt without measuring tapes at hand, estimated that social distancing rules were being ignored, a claim not borne out by reportage that Victorians were excelling in keeping their distance.

Surveillance and control reached new heights in social housing towers, revealing the Melbourne social, cultural, and political divide.

Punishing the Poor

Matters escalated on 4 July, just days before the second full-city lockdown. Some 3,000 social housing tenants living in high-rise towers were suddenly and totally subjected to home imprisonment without notice, surrounded and enforced by 500 armed police. With public health and compliance taking precedence, social health and wellbeing took a back seat. Residents were visibly shaken.

The daunting vertical buildings are home to diverse cultural groups. Refugees living in close quarters with their extended families are part of the multicultural landscape of Australia. Many speak little or no English, so messaging is always inadequate, and interpreters were not immediately mobilised. One woman spoke of her grandmother being suddenly confronted by police, forbidding her to leave, when unable to fully comprehend. The common thread of living in social housing is being poor. But even within the poverty paradigm, lived experiences vary.

The discourse of vulnerability alerts us to be mindful of the politics of care, and I use the term cautiously. Calling people vulnerable can be patronising. Social housing is buzzing with resourceful people who can tell us a thing or two about finding solutions to complex problems including Covid detection, prevention, and support. Despite poverty and all that flows, they call their modest accommodation home. They are not problems to be solved. These diverse communities are filled with strong people across the age and ethnicity spectra, something barely noticed by the middle classes who now inhabit these inner-urban locations but are largely segregated from life in the flats. Social workers and community workers know that top-down approaches that exclude those affected are incapable of making an impact. Drawing on people's strengths and not seeing them as deficits ought to be common sense.

This was not a war with bombs falling. Although the rapid spread of the pandemic within the towers was a serious problem resulting from design flaws conducive to spread, it was not instantly life or contagion threatening. You wouldn't think this was the case with the pandemic, with the use of military metaphors flourishing. On 13th July, in the first ten minutes of his briefing to the state and media, the Victorian Premier used the following terms: enemy virus, battle, war, frontline, fight, defeat.

What harm would have come from another hour or day? Police were readily mobilised. With more time and notification to tenants, health workers could have been in place and social and community workers could have been enabled to dispense a more caring approach. Coordination of food provision and allocation of necessary supplies would have been possible. It's highly unlikely that such impositions would have occurred for dwellers in closely proximate, stylish, and privately owned apartment blocks. Trust would have prevailed. Using force as the first line of action is devoid of humanity. We might instead have shared the knowledge and abundant resources to live up to the claims of the most liveable city. Most importantly, tenants and their supporters would have been called upon to build solutions from the grassroots, rather than bureaucratic impositions. Residents had asked for help in anticipation of the virus-spread, requesting more hand sanitisers and seeking ways to manage the few crowded and frequently broken elevators. Action eventuated from sheer panic after the virus had spread. The Chief Medical Officer referred to the towers as 'vertical cruise ships', alluding to the havoc wreaked on luxury liners. In a further punitive and humiliating measure, daily exercise was only permitted in a fenced-off enclosure. Lack of trust trumped humanity. As in many instances before, the disenfranchised were blamed for their plight.

Now, as residents increasingly break through the silence about what they witnessed and experienced, they can no longer be perceived as hapless and bereft of solutions but as people with agency and savvy. Consider refugees who have aspirations perhaps no different from the more affluent, to have a sustainable and secure life and to enable their children to have a fair go in this lucky country. Some have experienced the unimaginable, which we cannot truly fathom unless we have walked in their shoes. It is a source of great shame to people of conscience that the state created more of the unimaginable. Migrants in the lockdown flats are speaking to the media of their hopes and dreams. "I want to be a doctor', 'a teacher', 'Prime Minister." Years of system failures in social housing provision and maintenance are now coming into the open, and it took the pandemic to create awareness.

Food improved after some days, including culturally appropriate provision, after community groups, including Muslim organisations, rose to the challenge. In the meantime, residents had to suffice with minimalist supplies such as jam without bread, cereal without milk and items with expired use-by dates. There were people co-existing in the flats with serious health issues requiring medication, people with drug addictions likely to experience withdrawal symptoms, people with mental illnesses requiring support, and older people living alone. The working poor were unable to leave their homes for what were often precarious work situations. It's unlikely that any of the residents would not have been filled with dread in sudden captivity. The spectacle of policing, containment, and exercise yards for those living on the edge of society was thoughtless. Lived experiences are cumulative as revealed by targeting social housing residents. Community legal centres and young African people speak out about fracases with police. Just a few years ago, a minister of state wickedly declared that African gangs were terrorising Melbourne residents who were scared to go out. And if this were not enough, racism ascended during the lockdown, led by the notorious One Nation politician, Pauline Hanson, labelling those in the flats as drug addicts and alcoholics who do not speak English.

Calling on People of Conscience to Re-imagine a Just World

During Lockdown One, I was cautiously optimistic when observing neighbourliness in a busy city that I'd rarely seen before. I had hoped this might extend beyond people's comfort zones but with some exceptions, it seems that fear during Lockdown Two drove the populace to become more inwardly engrossed. The potential for consciences to be pricked waned and the question remains as to how this potential can be re-activated. As individuals perceive crises through their own lens, my clarion call is to summon people of conscience.

Might there be a space for increased questioning of the neo-liberal project that has benefited the rich and powerful and disadvantaged so many others? Now that the previously comfortable are faced with unemployment and narrowed lives, is there a prospect to extend concerns for self and family to those systemically victimised by market policies that diminish opportunities?

For those subject to time-limited quarantine, can we anticipate that empathy will evolve for others who are detained for longer periods and in harsher conditions, also without trial, namely asylum seekers who are subject to indefinite immigration detention in remote sites? Although whole populations experience border constriction, what would it take for critiques of border-thinking to be extended to those seeking asylum?

Questions can be asked about government spending. While applauding the injection of support to prevent pandemic-spread and to alleviate potential plunge into poverty, should we not challenge exorbitantly expensive government priorities of military hardware purchase, border protection to those 'othered', and the race to a vaccination in competition with many nations? Civil society ought to be called upon to partner in determining fiscal allocation that supports citizens and non-citizens reach their full humanity. One achievable short-term solution is to apply and adapt successful social housing approaches in other countries. By way of contrast, in Vienna, the government publicly acknowledges housing as a human right and provides subsidised public housing where more than 60 per cent of residents reside in social homes (Ball 2019).

Is there a chance that we could look outside our own wealthy nation by increasing foreign aid, without it being tied to our own interests as defined by the government? Before the pandemic, a significant proportion of the world's population lived on less than $1 per day. With many of us now fixated by our television screens, we can no longer ignore plights that were amplified by Covid, for example, migrant labourers in India, people living in the still segregated towns in South Africa, and minority ethnic groups in the United States. The United Nations has warned that post-Covid, global poverty will increase and that famine will take hold.

For those of us who work in social and community spheres, we can ensure that our voices are heard, while still applauding our fine health system in Australia and prudently recognising a role for community-oriented policing, where bureaucratic lines of control are replaced by inclusive, participatory approaches. Rather than being behind the scenes, we can vocally convey our contribution by condemning inequality – speaking out about vilification and dehumanisation and participating in truth-telling emanating from our witnessing.

Acting decisively on conscience is an urgent quest to re-imagining a new world order, where social justice prevails, social democratic ideals replace neo-liberal practices and the importance of community responses outplays top-down bureaucratic imposition. Recognising the role of non-health actors as partners in dealing with a crisis that is dominated by health paradigms alone is a crucial first step.

References

Ball, J. (2019) 'Housing as a basic human right: The Vienna model of social housing', *New Statesman*, 3 September [online]. Available at https://www.newstatesman.com/spotlight/housing/2019/09/housing-basic-human-right-vienna-model-social-housing [Accessed 7 July 2020].

Baxendale, R. (2020) 'Daniel Andrew's $3.5m cash splash on Covid consultants', *The Australian*, 6 July [online]. Available at https://www.theaustralian.com.au/nation/politics/daniel-andrewss-35m-cash-splash-on-covid-consultants/news-story/204952142d713449d9658cd25142e0e2 [Accessed 9 August 2020].

Szego, J. (2020) 'Council elections an opportunity for Melbourne's most vulnerable', *The Age*, 2 October [online]. Available at https://www.theage.com.au/national/victoria/council-elections-an-opportunity-for-melbourne-s-most-vulnerable-20201002-p561ck.html [Accessed 17 November 2020].

10

FEMICIDE AND VIOLENCE AGAINST WOMEN IN MEXICO

May 2021

Jackie Campbell

At the beginning of the global pandemic, I was surprised by a story my favourite aunt – who is now 90 – shared with me over the phone. Aunt Argelia lives alone and what she misses the most are the gym and the golf course, as she had to reluctantly give them up due to the pandemic. Back when she was 15 and her older sister had just gotten married, she often cried, but did not know why. Over the years she found out that her sister was mistreated and humiliated by her husband throughout her married life. She never said a word, but threats, infidelities, and physical, financial, and psychological control over her were evident to aunt Argelia even though she was able to identify the nuances only later. The incident that caught my attention as my aunt narrated the story happened in a mining town called Cloete in the northeast of Mexico, back in 1945, when as a young newly married woman-her sister (also my aunt) was at her father's (my grandfather) house because her husband worked as a doctor in a neighbouring town. While the doctor went to work, the young woman spent the day at her parents' house so as not to be alone at her own home. Her father heard that his daughter was not getting the respect she deserved and to my surprise, he did not tolerate this behaviour. My grandfather's response was an unusual one for the men of his times. In a one-to-one conversation with his daughter, he told her to return home and not endure such humiliation from her husband. I was given to understand that the young man used to shout at his wife, using expletives. I also found out that my grandmother did not get involved in the matter at that time, or at any other time. The reasons for her lack of involvement are not clear to me, but it could be that she did not observe the violence towards my aunt in the same way as my grandfather did. My aunt ignored my grandfather's advice. She created her life with her husband in the second-largest city in Mexico, Guadalajara, more

DOI: 10.4324/9781003320524-13

than 1,000 kilometres away from her parents. They had four daughters and three sons, and when her husband became ill in old age, she accompanied him, until the last day, in her role as a wife.

The sense of isolation during the pandemic probably opened the floodgates for aunt Argelia, who shared stories of how women had silently endured violence in Mexico, without any kind of community support.

Gender-based Violence against Women in Mexico

The situation that women have been subjected to in Mexico has not changed in the decades that have passed since the time of the story my aunt narrated. Although laws have changed with time, in the minds of people there are still these misogynistic customs that are reinforced by the messages that we consume every day through the media or through the judges or our teachers. Even today, some parents prefer that their daughters get married and start a family with well-earning professionals, rather than develop their own abilities and carve out an identity for themselves.

According to the data provided by the United Nations Population Fund (Arie Hoekman for UN News, 30 of April 2021), it is estimated that 24 per cent of the women in Mexico have experienced physical, sexual, or psychological violence from their current or former partner, a figure that increases to more than 33 per cent in the registers of adolescent women from 15 to 19 years. Overall figures reveal that Mexico closed the year 2020 with 3,723 violent deaths of women, where only 900 were categorised as femicides.

Gender inequality is prevalent within Mexican society, regardless of which social class people belong to, what career they pursue, or what kind of lifestyle they lead. It does not matter whether one has studied in a university or not, since everyone in Mexico gets 'educated' through the national television TELEVISA that has had a monopoly over media for decades. There are still popular songs, jokes, talks shows, news reports, and soap operas that make fun of the position of women in Mexico and continue to feed into a misogynist toxic culture that glorifies the permissiveness to attack women to subdue them, even to murder them for any perceived 'digressions'.

There are well-known Mexican soap operas such as *Forbidden Path* (1957), *Gutierritos* (1958), *Teresa* (1959), and *The Right to Be Born* (1966) that have been reproduced repeatedly on Mexican television and several generations can identify with them. In these television series and films, the roles of female characters were represented as poor, brunette, submissive, with no formal education, overly sexed, and treacherous. They gave a clear message that by not fulfilling a socially accepted role, women would have to pay for their mistakes or 'sins'. I offer three examples of songs whose lyrics are known to most people in Mexico. The third song ended in femicide, so the group who wrote the song had to change the words in 2017 in response to protests by feminists groups.

1. Rice with Milk, Children's song (Unknown author, 14th century, 3'12"). The song "Arroz con Leche," which can also be a Mexican rice pudding, is a Spanish-American folk song considered to be of French origin, its authorship is unknown and even today it is sung by children.[1]

   "Rice with milk,
   I want to get married
   with a lady from the capital
   who knows how to sew
   who knows how to embroider…"

2. Turn Around, song written by the Mexican famous composer José Alfredo Jiménez (1963, 2'14"). "La media vuelta" is a song that has managed to overcome the barriers of time to consolidate itself as one of the great exponents of the Mexican popular songbook in three different genres: *mariachi*, *bolero* or *ranchero*, interpreted and recorded by at least 15 singers.[2]

   "You're leaving because I want you to leave.
   Any time I want, I'll stop you.
   I know you need my love
   Whether you want it or not, I own you"

3. Ungrateful, song by the group Café Tacuba (1995, 3'35")[3]

   "That's why now I have to give you a gift
   A couple of bullets that hurt you
   And even though I'm sad to no longer have you
   I'm going to be with you at your funeral"

Discrimination against women is not only present in social and cultural spheres but also enforced through courts and law enforcement agencies. Legal practice impacts and in turn is impacted by everyday life, customs, and traditions. Law, power, and language are intertwined. Therefore, despite changing laws and regulations, the discrimination, oppression, and violence against women in Mexico continue. Crimes against women are trivialised. People responsible for executing justice, specifically for investigation and creation of criminal files, are not interested in cases of violence against women. Not only have they cynically declared it to the press, but it is also proven by the closure of cases without any investigation.[4] A robbery is denounced and generates discussion around citizens' security, since the perspective from which it is viewed is also part of the macho culture that does not prioritise concerns over the violence women endure both in the private or public sphere.

March 2021 became the most violent month against women in Mexico in the last six years. According to data from the Federal Government's National Secretariat of Security and Citizen Protection, March 2021 broke the record for the number of women killed, with 267 intentional killings reported in 31 days. However, it is presumed that only 92 of them will be investigated as femicides, since they have not considered the evidence that has been established to classify the murder of a woman as femicide if: *(1) The victim presents signs of sexual violence of any kind; (2) Inflammatory or degrading injuries or mutilations, before or after the deprivation of life or acts of necrophilia, have been inflicted on the victim; (3) There are antecedents or data of any type of violence in the family, work or school environment of the perpetrator against the victim; (4) There has been a sentimental, emotional or trust relationship between the asset and the victim; (5) There are data that establish that there were threats related to the criminal act, harassment or injuries of the perpetrator against the victim; (6) The victim has been held incommunicado, whatever the time prior to the deprivation of life; (7) The victim's body is exposed or displayed in a public place.* (National Commission to Prevent and Eradicate Violence against Women). Despite such clear guidelines, cases are not classified as femicides because perpetrators clean up the crime scene or flee so that they are not detained. Trials are not carried out, information is denied to the victim's family, or investigative folders are simply not opened.

The Costa Rican jurist Alda Facio[5] believes that a gender perspective allows us to examine the situation of women more succinctly. She argues that justice with a gender perspective is sought for those who have diverse needs and interests, not only to mention and draw attention to the reality of girls and women, the violence, abuses, and inequalities that they live with but to denounce and modify the context of suffering they live in. This perspective takes into consideration the understanding that all human action impacts women and men differently, due to how gender and power relations are configured. The androcentric perspective has been falsely projected as neutral, objective, and impartial, and therefore, there is a need to view reality from a new place. Making the context of women – their actions, feelings, and needs – invisible is retrograde and reflective of our very limited minds. Women's experiences are distinctly different from those of men. When a man marries a woman, his family does not fear that he will suffer violence; if a man walks alone down the street at night, he does not fear being harassed or raped. When women go to seek justice, they continue to be judged from an androcentric perspective and not from a gender-sensitive lens.

The widespread violence against women and the breakdown of the social net is the result of the silence of so many families who experience intra-family violence and of so many girls and boys, and adolescents, who have seen their mothers beaten, fractured, and bloody, and who have heard from them lies about what happened. They lie about having an accident and injuring themselves to hide their bruise and save themselves from further harm. This only leads the members of the family or the neighbourhood to have a mistaken idea about 'family', 'truth', and 'justice'.. The social net will remain fractured if impunity prevails. Therefore, as feminists have claimed, the personal needs to be seen as political.

The Pandemic That Precedes the Covid-19 Pandemic

The Covid-19 pandemic exposed the reality of poverty, inequality, violence and the effects of privatisation of rights, among others, on health and education. There are stark contrasts between those who live in the obligatory confinement the pandemic has introduced, luxuriously, in the comfort of their homes, and those who reside in a crowded and less privileged neighbourhood, who must live in proximity with many others while sharing resources. The privileged position of those who enjoyed the extended quarantine stands in stark contrast to the lives of individuals who must go out looking for food each day to survive and support their extended family, or those who must live on the streets. In this sea of uncertainties and anguish caused by Covid-19, the conditions of violence that must be faced at the highest levels of social inequality are evident.

Just as crises can bring hope to act creatively, raise voices, and build movements for rights – as seen after World War II, it is also true that pandemics have triggered xenophobia, racism, demagoguery, corruption, and the withdrawal of countries towards ultra-nationalist positions. What we are experiencing in these times of the pandemic is a phenomenon that unites us in the most basic way to the entire human species, regardless of who we are or what we do. This impact of the pandemic is of course compounded by intersections of disadvantages experienced by people.

As a result of this pandemic, we can find among the population, hunger, war, and death, three of the horsemen of the Apocalypse and evils that imply the end of humanity. This can generate a justified fear if we conjure up the historical memory of similar events. However, violence against women is an ancestral pandemic, a perpetual threat, where the risk presents itself to half of the world population and yet that does not seem to interest the heads of states. For this reason, it will not end if we do not act against it with transformative actions in all fields, every day.

Physical mobility restrictions have contributed to the increase in gender-based violence. Girls and women who already lived in environments of violence are now confined with their aggressors, with more provocations and less support. Therefore, there is a lot of distress, pain, and fear in women. According to the executive secretariat of the National Public Security System, before the pandemic, ten women were murdered in a day in Mexico.[6] The pandemic has caused an increase in violence against women. According to the National Network of Shelters, women's and children's calls and texts to helplines increased by 55 per cent between March and June 2020, when compared to the previous year.[7]

A year after the pandemic began, in April 2021, Maria Fabiola Alanís Sámano, the head of the National Commission to Prevent and Eradicate Violence against Women (Conavim), spoke of the declaration of emergency for violence against women in Mexico City by noting that in Mexico every hour 11 crimes are committed against women. In addition, three out of ten illegal acts reported nationally are in grievance to the female population, the national average of femicides is 36 per 100 thousand women, and 100 per cent of the femicides is concentrated in 6.9 per cent of the country's municipalities.[8] According to the executive secretariat of the National Public Safety System data, by the end of 2020, 54,314 crimes against sexual freedom were reported. It is the highest number since 1997 when 20,695 were registered; in 2010 they were 34,086 cases.[9] Feminists claim that the numbers reflected in the 2020 data are probably lower than the actual numbers because a number of women were unable to report crimes against them.

According to data from Mexico's National Network of Human Rights Defenders, of which I am a member, assaults on defenders tripled in March 2021 compared to January and February of the same year, with a total of 84 being recorded. Repression of protest, defamation, limitations on the right to report, arbitrary detentions, and digital violence were some of the main assaults recorded.[10] The assaults on demonstrations occurred in different parts of the Republic and by different security forces of local and state order. This is taking place in the context of stigmatisation and criminalisation of the feminist movement by authorities and anti-rights groups.

For almost 20 years, I have suffered harassment, threats from police or officials, and smear campaigns in the media for my activism or for being a woman. In 2008, I needed to go into exile for the defence I made for women sexually assaulted by the military (at that time the president of Mexico ruled the country with military force). But in January 2020, I was criminally sued by the municipal president of Saltillo, the city where I have been living since the year 2000, for painting the first mural that in the state of Coahuila refers to femicides.[11] In February 2021, I suffered a break-in inside my apartment where the man that came in left me a symbolic message over my bed. Also in that month, my iCloud account was hacked and I was stripped of all kinds of documents, photographs, data, agenda, etc. Violence has been constant and more aggressive, as has the damage it causes. Neither these nor the earlier threats on me have been investigated or sanctioned, even though I have presented lawsuits before the authorities.

On the night of 7 May 2020, in the city of Torreón, Coahuila, the bodies of three women (48, 56, and 59 years old) were found inside a home; they were sisters and nurses. The police report indicated that the bodies were "in a state of decomposition … they would have died from strangulation," "they showed signs of violence and were handcuffed." National Victimization and Perception Survey on Public Safety for 2019 indicates that of the crimes that were made public, there was impunity in 95 per cent of the cases, including cases of femicidal violence. Despite these figures, one day after the event, state authorities announced the arrest of two people as responsible for the femicide and the motive for the triple murder was recorded as robbery. It was obvious that the authorities had to present scapegoats if the health sector was being observed by the whole country during this pandemic. The federal authorities publicly called for the crime not to be left in impunity. But to title the case folder as robbery was an absolute mockery of society and a lack of respect for the victims; closing the case in this manner is akin to not doing justice at all.

On 8 May 2020, the National Human Rights Commission (CNDH) confirmed in a statement that domestic violence had increased in Mexico during the lockdown periods of Covid-19. Unlike what the President declared in his morning homilies,[12] the home is *not* a safe space for women.[13] On 15 July 2020, the Governing Board of the National Women's Institute authorised a 75 per cent reduction in its budget by an austerity decree. The cut is an unnecessary dismantling that will affect the development of equality policies in states and municipalities in the country that fight against gender violence and will be left without adequate resources to act. In July 2020, Mexico presented its report to the Convention on the Elimination of All Forms of Discrimination against Women (CEDAW), which mandates that state members must strengthen resources to eliminate sexist violence. At a time when Mexico tries to stand out in the international arena for its feminist policies,[14] its budget cuts suggest the opposite. In addition, these financial cuts should not be approved within the national body but in the Chamber of Deputies of Mexico. This is a double violation because on the one hand it limits a budget necessary for the safety of women and on the other hand, this measure was a presidential decree, without respecting the National Constitution that indicates that the budget must be approved by the legislature, not the executive. Once again, the president of the Republic gives his point of view and suggests: "There has not been a more feminist government than this one,"[15] and once again women say: "We have other data."[16]

During the first year of the pandemic, I was involved in activities of the communication team that I have been advising for years for the Catholic Diocese of Saltillo, especially in the transmissions of events that, given the impossibility of doing them in person, had to be carried out virtually. Last July 2020, tests had to be done for the live broadcast of an event in a catholic temple. Two days before the event, a location had to be found to place cameras and draw direct sound from the audio of the venue. I sat on the main chair of the temple, to show that the height of the chair and the unevenness of the enclosure would not capture the face of the one who would preside. The priest began to scream. I was astounded as I did not understand why the priest was screaming. The screaming continued and he came up to me and said that I was a woman, a secular, and I should not sit on the main seat of the temple; suggesting my inferiority a power that did not correspond to me and the impurity of my gender. He moved the 'contaminated chair' and sat down on another, assuming he was helping us. I left the temple with the team. Many centuries have passed (or perhaps not) since the *Malleus Maleficarum* (1486) manual that detailed persecution, torture, burning, prosecution, condemnation, and punishment for women considered witches.

The church is built by people, not objects nor the construction of the temple. The wooden chair, if it's not for the poor to use and have a place, is worthless. It is better that the chair offers a fire that provides warmth to a family or a campfire that produces food for a group of migrants; suffice it to remember that there is no Lord's Supper without community. The important thing about this fact is not that the Bishop, the Superior of the violent priest, cancelled the celebration in the 'man's' temple and made the first priestly ordination in times of pandemic in the cathedral (behind closed doors), emphasising during the homily (a real one in a church) how a priest should serve the community, be part of it, and build as brothers and sisters a better place to live, without pretending special places or differential treatment. The transcendental thing is to recognise that those who witnessed the humiliations by the priest towards me did not place the fact as violence, and to let it pass is to wait for the hatred in the heart of that man to destroy entire lives. It is terrible to know that there are a lot of institutions that do not punish acts of violence against women. There should be no tolerance for violence against women in any of its manifestations. Neither humiliation nor murder. The difference does not exist in those acts. This happened in the state of Coahuila, in Mexico. While Coahuila is not the state of the country where the most number of women are killed, but just in 2019, femicides increased by 600 per cent. No more violence against women. If we do not make the facts visible, if we do not make them public, if we do not change the misogynistic culture, we are not going to wake up the day after, with a life without violence. Sororal networks must be activated to ignite hope in our generation and those to come.

What Must We Do?

The contempt for the feminine and for the various ways in which we manifest ourselves, violating us, denigrating us, discriminating against us, objectifying us, or eliminating us physically or verbally, will not impede our awareness nor the recovery of our dignity.

One of the articles of the Spanish writer Gemma Lienas[17] included in the book "Rebels, No Whores No Submissives" invites to teach women how to fish:

> The most important investment a nation can make to overcome poverty is to educate girls and women. If women have access to

training, if they can get out of the situation of sexual, economic, and labour subordination in which they find themselves, they become the main factor of success in eradicating poverty.

Hopefully, this pandemic will not only find us washing our hands (those of us who have soap and water) but make us more supportive of each other, especially the most disadvantaged and marginalised. Let us work with women survivors of violence to help them turn their lives around, share information and stories of experiences of women who have survived, create spaces of trust to talk, ask for and give help, and integrate networks. Let us remember that together our voices have more power to make those in control, uncomfortable. Let us teach ourselves to be alert, train ourselves, detect violence, take care of ourselves, make visible all manifestations of violence, and reverse individual situations of violence and influence collective ones as well. It is important to disrupt the uneven distribution of patriarchal power and grab the attention of our communities and authorities towards issues of gender inequity. Women must have education, economic freedom, and control over their bodies to stay alive and advance in the conquest of rights.

The health crisis reveals a global model that disdains solidarity and turns its back on humanism. It has evidenced that we must take advantage of and invest in it to create social objectives and policies that benefit both the middle and lower classes, especially women. Social and political mobilisation is always required to advance towards the conquest of rights and happiness; we have never won rights as gifts from states, and the elimination of violence against women will be no exception. Human rights are the harvest of struggles, sometimes peaceful, but many others have cost lives, deprivation of liberty or torture, to say the least. Investing in people is required, not experiments with privatised services. People-centred societies should be created, where all rights can be accessed, regardless of class, disability, age, sexual orientation, nationality, or any excuse that has historically been given to exploit and discriminate majorities. Some people will call it creating awareness of collectivity or humanity building. As the French economist Thomas Piketty[18] narrates: "Stop defending extreme inequality (ranging from basic needs, the right to property and fundamental rights, to new slaveries) and distribute wealth equitably, having a new narrative." The deficiencies in the way of thinking, coupled with the unquestionable hegemony of an unbridled thirst for profit, are responsible for innumerable human disasters. This has been evidenced during the Covid-19 pandemic as well.

We cannot leave this pandemic indifferent. We must transform and multiply our actions for the benefit of women and modify our reality so that we can have access to education and rights. We must create spaces for women to talk about our needs and desires but also to receive training, not just about feminism, self-care, or self-defence but also to attain financial independence. The support of sisterhood networks can help us, women, out of a situation of violence, as well as the inability to feed ourselves and support our daughters and sons. When women support other women, a community of unsurpassable strong relationships is created. And this is what we need to do in these dire times of loss, dispossession, and layoffs from family and friends. I think that if we contemplate ourselves mutilated, we will not advance, but if we complement ourselves with other women, together we can make our society a more humane and liveable place, that could allow anyone to be happy and live a life with dignity and rights, and not just continue to resist for mere survival. Our participation in decision-making and access to power is the way forward. The change in course that we want to achieve for the planet, after this pandemic, is ours. No one will stop us now. When they silence one, they expose the shout of all.

This chapter was first written in Spanish and then translated by the author.

Notes

1 Unknown author (14th century) [Arroz con leche]. https://youtu.be/4STiEqI4Vtk
2 Jiménez, José A. (1963). [La media vuelta]. On the album *"La media vuelta" by Javier Solís*. Universal Music Publishing Group. https://youtu.be/eVWXKlWpo5Y
3 Café Tacuba (1994). [Ingrata]. On the album *"Re."* Warner Chappell Music Mexico. https://youtu.be/kIr8hsVTCzg
4 With data from 2017 to 2018, a newspaper notes the impunity in cases of femicides: https://www.animalpolitico.com/2020/11/el-50-de-las-investigaciones-de-feminicidio-en-mexico-no-se-resuelven-dice-reporte/
5 Alda Facio is a lawyer, writer, and feminist activist. She is an international expert on women's human rights, violence between the sexes and the gender perspective; she is one of the founders of the Women's Caucus for Gender Justice at the International Criminal Court.
6 https://www.milenio.com/policia/en-enero-de-2020-cada-dia-10-mujeres-fueron-asesinadas
7 https://www.aljazeera.com/news/2020/7/24/number-of-women-seeking-help-from-mexico-lockdown-violence-surges
8 https://www.jornada.com.mx/notas/2021/04/27/sociedad/cada-hora-se-cometen-11-delitos-contra-mujeres-en-mexico-conavim/
9 https://digismak.com/sexist-violence-the-pandemic-exposes-the-plague-of-sex-crimes-in-mexico/
10 Joint communication of several networks of Human Rights Defenders in the region. Available at: https://im-defensoras.org/2021/05/marzo-el-mes-mas-peligroso-para-las-defensoras/
11 There is a phrase in the mural: "Patriarchate is a judge who judges us to be born, and our punishment is the violence you do not see," taken from the performance of the collective "Las Thesis" from Chile. There are three faces of women from the state of Coahuila who were killed at different times and whose investigation folders, were different as well, despite having the characteristics of femicide. Serymar Soto Arzúa, originally from Torreón (southwestern area of the state), was killed by her fiancé on 28 January 2017; thanks to her family's struggle, her perpetrator serves firm sentence for femicide in Piedras Negras. Brenda Nail González Montelongo, originally from Piedras Negras (north of the state), was found dead on 21 October 2018, ten days after her disappearance, murdered the day her firstborn turned 15 years old. There's no investigation, just threats

to her family that had to leave the country. Elisa Loyo Gutiérrez, originally from Saltillo (southeastern of the state), was murdered at her workplace (Fontana Leisure Park and Casino in the Philippines) on December 23, 2008, where they led to the belief that it had been a suicide. The night she was killed, a restaurant would open where the head chef would be Elisa. Her crime is still unpunished.

12 A homily is a religious discourse, and it is a commentary that follows a reading of scripture. It is more importantly moral and hortatory. In Catholic, Anglican, Lutheran, and Eastern Orthodox Churches, a homily is usually given during Mass at the end of the Liturgy of the Word. The President of Mexico has a daily Press Conference at 7 am, and what he says there, is taken by the media, as if it were the word of God, without criticism or filters, that is why the mockery that people are not receiving a political speech, but a spiritual edification.

13 The picture gets worse as the pandemic progresses. https://www.eleconomista.com.mx/politica/Violencia-feminicida-en-el-territorio-nacional-se-expande-20210512-0018.html

14 The issue of the elimination of gender-based violence is part of the speech of the President of Mexico and his cabinet; he has presented programs in conjunction with some countries seeking to curb violence, but meeting the objectives takes budget and training, as programs cannot be implemented only with good intentions and his very repeated phrase that he wants "hugs and not bullets" during his rule https://foreignpolicy.com/2020/12/30/mexico-feminist-foreign-policy-one-year-in/

15 On different occasions, the President of Mexico has discredited movements and collectives of women, minimising national campaigns, and even dismissing the causes of femicide, unlike a homicide. "Of course, it's the right tucked in, the conservatives. Just as there are women who, out of conviction and freely, protest and will continue to do so, so are opportunists" (Press Conference, February 21, 2020). "Conservatives disguise themselves as feminists because they saw it was a chance to attack us" (Press Conference, March 6, 2020). "It is very regrettable that the feminist movement is used for other purposes, since when does conservatism sympathize with the feminist movement?" (Press Conference, March 2, 2021). However, multiple women with federal positions in the government have defended the President and interpreted his words. https://elpais.com/mexico/2021-03-08/las-mujeres-del-gobierno-salen-a-defender-a-un-presidente-acorralado-por-la-polemica-con-las-feministas.html

16 The citizen and feminist movement "We have other data" is made up of defenders of Women's Rights, academics, artists, researchers and politicians who demand that the federal government ensure that women are present in all government decisions and ensuring that a public policy complies with equality.

17 Spanish writer, feminist activist, and politician; very active in defence of women's rights, she has developed a notable political career in recent years linked to leftist positions.

18 French economist who is Centennial Professor of Economics in the International Inequalities Institute at the London School of Economics. He is a columnist for the French newspaper Libération and occasionally writes op-eds (opinion articles) for Le Monde. His work focuses on public economics, in particular income and wealth inequality.

References

Arteta, I. (2020). 'El 50% de las investigaciones de feminicidio en México no se resuelven, dice reporte', *Animal Politico*, 10 November [online]. Available at: https://www.animalpolitico.com/2020/11/el-50-de-las-investigaciones-de-feminicidio-en-mexico-no-se-resuelven-dice-reporte/ [Accessed 3 January 2021].

Brena, C. M. (2021). 'Government Women Come Out to Defend a President Cornered by a Controversy with Feminists', *El Pais*, 8 March [online]. Available at: https://elpais.com/mexico/2021-03-08/las-mujeres-del-gobierno-salen-a-defender-a-un-presidente-acorralado-por-la-polemica-con-las-feministas.html [Accessed 10 March 2021].

Deslandes, A. (2020). 'Checking In on Mexico's Feminist Foreign Policy', *Foreign Policy*, 30 December [online]. Available at: https://foreignpolicy.com/2020/12/30/mexico-feminist-foreign-policy-one-year-in/ [Accessed 2 February 2021].

Mesoamerican Initiative of Women Human Rights Defenders. (2021). 'March, the Most Dangerous Month for Women Defenders?' *Mesoamerican Initiative of Women Human Rights Defenders*, 4 May [online]. Available at: https://im-defensoras.org/2021/05/marzo-el-mes-mas-peligroso-para-las-defensoras/ [Accessed 12 May 2021].

Perez, M. (2021). 'Feminicidal Violence in the National Territory Expands', *El Ecconomista*, 12 May [online]. Available at: https://www.eleconomista.com.mx/politica/Violencia-feminicida-en-el-territorio-nacional-se-expande-20210512-0018.html [Accessed 15 May 2021].

GOVERNANCE

11

DOMESTIC VIOLENCE DURING THE COVID-19 LOCKDOWN

Interventions by the Special Cell for Women Located at Police Stations November–December 2020

Trupti Jhaveri Panchal and Aarthi Chandrasekhar

The recent outbreak of the Covid-19 pandemic made governments around the world adopt various preventive measures to contain the contagion. These measures included the imposition of lockdowns, travel restrictions, the mandatory wearing of masks in public, maintaining physical distance, and so on. Though these measures curtailed individual freedoms, they were considered to be essential to protect public health. These unprecedented changes also resulted in unintended negative consequences, such as generating multiple new stresses, including physical and psychological health risks, isolation and loneliness, and those associated with the closure of schools and businesses, economic vulnerability, and job losses (Bradbury-Jones and Isham 2020).

The massive efforts taken by governments to stop the spreading of the virus and save lives paradoxically put women living in abusive relationships at risk. Multiple reports have shown that there has been a surge of domestic violence cases around the world, challenging the popular perception of the home as a safe haven, rather showcasing it is as a place where domestic and familial violence takes place in the form of physical, psychological, financial, and sexual abuse.

The Covid-19-induced quarantine forced vulnerable people to share space with the aggressors. The already distorted dynamics of power in the homes of abusive or controlling individuals can easily intensify during a crisis, as the abuser gets more freedom to act, while the survivor's movement is restricted. Away from any kind of scrutiny from the outside, one of the major implications of stay-at-home from the perspective of violence against women is the range of difficulties faced by survivors to seek help or escape (Telles et al. 2020).

DOI: 10.4324/9781003320524-15

Prevalence Data on Domestic Violence during Covid-19

The cases of domestic violence have increased around the world during the lockdown period. According to the UN Women (2020), multiple reports from parts of Asia, North and Latin America, Australia, and Europe have shown a significant rise in the number of women seeking help by calling crisis helplines and reporting abuse during the current pandemic; in France, for instance, reports of domestic violence have risen to 30 per cent after the onset of lockdown. The WHO (2020) referred to reports of an increase in domestic violence in China, the United Kingdom, and the United States, among other countries, since the outbreak of Covid-19.

According to an article published in June 2020 in the Indian daily, *The Hindu*, since the national lockdown, there was a 2.5-fold increase in the number of complaints of domestic violence registered by the National Commission for Women (NCW) (Jagriti Chandra 2020). The following week, *The Hindu* carried an article about 1,477 complaints of domestic violence having been reported between the first phase of lockdown in India, between 25 March and 31 May 2020, higher than those received in previous years during the same months (Radhakrishnan et al. 2020). With rising numbers, survivors' access to support was of crucial importance.

The Role of Special Cell for Women and Children in Police Stations during the Pandemic

Special Cell for Women and Children[1] (hereafter, Special Cell) is an effort aimed at eliminating violence against women. The Special Cells are located within the police station and offer psycho-socio-legal services to women survivors of violence. Its strategic location within the police system allows for support in navigating the criminal justice system, while also building the support system of the survivor, negotiating non-violence with various stakeholders, working with men in the interest of violated women, and engaging with stakeholders for a multi-agency coordinated response. These services are facilitated through trained, professional social workers who operate within a feminist social work framework.

The first Special Cell dates back to 1984 as a collaboration between the Mumbai Police and the School of Social Work, Tata Institute of Social Sciences, Mumbai. Having been institutionalised as a state programme in Maharashtra in 2005, Special Cell for Women has since expanded to other parts of the country. States such as Haryana, Gujarat, and Rajasthan have also adapted and institutionalised it as a state programme.

The pandemic and subsequent physical distancing norms had a severe impact on the provision of essential health, justice, policing, and social services for women and girls experiencing violence. This also resulted in several Special Cells shutting their physical operations, depending on whether or not the area they operated in had been declared a containment zone. This prompted the Special Cells to open up other channels of access to their services for survivors, for instance, telephone, among other organisational strategies to increase their reach. This chapter draws upon the collective effort of the team at Special Cell for Women and Resource Centre for Interventions on Violence against Women (RCI-VAW)[2].

A Glimpse into Data on Domestic Violence Cases in Maharashtra State during the Lockdown

During the period of total lockdown (April–June 2020), 123 Special Cells for Women in the state of Maharashtra and the helpline – Mala Bolaycha Aahe[3] received 8,698 calls, of which 4,801 were calls pertaining to VAW. Once the helpline was launched, there were not only callers seeking support to address violence but also those who were stranded and needed access to support including ration/food, those who wanted information related to the pandemic, and some who wanted to know more about the helpline. Given the situation, the helpline responded to all such calls. The high number of reported cases may be attributed to several factors, including strategies that were specifically adopted during the lockdown period to increase visibility and accessibility of the service.

Programmatic Strategies Adopted by Special Cells during Covid-19 Pandemic

The new context of the pandemic demanded new strategies of service provision, and the Special Cell drew upon its long and rich experience of working with women to come up with appropriate mechanisms and systems to make the service accessible to survivors.

Domestic Violence Helpline

During the lockdown, many survivors were locked inside their homes, forced to live continuously in proximity to their abusers. They lacked privacy or the space to seek outside help and found themselves carrying the increased burden of household work. In such a situation, it became imperative for the Special Cells to respond to the emotional distress suffered by the survivors and extend their services telephonically. However, social workers facilitated in-person meetings with the survivors and their abusers at the police stations in the pre-Covid-19 time and did not have the training to do the same telephonically. The Special Cell, therefore, first facilitated training sessions for social workers as well as Protection Officers[4] to equip them with skills to navigate through the new way of working, while prioritising the safety of the survivor. The Special Cells in Maharashtra and other states, in collaboration with the police, synergised their efforts to ensure that the police reached the location to stop the violence and extend need-based assistance to the survivors by relocating them to a safe space or helping them access medical care and treatment.

Information about the domestic violence helpline was advertised on multiple platforms. Flyers and pamphlets in local languages were disseminated within local networks at the community level. Stakeholders such as the state authorities, women's groups, and multiple NGOs across the country played an important role in spreading the word. This extended the Special Cells' reach beyond their physical location, and they received calls from neighbouring districts and states. Below is an example of the coordinated efforts between the social workers and the police:

> *A 32-year-old woman called Special Cell's helpline number after learning about it from a local newspaper. Her husband had beaten her with a stick and her leg was bruised. He had been violent with her throughout their six years of marriage, and it had only worsened during the lockdown. She needed immediate medical attention and also wanted help in leaving the violent space of the home. The social worker coordinated with all the parties involved to ensure that the survivor received immediate medico-legal care at the local primary healthcare centre. The social worker spoke to the woman and explored safe spaces that she could go to. Her natal home was about 20 kilometres away. The social worker contacted the survivor's parents and conveyed the situation. They wanted to bring their daughter home but were uncertain about transportation owing to the lockdown. The social worker harnessed local police support through the station house officer, who ensured that a patrol van was sent to rescue the survivor.*

Focused Advocacy Campaign on Putting an End to Domestic Violence

When the lockdown was announced, it became imperative for violence against women interventionists, especially the ones working in the service-delivery space to think out of the box to respond to women who were experiencing violence, engage men who were perpetrating violence, and bystanders who were witnessing violence. It was high time that anti-domestic violence campaigns were not only active but effective in how they addressed the issue.

The Special Cell in collaboration with Akshara Centre, a non-profit women's organisation and resource centre working for the empowerment of women and girls, engaged with the Government of Maharashtra to respond to violence against women by making a formal, written request to the Chief Minister and Director General of Police of Maharashtra that they issue directives to state helplines to continue responding to women in distress. The need was identified for police and district administrations to provide vehicular support to social workers for the facilitation of rescue efforts and transfer the woman to safety.

As a result of this engagement and advocacy, the Chief Minister's Office in Maharashtra released a tri-lingual public service announcement in the month of April. This included showcasing individuals from the sports and entertainment industries on the screen appealing to women to have zero tolerance against violence and encouraging citizens to report violence. The corresponding social media campaign #LockdownOnDomesticViolence[5] received 5.5 million views on various social media and received extensive press coverage. This campaign was mainly designed to make 'domestic' issues a mainstream concern.

Strengthening Systemic Responses

The Special Cell along with Akshara Centre also created a web application (standupagainstviolence)[6] for the survivors to get in touch with services directly on their mobile phones. This app contains a list of over 450 mobile numbers of state services from the districts and sub-districts of Maharashtra, including those of the Special Cells, One-Stop Centres,[7] helplines, Protection Officers, and Service Providers[8] registered under the Protection of Women from Domestic Violence Act, Family Counselling Centres, and shelter homes. This is a unique directory of people and services, especially for pandemic times, when restricted mobility has severely hampered access to justice for survivors. This app was circulated among all state and non-governmental stakeholders working with women.

Another helpline '*mala bolaaycha aahe*' (I Want to Speak) was created by the team working at the Special Cell in collaboration with the Women and Child Development Commissionerate, Maharashtra. The helpline was named thus, because of the recognition that women want a safe space to voice their concerns, in the context of limited access to safe physical locations. Through this helpline, the coordinating team of the Special Cells connected the Protection Officers, Police, crisis interventionists, and survivors in Maharashtra with the corresponding Special Cells located in the sub-districts.

Facilitating a Multi-agency Coordinated Response

The Special Cell recognises the importance of a multi-agency coordinated system to provide a comprehensive response to survivors, involving all relevant agencies, such as the police, health system, legal system, and social services. Each has a significant role to play within the synergistic response framework. Social workers of the Special Cells play the role of providing emotional support to the survivor, work with them to draw up a safety plan, and coordinate with various agencies based on the requirement of the survivor.

Some of the women survivors who reached the Cells directly or telephonically had faced extreme physical violence. Many of them, who had approached the Cell before the pandemic for support, contacted the social workers sharing recurrence of violence during the lockdown. The social workers coordinated with the police for rescue, accompanied the survivors to medical facilities as well as successfully advocated for electronic-FIRs[9] to be filed.

> *In one instance, an organisation working on prisoners' rights sought the help of the Special Cells' team in the case of an undertrial man who was let out on parole in response to the government's policy of containing the pandemic spread by reducing crowding of prisons. The man in question had been physically violent towards his wife and children and had forced them out of the house citing fear of contracting Covid-19. In this case, the Special Cell team was able to coordinate for the provision of temporary shelter for the woman and children in an NGO-run home, while also harnessing police support for future intervention with the man, so that the woman and children may go back to live in their home.*

Because of the work that the Special Cell has done with the police system over several years, it was able to facilitate escalation of cases of survivors directly to senior police officers for on-ground intervention, after which the violence would reportedly stop. Women survivors, who were not staying in their marital homes at the time of the lockdown, due to a preceding violent incident that had forced them to leave, contacted the Special Cells worrying about their children as well as belongings that they had left behind. Many of them also shared the discontinuation of maintenance payments or contribution to household expenses by the estranged spouse. In such cases, social workers of the Special Cells helped survivors record as much evidence as possible of the violence, prepare and plan legal steps to be taken post the lockdown. Planning for the safety of the survivor was prioritised during the lockdown.

> *A 30-year-old woman married for five years called the Special Cell to complain about her husband, who physically and sexually abused her. He was in an out-of-marriage intimate relationship. The woman had gone to spend a few days with her natal family but was unable to return to her matrimonial home until the end of the lockdown. On her return, her husband did not allow her and the children to enter the home and told them to go back to her natal home. She called the helpline number of the Special Cell. The social workers harnessed police support and ensured her right of residence to her matrimonial home. The social worker has contin-*

ued to follow up to carry on the support and assist her with legal procedures.

Access to medical care, including maternal healthcare was a challenge during the lockdown, especially for women facing domestic violence, with little support from the natal family.

A 32-year-old woman was referred to the Special Cell social worker. She was nearing the ninth month of pregnancy. Owing to severe violence in her marital home, she had left for her mother's house before the lockdown had been announced. At her natal home, she faced violence from her brother. She conveyed to the social worker that she wanted to move to a shelter home for the time being. The social worker tried coordinating with several shelter homes but all of them refused to admit her due to the situation of lockdown, stating the Covid-19 test as one of the eligibility criteria for admission. The social worker tapped into her network with the One-Stop Centre personnel to explore the option of temporary shelter as well as support for admission to the hospital. The hospital admitted her and two days later, she delivered her child without many complications. After a discussion with the woman, the social worker also engaged with the survivor's husband for ensuring his financial support. The requirement at that point in time was strengthening support for the woman. The social worker used all possible resources she had access to, for a timely response to the survivor.

There were instances where supportive family members called on behalf of the survivor, worried about the latter's safety, and the social worker coordinated the survivor's transfer to safety.

A mother called the Special Cell telephone line with concern for her 21-year-old daughter's safety. A few months into the marriage, her daughter had shared that she was facing violence at her marital home. She had called one night sounding terrified. When the social worker contacted the survivor on the phone, she replied saying she was fine and that there was no need to call her again. The next day the survivor called back explaining that she had been unable to speak then and needed help in leaving the violent space. The social worker coordinated with another helpline number as well as with the police to ensure that the Police Control Vehicle (PCR) reached the spot. Upon the arrival of the police, her husband assured her that he would not be violent with her in the future. With this assurance, that too in the presence of the police, the survivor decided to stay back in her matrimonial home. The social worker reiterated

*to the woman that her safety could be in jeopardy if she decides to
stay on in her marital home, as the violence may recur. However,
in the subsequent follow-ups, the survivor shared with the social
worker that violence had stopped after the intervention of the police. The social worker assured the woman of continued support.*

In this case, the social worker facilitated coordination and harnessed police
support based on established networks, by way of being located within the
police system, thus underlining the importance of the location of the Special
Cell within the police station premises. This case highlights the importance
of reaching out to survivors – the social worker called up the survivor
immediately after being informed by her mother. The call opened up the
possibility for her to call back at the first opportunity.

Through the collaboration and coordination with the police, Special Cell
social workers were able to assist survivors in filing formal complaints in
the form of FIR and NC[10], facilitate access to medical care, transfer survivors to safety, assist in retrieving economic assets and financial entitlements
and where required, coordinate to ensure police intervention to stop violence, while also extending psycho-social support to reduce distress. During
the lockdown, the Special Cells harnessed its existing network and collaboration with state and non-governmental stakeholders to coordinate appropriate responses in the interest of the survivor.

Preparedness for Such a Pandemic

The pandemic and the subsequent lockdown demanded the Special Cells
to adapt to the new context promptly, which involved adapting its intervention strategies. While working with the perpetrator to stop violence is a
part of the long-term intervention with women survivors, such an intervention was not feasible in a lockdown situation. Initially, it posed a challenge
but continued work on building a support system for the woman through
engagement with local stakeholders went a long way in formulating and
operationalising appropriate response. The pandemic was seen as a limiting
factor by several stakeholders, yet engagement and coordination had to be
carried out to facilitate an effective response.

Integrating Response to Violence against Women within
State Systems

The experience of the Special Cells has underlined the need to have response
services working at various locations, not only in terms of the geographic
spread but also within multiple state systems, such as the health system,
police system, and others, as the profile of women approaching each of these

state systems varies. Those survivors, who need medico-legal care, are more likely to come in contact with the hospital, while those considering action through the criminal justice system are likely to access the police. Hence, both state systems would benefit from having trained social workers, who can provide requisite support to survivors based on their specific needs, which may differ depending on the particular state system they approach. Each of these systems and spaces is important in making support accessible to survivors of violence, especially during a pandemic or lockdown, when resources are limited, and mobility is restricted. This builds the case for such psycho-social-legal support services to be recognised as 'essential services'. It also highlights the urgency for the state to make financial resources available for carrying out such crucial work.

Notes

1 https://tiss.edu/view/11/projects/all-projects/special-cell-for-women-and-children-maharashtra/
2 The Resource Centre for Interventions on Violence Against Women (RCI-VAW), was set up in 2007–2008 as a field action unit of the School of Social Work, TISS, Mumbai, to resource the Special Cells and inform the larger discourse and praxis in responding to VAW in India. https://www.tiss.edu/view/11/projects/rci-vaw-resource-centre-for-interventions-on-viole/
3 Helpline created by the coordinating team working at the Special Cell in collaboration with Women and Child Development Commissionerate, Maharashtra, to respond to calls during the lockdown.
4 Protection Officer is an officer appointed by the state government to facilitate access for survivors to reliefs under the Protection of Women from Domestic Violence Act, 2005.
5 https://www.youtube.com/watch?v=v2e3JwxFmw8
6 http://standupagainstviolence.org/maharashtraApp/index.html
7 The One-Stop Centre, Family Counselling Centre, and Swadhar Greh are national schemes implemented by the Ministry of Women and Child Development (MWCD) introduced in 2015, 1983, and 2001, respectively, to support women facing violence. OSCs offer medical assistance, police assistance, psychosocial support, legal aid, and temporary shelter within a single unit located in the proximity of a medical facility. Family Counselling Centres (FCC) offer counselling, referral and rehabilitative services to women and children facing violence. Shelter homes under the Swadhar Greh Scheme offer shelter, food, clothing, counselling, training, clinical and legal aid with the aim of rehabilitation of women in distress.
8 Service Providers registered under the PWDVA can record a Domestic Incident Report in the prescribed format and forward it to the concerned Protection Officer for further process. They are also in a position to provide necessary support such as facilitation of medical examination and shelter to survivors of violence.
9 First Investigation Report (FIR) refers to the formal record of information that sets the criminal law in motion.
10 NC or non-cognisable complaint is a record of a non-cognisable offence; however, it does not initiate an investigation.

References

Bradbury-Jones, C., and Isham, L. (2020). The pandemic paradox: The consequences of COVID-19 on domestic violence, *Journal of clinical nursing*, 29, 13–14.

Jagriti Chandra. (2020, June 15). 'NCW records sharp spike in domestic violence amid lockdown', *The Hindu*. 15 June [online]. Available at: https://www.thehindu.com/news/national/ncw-records-sharp-spike-in-domestic-violence-amid-lockdown/article31835105.ece. [Accessed 28 April 2021].

Radhakrishnan, V., Sen, S., and Singaravelu, N. (2020). 'Data | Domestic violence complaints at a 10-year high during COVID-19 lockdown', *The Hindu*, 22 June [online]. Available at: https://www.thehindu.com/data/data-domestic-violence-complaints-at-a-10-year-high-during-covid-19-lockdown/article31885001.ece. [Accessed 9 September 2020].

Telles, L. E., Valença, A. M., Barros, A. J., and da Silva, A. G. (2020). Domestic violence in the COVID-19 pandemic: A forensic psychiatric perspective, *Brazilian Journal of Psychiatry, (AHEAD)*, 43, 3.

UN Women. (2020). 'COVID-19 and essential services provision for survivors of violence against women and girl' [online]. Available at: https://www.unwomen.org/-/media/headquarters/attachments/sections/library/publications/2020/brief-covid-19-and-essential-services-provision-for-survivors-of-violence-against-women-and-girls-en.pdf?la=en&vs=3834. [Accessed 9 September 2020].

World Health Organization. (2020). 'COVID-19 and violence against women: What the health sector/system can do' [online]. Available at: https://www.who.int/reproductivehealth/publications/emergencies/COVID-19-VAW-full-text.pdf. [Accessed 9 September 2020].

12

RE-IMAGINING GOVERNANCE IN POST-COVID-19 BIHAR[1]

May – June 2020

Harshita Jha

The limitations of existing governance mechanisms have come to glaring visibility in the pandemic-struck world. Governance at all levels – international, national, provincial, and local – has been stretched to the extent of their breakdown. Overwhelming the system to an unparalleled extent, Covid-19-induced challenges have caused disruptions in all spheres of human life. From being a public health emergency, it has led to the disruption of the economy, the political order, and administrative processes and wreaked havoc in supply and logistical chains. When businesses were shut down and movement of people curtailed to stop the spread of the virus, the economy collapsed, and people became jobless overnight. Governance systems crumbled, hospitals were packed to the rafters, and human life came to a virtual standstill in all parts of the globe. For this reason, the World Economic Forum has rightly called the crisis the 'Great Reset', as the pandemic has revealed inconsistencies, inadequacies, and contradictions of multiple systems – from health to finance to education – amid concern for life, livelihood, and the planet (WEF 2020). It has also thrown open unprecedented challenges to global leaders and policymakers who have been forced to make several trade-offs for tiding over short-term pressures amid protracted long-term uncertainties.

According to the World Health Organization (WHO) Director-General, there will be no return to the 'old normal' for the near foreseeable future (Guardian 2020). Therefore, the Great Reset is being seen not only as a complex challenge but also as a window of opportunity to reimagine the world. As it laid bare the rot in the system, intellectuals, politicians, newspapers, and public discussions are preoccupied with the question of what should change in the post-Covid-19 world. In the Indian context, one recurrent theme that comes up in the discussion is the limitation of a centralised state in dealing with a pandemic-like situation, hence calling for

DOI: 10.4324/9781003320524-16

strengthening local governance institutions (Oommen 2020; Sridevan and Currimbhoy 2020; Aiyar 2020).

In India, the 73rd and 74th[2] amendment in the Constitution was brought into effect in the early 1990s. It paved the way for deepening democracy through decentralisation, which was not merely the devolution of administrative power from a centralised state to a local state but also involved the transfer of political decision-making power to the local bodies. The 74th Amendment democratised towns and cities and the 73rd Amendment, the villages. As the statement of objectives of the 73rd Act states, this amendment was brought to life to address the problem of unresponsive local bodies in villages due to the absence of elections, prolonged supersessions, insufficient representation of disadvantaged sections of society such as people belonging to the Scheduled Castes, Scheduled Tribes,[3] and women, as well as lack of financial resources. The Act was to also provide for institutional designs for local governance in villages. Thus, it aimed to vest power and authority in Panchayats and municipal bodies[4] that would enable them to work as units of self-governance.

In India, Covid-19 has brought to the fore the problem of incapacity of the state – unevenly spread across the country. While some southern states such as Tamil Nadu and Kerala have built state capacities over the years, states such as Bihar are infamous for their incompetence. Undoubtedly, there is a deep historical background to the existing political and economic problems in Bihar. A lot has also been written about the worsening of state infrastructure in Bihar, a fact that many attribute to the downward turn in administrative politics after 1991 (Mathew and More 2011). It is believed that the absence of functional law and order led to a decline in private investment, which resulted in low growth performance. Rampant corruption in the implementation of central and state-sponsored schemes hindered the poverty reduction of poor households. It is also believed that since Bihar was politically out of sync with the government at the centre from 1992 to 2004 it was systematically starved of funds. The division of the state into two in the year 2000 for administrative purposes left Bihar with most of the liabilities, whereas the new state of Jharkhand (a state in eastern India, carved out of Bihar) received profit yielding industrial and mineral resources. Today, Bihar remains one of the poorest and most 'backward' states in India, if measured using conventional development indicators. This became amply evident when Bihar was declared the worst performer in the NITI Aayog[5] Sustainable Development Index (SDI) 2019 (NITI Aayog 2019). Covid-19 has put tremendous stress on the best performing states, and therefore, it becomes important to understand how a 'backward' state like Bihar has tried to cope with the pandemic.

Most of the Covid-19-related state response was implemented at the grassroots level, whether it was mobilising frontline health workers, providing relief to communities, ensuring that lockdown norms are being followed, preventing the spread of the virus, and making people aware of physical distancing rules. Therefore, the effectiveness of the response was entirely dependent on the capability of institutions at the grassroots level, which includes mainly local government bodies. In this context, this chapter explores the question of how local government institutions in Bihar have responded to the Covid-19 crisis.

The chapter draws from primary data based on telephonic interviews carried out with key informants (community workers of an NGO in the region, teacher of a government school, correspondent of a daily local newspaper and *Anganwadi*[6] workers) from Rattipur Baria Panchayat, Raghopur Panchayat, and Gosaidaspur Panchayat of Nathnagar block[7] in the Bhagalpur district[8] of Bihar. For analysis and discussion, it draws on resources such as academic articles, newspapers, and online media reportage.

The first part of the chapter looks at the importance of decentralisation and its relevance in dealing with a crisis induced by the pandemic. It also attempts to argue why the decentralised state, as opposed to a centralised state, should be a norm in the post-Covid world. In the second part of the chapter, the findings of the study are discussed in detail. The chapter concludes that the Covid-19 response of the local government in Bihar was inefficient and ineffective and argues that the state needs political will and vigour to build the capacity of local government institutions.

Decentralisation and Covid-19

The 73rd Amendment Act sought to create three-tier local self-government institutions – at the village, intermediate, and district levels. Additionally, it has mandated reservation (affirmative action) for persons belonging to the Scheduled Castes and Scheduled Tribes in these bodies, proportionate to their population, and one-third of all seats are reserved for women. These bodies were mandated to prepare plans for economic development and social justice as well as carry out the implementation of development schemes. The state government was also supposed to ensure the economic independence of these bodies by proper financial devolution and by allowing Panchayats to raise revenues.

Twenty-eight years down the line, however, local governments have not become independent units of self-governance (Raghunandan 2018). The implementation of the Act remains uneven, with some states like Kerala having established a strong decentralised institution. Devolution is a state subject.[9] The various states of India have absolute control over the funds, functions, and functionaries of local governments. This has resulted in Panchayats being at the mercy of state governments, which has hampered their emergence as empowered bodies capable to carry out their constitutionally mandated task. Although 29 subjects are mentioned in the 11th Schedule[10], only a handful of core functions like water supply, sanitation, roads and communication, streetlight provision, and the management of community assets are mainly devolved by the state. Along with it, local bodies are financially constrained due to reduced allocation; their access to funds is made conditional; and they are not empowered to raise tax revenues. Election to the local bodies is often delayed unduly and indefinite supersessions[11] have become a norm in many places. These structural issues have hampered Gram Panchayats from becoming strong units of self-governance. In most states, local government bodies are abysmally lacking the capability to even carry out the routine functions of government, viz. the implementation of development schemes.

Now, let us understand decentralisation conceptually and see how it helps in managing a crisis like Covid-19. This can be answered by looking at the economic implications of decentralisation on the ground. As we have seen during Covid-19, the state machinery was expected to quickly respond to public health crises occurring locally, by stopping the spread of the disease and providing respite to the people in terms of distributing welfare measures. One of the greatest advantages decentralised bodies have over the centralised state is the information edge it gives to the decision-maker (Bardhan 1996). At the community level, the decision-maker may be fully aware of the nature of demands that are occurring in the community, and this allows them to mobilise local resources to meet those demands. This is also applicable to the public delivery system, where the information advantage ensures effective, time-bound distribution of services. This will be more efficient than a traditional centrally sponsored, one-size-fits-all service delivery system, which is limited by uniformity constraints and is, therefore, unable to satisfy the diversity of locally occurring preferences.

The management of the Covid-19 crisis depended on decentralised responses, and local governments possessed the information advantage that enabled them to monitor and take immediate action to contain the spread of the virus. This is true for any other crisis, like managing floods or other natural disasters. The informational advantage also ensures better coordination and enforcement by local systems. If the local institutions are established and function properly, they can rely on information about the local needs of the public that they can collect in less time. The Covid-19 response especially involved coordinating with different departments and civil society stakeholders.

Another aspect of decentralisation is the enhanced accountability it ensures (Bardhan 1996). When political decision-makers hail from the local community itself, they usually have more incentive to act, as compared to agents of the central institution. The periodic electoral review that local leaders are subject to, ensures political accountability.

However, the idea is not to offer decentralisation as an alternative to centralisation, but about finding the right balance between the two. This is because decentralised bodies do not have the advantage of economies of scale that a centralised economy has.

In the discussions around Covid-19 management, the example of Kerala[12] is often talked about. The key agents of managing Covid-19 in Kerala have been the local government agencies (Vijay an 2020; Isaac and Sadanandan 2020). Kerala's local government had been strengthened over the years with a substantial allocation of funds, wider devolution of functions, as well as clearly marking the responsibilities and duties of functionaries. Ever since participatory planning[13] started in Kerala in 1996, it began to involve communities in the local governance, thus inching closer to the dream of self-government. Kerala had already devolved much of its health-related functions to local bodies and by the time Covid-19 struck, it was already prepared to tackle the crisis (Isaac and Sadanandan 2020). The local governments have been mandated to implement the important functions of improvement and maintenance of the buildings of primary healthcare centres and sub-centres; employ doctors, nurses, and paramedical staff on contract; supplement the honorarium of Accredited Social Health Activist (ASHA)[14] workers; purchase drugs; and medical equipment. They have also played an important role in geriatric care, supporting persons with disabilities, financing special schools for children with cognitive disabilities, and overseeing the prevention of vector and waterborne infectious diseases.

All this has allowed local governments in Kerala to leverage their full potential during the Covid-19 pandemic (Isaac and Sadanandan 2020). As an institution which is very much rooted in the community, local governments were mobilised for generating awareness about Covid-19 and spearhead the 'Break the Chain'[15] movement, carry out sanitation activities, support persons in isolation, ensure availability of essential items, and document prevention efforts, including preparing an inventory of medical and other resources and a list of the number of persons who needed additional support. The local government along with decentralised bodies like Kudumbashree[16] volunteers and frontline health workers took up the responsibility of alleviating distress by setting up community kitchens that provided free meals to migrant labourers, homeless, disabled, and other sections of the society. There was also the option of home-delivery of cooked food through volunteers as well as that of reaching raw material of the mid-day meal[17] through ASHA workers to pupil's homes.

The Kerala example shows that the state or central government can give broad directions and guidelines, but people's participation under the leadership of empowered local governments seems to be the most effective strategy to contain the spread of the pandemic. At the same time, a strong public sector in health and education, which is not possible without economies of scale, is necessary for this decentralised model to work well.

Assessment of Welfare Measures Post-Covid-19

A large section of the population relied on social protection measures by the state to cope with the life course risk as well as the economic downturns that the pandemic brought in. Several relief measures had been announced by the state government of Bihar for Below Poverty Line[18] households/individuals post the lockdown. It mostly included reaching benefits of pre-existing schemes and programs to these households/individuals. Accessing these welfare measures and schemes has been a serious challenge for these households in Bihar. So, what happens to the implementation of these welfare measures at the local level with the onset of Covid-19?

Food Security Measures

The informants reported that there was an unexpected increase in the prices of basic food items during the first phase of the lockdown. For instance, the price of a small packet of salt increased from INR 5 ($0.068) to INR 15 ($0.20), the price of mustard oil rose from INR 20 ($0.27) for 250 millilitres to INR 30/$0.41 (from INR 80/$1 per litre to INR 130/$1.76 per litre), and the price of rice also rose by more than INR 10/$0.14 per kg. While the price of salt eventually fell to the pre-lockdown rate, prices of other items remained high. Vegetables have either been unavailable or are expensive, and the rise in the price of cooking oil has forced many to subsist on meals consisting solely of rice with a bit of salt. With the high price of rice and other essentials and no source of income, many households in the Panchayat who were not covered under the Public Distribution System[19] were pushed to solely depend on the free ration being provided by the Panchayats.

Most households had almost exhausted the rations they had received under the Public Distribution System in mid-May and are awaiting the next instalment. At the time of the interview, there was no information as to when the next instalment of rations would arrive. In addition, many households did not receive the quantity of ration they are entitled to. The *Anganwadi* centres in the source Panchayats have been shut since the announcement of the lockdown. *Anganwadi Sevikas*[20] have been distributing only *Sattu* (roasted gram flour) to pregnant/lactating women every week, as there are no funds to procure other food items. Mid-day meals were not provided to school children after the schools were closed due to the lockdown.

> I am a teacher at the primary school, and I know that in each class, there are 10-20 students who belong to families of daily wage labourers. They attend the school only to get a mid-day meal. They must have struggled to get food due to the lockdown.
> – Narendra Sharma[21], Primary school teacher,
> Raghodaspur Panchayat

The irregular ration distribution and non-accessibility to mid-day meals and food essentials from *Anganwadis* have led to reduced food consumption among members of these households, which has put them at high risk in terms of contracting Covid-19, as well as other diseases. Realising the immediate value of food security, the Public Distribution System, backed by accumulated food stocks should be revamped, as part of the post-covid economic recovery plan of the government. The capacity of local institutions responsible for implementation, in the long run, should be strengthened.

Issues in the Implementation of the Mahatma Gandhi National Rural Employment Guarantee Scheme (MGNREGS)

The objective of MGNREGS[22] is to provide a secure source of income for the poor, vulnerable, and marginalised. Since the very beginning, the implementation of MGNREGS has suffered from gross violations of guidelines, irregularities, and delayed payments in the state of Bihar. On an average, the human-day of work generated has been around 40 to 45 days in a year as per one of the research informants. After the lockdown was announced, not a single human-day of work has been generated in any of the three source Panchayats; in fact, the wages for at least 7 to 12 human days of work (on average), for the months of December and January 2020 were yet to be paid at the time of the interview.

> Everyone is aware how MGNREGS operates here, the job cards[23] are not with people who are job cardholders; someone does the work and someone else gets the money. But even when a person does end up getting five to ten days of work, the wages for the same are not given on time.
>
> – Community worker, NGO

The unplanned lockdown has led to a situation in which vulnerable sections of the rural population such as daily wage labourers, small self-employed households, and farmers with small or no landholdings are under severe duress. The near absence of other employment opportunities in the area may give rise to the demand for work under MGNREGS. The issues of non-generation of work or delayed payment of wages will push the dependent households into further marginalisation.

Agriculture-related Welfare Measures

Agriculture-related work requires workers to leave their houses, and this work is only seasonal in nature. In the *rabi* season[24], though wheat is the main crop, mustard, potato, pulses, and peppermint are also grown in the source Panchayats. When the lockdown was announced, the standing wheat and mustard crops were ready to be harvested. Pulse crops such as gram and *masoor*[25] got damaged due to bad weather (excessive untimely rains).

The informants reported that the production of gram and other pulses sown in the season was adversely affected, and there was no surplus for selling in the market. Farmers found it difficult to sell their grain and produce. The farmers did not receive any support from their Panchayats to overcome these difficulties. Only a fairly small number of farmers had received INR 2,000/$27 under the Kisan Samman Yojana[26] (a welfare scheme for farmers) in one of the three source Panchayats. With the absence of any handholding from the local government as well as the state government's Department of Agriculture, farmers in the region are in a vulnerable situation. More vulnerable than ever.

National Social Assistance Programme

The social assistance program aims to provide benefits to poor households in specific cases such as old age, disability, widowhood, death of the bread-winner, and maternity. As per the informants, beneficiaries of these social assistance programs have always witnessed delayed payments of pensions, arbitrary striking off names from the beneficiary list, and non-payment for unknown reasons. Due to a lack of access to any database on the monthly payments received by the beneficiary, it is difficult to analyse if the individuals received the assistance on time, at least in the period of the lockdown. But the informants complained about non-payment of pensions in the source Panchayats. Such negligence of the local institutions towards assisting individuals dependent on this program for their subsistence, even in these extraordinary times, shows the apathy of the local government.

> Pension schemes here are given to the allies of the people in power who may not even be eligible. If one verifies the beneficiary list of the various pension schemes, many such discrepancies will be exposed.
>
> – Community worker, NGO

Welfare Measures for Healthcare

As per the informants, the Panchayats ensured the sanitisation of public places after the outbreak of Covid-19. Masks and sanitisers were also distributed to all households in the Panchayats. Buildings of the government schools were turned into quarantine facilities for the migrant workers returning to the Panchayats. But non-availability of medical professionals at the primary healthcare centre even during this pandemic posed a serious challenge. People suffering from diseases other than Covid-19 found it difficult to receive medical care. In case of health-related issues, residents of the Panchayat rely upon private clinics or else travel to hospitals located at the district level. Due to the lockdown, doing the same was not possible, and this added to the challenges faced by the people. It is the consequence of existing poor infrastructure and poor planning of healthcare facilities at the local level, which needs to be addressed in a major way post-Covid-19.

The primary schools were turned into quarantine centres and teachers were given the responsibility of supervising these centres but there was no provision for medical care of any kind at the block or Panchayat level.

– Narendra Sharma, Primary School Teacher

Our village is highly populated. But we have only one ASHA *Didi*[27] appointed here who looks after more than 1000 households. The medical officer is rarely found at the primary healthcare centre. Usually, everyone goes to Bhagalpur or Patna (other district head-quarters in the state) in case of any health-related issues but due to COVID-19, mobility is restricted. Lack of healthcare services in nearby places has left people feeling helpless.

– Community worker, NGO

Towards Re-imagining Governance in Post-Covid Bihar

The crisis that Covid-19 has posed has laid bare many questions regarding the state's capability to address the issue of poverty as well as those of service and infrastructural lapses. The ability to tide over the crisis has depended on how responsively the state has taken decisions and how timely it has executed the implementation of social securities and welfare measures to provide support to the vulnerable.

In Bihar, with poor state capacities, decaying and unresponsive institutions, and entrenched corruption, Covid-19 has thrown open complicated challenges that are reflected in the assessment of the delivery of welfare measures. Notwithstanding the fact, the whole state machinery has been engaged in efforts to contain the spread of this pandemic. But due to the deplorable condition of the primary structure of governance that is the Gram Panchayat, it could not be efficiently mobilised to address the ongoing crisis.

It has been argued time and again that decentralisation is a step in the right direction when it comes to increasing the capacity of the state to address poverty in the so-called Third World countries. Decentralisation is the best possible institutional arrangement that can solve the notorious problem of 'last-mile delivery'. In times like this, the health of its institutions of governance, effortless transmission of commands, and swift action are necessary at the local level.

However, a state's performance during a pandemic cannot be better than during other times. For this reason, in an extraordinary situation like a pandemic, it is important to assess how the implementation dynamics have played out in the scenario of an already weak state system and pave a way forward. If we look at the state of Bihar, there are 8,463 Gram Panchayats, 534 block panchayats, and 38 district Panchayats catering to more than 80 per cent of the state's population. The scope and outreach of the Panchayati

Raj Institutions is massive.[28] To address the denied or deprived social protection of the poor, there is an urgent need to accelerate the capability of the local institutions first. This must be supplemented with re-thinking of the Bihar Panchayati Raj Act,[29] with an emphasis on devolution of both administrative and fiscal power.

Re-imagining governance in Bihar would require a critical analysis of the Panchayati Raj Act of Bihar. After the 73rd amendment to the Indian Constitution, the Panchayati Raj Act, 1993 was enacted and the three tiers of the Panchayati Raj became functional. However, in 2006, the new government led by Chief Minister Nitish Kumar replaced the 1993 Act with a new Panchayat Act of 2006. As per the Bihar Panchayat Act, 2006, 20 departments have on paper devolved their functions to Panchayati Raj Institutions.[30] But the major limitation that holds back the Gram Panchayats and the various standing committees[31] in the Panchayat to implement various actions is that they have not augmented their own sources of revenue so far, even after the amendment made to the Panchayati Raj Act. This is because the state government has not notified the maximum rates of taxes, tolls, and fees to be imposed by them yet. Broadly speaking, the Panchayati Raj Institutions have failed to raise their own resources and thrive largely on central and state government grants. Thus, revenue assignment – one of the hallmarks of local government's autonomy – works out to almost zero for Bihar's Panchayats. The devolution of functions without the devolution of functionaries and funds has resulted in no change in the Panchayati Raj Institutions even after the amendment in the Act. Usually, when a new act is passed, it is required to mend relevant existing acts to acknowledge the new act. This facilitates in clearing the operating ground for the new act. For instance, In Kerala after the Panchayati Raj act was revised, around 130 existing acts were amended to enable the implementation of the new Panchayati Raj Act in the state.

To overcome this, there is a dire need for devolution of the three Fs – funds, functions, and functionaries, not just on paper but on the ground as well. The Panchayati Raj Act must lay down specific rules which prescribe how devolution of functions and functionaries is to be implemented in the Gram Panchayats. It must include revenue sources for Panchayati Raj Institutions so that it enables the Panchayat's ability to generate its own funds.

The absence of any sense of accountability is the root cause of the failure of these structures. To ensure the fair functioning of Gram Panchayats, accountability is much required. The community-based organization (CBO) of the poor set up by the State Rural Livelihood Mission[32] (SRLM) can play a dynamic role in establishing accountability through community monitoring of the implementation of welfare measures. The mobilisation of the organisation of the poor built by the SRLM will allow the community to understand the causes of poverty, different variables of poverty, and the magnitude of poverty, as well as the loopholes in the implementation of welfare measures. It will empower them to identify their entitlements and utilise the common platform (i.e. Gram Sabha)[33] to demand and ensure efficient and effective implementation of development programs.

Based on the Kerala model[34] of governance, if community-based organisations and Panchayati Raj Institutions collaborate to work for the development of Gram Panchayat in post-Covid Bihar, livelihood and social security of the poor and marginalised can be created and sustained in the long term. The state must take the post-pandemic scenario as an opportunity to act upon its long-term goals. It's now or never.

Notes

1. Bihar is a densely populated state in the east of India with a population of 128 million; it shares its northern border with the southern border of Nepal.
2. The 73rd and 74th constitutional amendments give recognition and protection to local governments and, in addition, each state has its local government legislation.
3. Scheduled Castes are located at the lowest rung of hierarchy in the Hindu caste order. They were considered as 'untouchables'. Scheduled Tribes refers to the Tribal communities that are deemed under the Constitution of India to be scheduled tribes. The reason behind including these communities under the respective schedules was to provide them with constitutional safeguards for their socio-economic upliftment, such as reservation of seats in educational institutions and public offices and protection against violence and various forms of discriminations.
4. Panchayat refers to the rural local body of governance in India. The Indian urban local structures are known as municipal bodies.
5. The public policy think tank of the government of India is known as Niti Aayog. It was established in the year 2015 by the NDA (National Democratic Alliance Government) government by replacing the planning commission which formulated India's Five-Year Plans. http://niti.gov.in/
6. The government-run rural child care centre in India is referred to as Anganwadi. It was started by the government of India in the year of 1975 as part of the Integrated Child Development Services Programme to alleviate child hunger and malnutrition.
7. It is an official administrative unit in India. A block consists of several Gram Panchayats, which varies from block to block across the country.
8. Province. It is an official administrative unit within a state of India.
9. The 7th Schedule of the Indian Constitutions includes three lists of subjects that specify the division of power related to the subject between the central and the state government. The centre has exclusive powers to design laws on the subjects included under the union list of the Indian Constitution such as Defence, International relations, Railways, etc. The states can exclusively make laws regarding the subjects mentioned under the state list such as Police, Public health and sanitation. Also, there are subjects regarding which both central as well as state government can legislate.
10. The 11th schedule in the constitution of India refers to the section where power, authority, and responsibilities of the rural local self-government are mentioned.
11. The tenure of an elected member of the Gram Panchayat is of five years. It is mandated that fresh elections should be conducted before the expiry of the five years. If fresh elections are not conducted and the elected representative continues to hold the office beyond the tenure, it is known as supersession.

12 It is a state situated on the south-western Malabar Coast of India.

13 Participatory planning is a process by which a community undertakes to reach a given socio-economic goal by consciously diagnosing its problems and charting a course of action to resolve those problems. The Left Democratic Front-led government in Kerala under the leadership of E.K. Nayanar decided to implement the Ninth Five Year Plan as People's Plan, giving the local self-governments powers in the process of plan formulation and implementation, to realise the true spirit of the Constitutional amendments. The People's Plan campaign was launched by the state government on 17 August 1996 by ensuring people's participation in the decentralised planning process, starting from the stage of preparation of the plan itself. The government also took the most significant decision to devolve 35–40 per cent of the state plan funds to the local level plans. Such devolution of funds coupled with decentralisation of powers was the first of its kind in India.

14 ASHA is the abbreviation for Accredited Social Health Activist (ASHA). They are the community health workers at the village level appointed by the Ministry of Health and Family Welfare as a part of the National Rural Health Mission in India.

15 'Break the Chain' refers to the mass campaign initiated by the Kerala state health department to sensitise the public about the importance of public and personal hygiene in the wake of the COVID-19 outbreak.

16 A network of women Self Help Groups in Kerala that are integrated with Local Self Governments in India.

17 The mid-day meal is a scheme that aims to provide hot cooked meals to children of primary and upper primary classes in government-run/aided schools for improvement of nutritional status of school-age children.

18 It refers to the level of income that is required to meet minimum living conditions for an individual.

19 PDS is an abbreviation for the Public Distribution System, which is a system of distribution of food grains at affordable prices by the government of India. Presently, under the PDS, the commodities namely wheat, rice, sugar, and kerosene are being allocated to the States/Union Territories for distribution.

20 Anganwadi Sevika is the worker at the Anganwadi, which is the rural childcare centre in India. The role of the worker is to execute the Integrated Child Development Services programme at the primary level. Their responsibilities include conducting regular quick surveys of all families, organising preschool activities, providing health and nutrition education to families, encouraging families to adopt family planning, educating parents about child growth and development, etc.

21 Name Changed.

22 Mahatma Gandhi Employment Guarantee Scheme is a social welfare measure that aims to guarantee the 'right to work'. It was initiated in the year 2005 to enhance livelihood security in rural areas by providing at least 100 days of wage employment in a financial year to every household whose adult members volunteer to do unskilled manual work. Employment is supposed to be provided to the applicant within 5 km of his/her residence, and minimum wages are to be paid which varies from state to state. If the applicant does not get the work demanded within 15 days of applying, they are entitled to an unemployment allowance. That is, if the government fails to provide employment, it has to provide certain unemployment allowances to those people.

23 It is a document that is provided to eligible beneficiaries of MGNREGS, which records workers' entitlements under the scheme. It legally empowers the registered households to apply for work.

24 The Indian cropping season is classified into two main seasons: (i) *Kharif* and (ii) *Rabi*, based on the monsoon. The *Kharif* cropping season is from July to October during the southwest monsoon and the *Rabi* cropping season is from October to March (winter).

25 Red Lentil.

26 It is a central government sponsored scheme with 100 per cent funding from the government of India. It became operational in 2018. Under the scheme, income support of INR 6,000 per year ($82) in three instalments will be provided to small and marginal farmers having combined land ownership/holding up to 2 hectares. Available at: https://pmkisan.gov.in/

27 The ASHA or the community health workers are commonly referred to as ASHA didi (Sister) in the villages.

28 Available at: https://state.bihar.gov.in/main/SectionInformation.html?editForm& rowId=13

29 Bihar Panchayati Raj Act provides for the constitution of the three-tier Panchayati Raj system in the state – at the village, intermediate, and district level.

30 The amended Panchayati Raj Act of Bihar was enacted in the year of 2006 after the state was divided into Jharkhand and Bihar, and a separate Panchayati Raj Department came into existence in 2007. The amendment in the Panchayati Raj Act, 2006 included a provision for under 50 per cent reservation in all categories. It mentioned that up to 50 per cent of reservation would be provided for women in all categories. The reservation for SCs and STs would be in proportion to their population and a maximum of 20 per cent of seats would be reserved for the backward classes. It also had a unique feature of establishing Nyaya Panchayat known as Gram Katchaharies (Village courts), which aimed to ensure access to justice delivery at affordable costs to the rural population. According to the Panchayati Raj Act, 2006 20 departments had devolved functions to Panchayati Raj Institutions.

31 A Gram Panchayat constitutes various standing committees by election from among its members for effective discharge of its functions such as Education Committee, Social Justice Committee, etc.

32 SRLM is an abbreviation for State Rural Livelihood Mission. SRLM has been established in the states of India for the implementation of the National Rural Livelihood Mission, which is the poverty alleviation project. It is implemented by the Ministry of Rural Development, Government of India. It is primarily focused on promoting self-employment and the organisation of the rural poor.

33 Gram Sabha (Village Assembly) is the primary body of the Panchayati Raj system.

34 Decentralised governance and community engagement in the decision-making process in Kerala.

References

Aiyar, M. S. (2020). 'The panchayati front: Tap potential of local self-government to fight COVID-19', *The Indian Express*, 6 May [online]. Available at: https:// indianexpress.com/article/opinion/columns/coronavirus-pandemic-panchayati-front-6395715/ [Accessed 8 May 2020].

Bardhan, P. (1996). 'Decentralized Development', *Indian Economic Review*, 31(2), 139–156.

Guardian. (2020). 'Coronavirus: no return to normal 'for the foreseeable future, says WHO Video', *The Guardian*, 13 July [online]. Available at: https://www. theguardian.com/world/video/2020/jul/13/coronavirus-no-return-to-normal-for-the-foreseeable-future-says-who-video [Accessed 2 August 2020].

Isaac, T. T., and Sadanandan, R. (2020). 'COVID-19, Public Health System and Local Governance in Kerala', *Economic and Political Weekly*, 23 May, 55(21), 35–40.

Mathew, S., and More, M. (2011). 'State Incapacity by Design: Understanding the Bihar Story', *IDS Working Paper*, 366, 1–31.

Niti Aayog. (2019). SDG India Index & Dashboard. Available at: https://niti.gov.in/sdg-india-index-dashboard-2019-20 [Accessed 11 May 2020].

Oommen, M. (2020). 'The critical role of decentralized responses', *The Hindu*, 8 June [online]. Available at: https://www.thehindu.com/opinion/op-ed/the-critical-role-of-decentralised-responses/article31782116.ece [Accessed 9 June 2020].

Raghunandan, T. R. (2018). Introduction. In T. R. Raghunandan, *In Decentralization and Local Governments: The Indian Experience*. New Delhi: Orient BlackSwan, 1–20.

Sridevan, S., and Currimbhoy, A. (2020). 'The social contract needs to be rewritten', *The Hindu*, 9 July [online]. Available at: https://www.thehindu.com/opinion/lead/the-social-contract-needs-to-be-rewritten/article32025342.ece [Accessed 10 July 2020].

WEF (2020). 'The Great Reset', *The World Economic Forum*, 14 July [online]. Available at: https://www.weforum.org/agenda/2020/07/covid19-this-is-how-to-get-the-great-reset-right/ [Accessed 10 August 2020].

13

COVID-19 STORIES
Imaginations of the Local

Artwork by Danalakota Vinay Kumar Nakash and Commentary by Chandan Bose

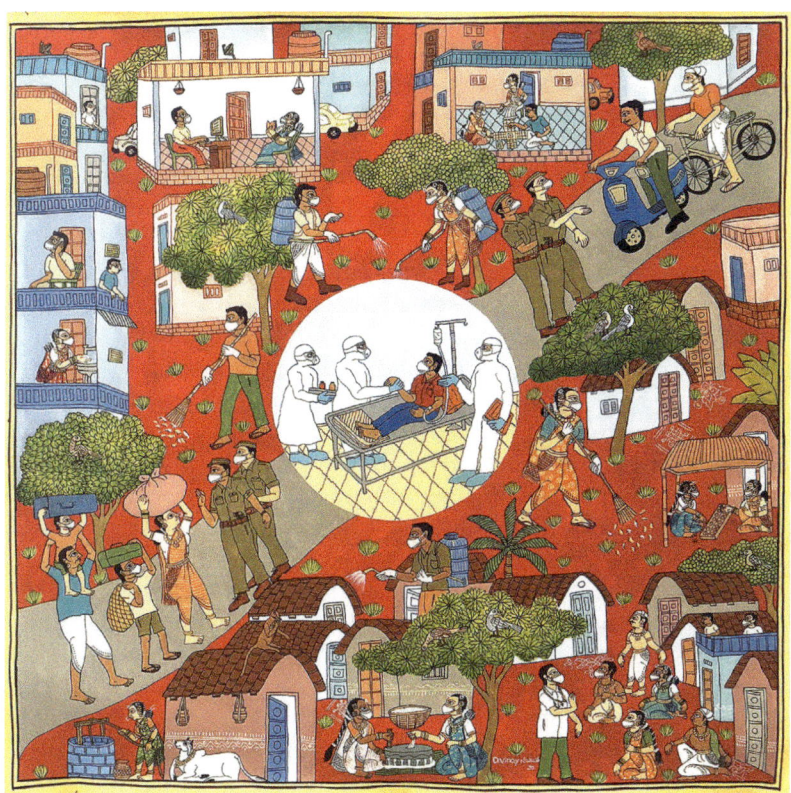

Artwork 13.1 Covid-19 Stories.

How do artists see? Is their art a reflection of the way they cope with their local environments? How can artistic and local perspectives reconfigure

DOI: 10.4324/9781003320524-17

knowledge about the world? These are some of the questions that scholars and practitioners alike have been posing in order to democratise not just institutions of art but also methods through which new knowledges and new worlds are constantly emerging. The world during Covid-19 has drawn our attention to the need for local perspectives to a global problem. Simply put, Covid-19 has changed the world and the way it is conceived, thought of, spoken about, and represented. Reading about, listening to, and looking at the myriad ways in which equally myriad locales are changing, coping, and adapting are central to understanding how living with Covid-19 is affecting our potential as humans and to be human.

Featured here is the work of Danalakota Vinay Nakash, a 25-year-old artist living in Hyderabad, Telangana, the hub of India's IT industry. Vinay belongs to a long lineage of traditional artisans of the Telangana region, *nakash*, who specialise in mural-making, wood sculptures, narrative scrolls, and decorative items of everyday use. Historically known for producing images that narrate folk mythologies, particularly of marginal and occupational communities in the region, the *nakash* artform of Telangana has developed its own unique visual vocabulary that is extremely powerful, both materially and viscerally. Landscapes, events, and actors are set against a rich red background, meant to bring everything happening in the forefront to life through a brilliant choreography of colours and dextrous brushwork. Created on canvas made of coarse cotton and executed in watercolours, both of which are locally sourced, *nakash* artform ought to belong to a directory of global practices that are tied to the sustenance of local ecologies and economies. At the outset, these images tell stories; stories of resilience, of how communities were formed and struggled to survive, and of how they practice their knowledge and moral codes in everyday life. Historians have appreciated how these narrative artworks should be perceived as constitutions of communities whose identities and struggles have been denied a voice and agency in history textbooks and institutional archives. Aesthetically, these images have always been relegated to the category of 'folk', 'tribal', 'traditional', and 'Indigenous', whose distinction from 'modern' and 'contemporary' art is based on the former's supposed inability to address themes that are universal and transcendental.

Where then do we locate folk artists like Vinay who address universal phenomena like Covid-19 through their work? Does the visceral quality of folk representations depreciate outside of their local contexts? Is there something more fundamental about the human experience of Covid-19 that we can glean from local imaginations? My interaction with Vinay began during my doctoral fieldwork in 2012 when I was enrolled in a PhD program in New Zealand, and he was pursuing an undergraduate degree in Fine Arts from one of the leading Fine Arts institutes in Hyderabad. At the time it was Vinay's father Danalakota Vaikuntam Nakash and his narratives of work and identity that formed the thrust of my ethnography. As a young adult still learning the ropes of a family-based work and enrolled in an urban educational institution, Vinay's imagination of his own future has been drawn from multiple and intersecting locations – his socialisation and training within the household, his engagement with the 'folk' and 'artisanal', 'traditional' status of his family's home-based work, the discourse around 'art' as part of his modern academic pedagogy, and as part of a young demographic within contemporary India, and his expectations from digital platforms and information technology. I am very aware that my own journey from being a graduate student to having a tenure-track academic post is probably one of the numerous representations of aspirational mobility that Vinay constructs for himself.

This politics of location of both the research and the researcher has been fairly employed as a critique of the way in which ethnographic texts have been historically written. However, over the course of nine years that I have known Vinay, I have seen him grow not only into an independent artist but also as an entrepreneur taking the reins from his father and introducing new innovations within the management of the business, such as a robust online presence. In an integral way then, this piece is my own acknowledgement of Vinay as a new protagonist, a young artist who is currently charting his own trajectory to amalgamate the universal promises of modernity and faith in his particular histories. Through this piece, I would like to initiate a discussion about the kind of potential selves that young artisans like Vinay are exploring and creating through their relationship with their work, their inheritance, and their environment. Vinay has always maintained,

> My centre has always been and will remain to be the regional style that my family has specialized in and preserved. Formal training has helped me to take this skill forward in different directions – like printmaking, use of different materials and technologies, trying out different formats. This is what I tried to achieve in this *Covid-19 Stories* painting. I wanted to introduce a new style of telling stories; after all that is what our paintings are historically about – communicating stories.

The title *Covid-19 Stories* is a name that Vinay chose for his creation. Its surface, as one can see, contains a plethora of diverse characters, places, and activities that made up everyday life specifically during the Covid-19 lockdown, which extended in India from the end of March to the end of May 2020. Rendered in a scale that is two-dimensional and panoramic, the events in the painting are also spatially segregated – the upper half depicting an urban neighbourhood and the lower half a rural setting. Interestingly positioned in between these two locales are two profound visuals. One, the images showing migrant workers returning to their homes in villages from the city, and two, the image of a Covid-19 patient receiving treatment from medical staff dressed in Personal Protective Equipment (PPE). The placement of these two events and spaces between urban and rural life-worlds indicates how Vinay perceives the migrant worker and the Covid-19 patient as bodies in transition – from homelessness to home and from disease to health. It is his imagination of place and placelessness, of belongingness and the lack of it that is translated into the visual structure of the painting. It is through his imagination that the different associations and relationships within the text are mapped through images. But how did Vinay conceptualise this world?

> These are images I saw on the television. Everyday news channels would be flooded with images of migrant workers walking hundreds of kilometres, of policemen having to manage the traffic of migrant workers, of ICUs in Covid-19 speciality hospitals, of how people residing in apartments in the city would spend their time. That is what gave me the idea. There was so much hype around work-from-home and different technologies people were using to do that. But there was this one report that mentioned how during the lockdown, many families would spend time playing board games like Ludo; of how old and pre-internet ways of having fun were returning. That is how I thought of showing a family playing a dice game. You get to see the urban folk through the windows and balconies in their homes. Whereas in the villages below, you see most activity happening outdoors. That is how village life is, open. What is common to both the urban and rural scenes is that everyone is wearing a mask and ensuring general cleanliness.
>
> I placed the migrant workers in the middle to show their journey from the city to the village. I also made a policeman instructing a motorcyclist to wear a mask, and similarly a local doctor offering advice to women in a village. These are all stories and images I saw on television.

Where would we claim lies the source of this painting? In the digital circulation of images? Or, in Vinay's imagination? But isn't this question superfluous? For the artist, their art is always sourced from somewhere or something. That is how their art becomes the story of that place or object. Vinay calls his painting *Covid-19 Stories*; apart from curating excerpts of everyday life during Covid-19, this is also the story about how knowledge is created in a hyper-networked society. More critically, Vinay is archiving the representational practices of global media in the creation of places, identities, and practices. It is through Vinay's imagination however that the relationships between these places, identities, and practices find a visual field to manifest. The division between the upper-urban and lower-rural is bridged by the movement of migrant labour. Private lives of city-dwellers open up as showcased exhibits, whereas communal living becomes the defining character of the rural. Central to all these narratives is the one around science and health that is distinctive in its pristine and near-blinding white hue, almost like a sacrosanct object desired by all.

Folk art in India, as expressive practices of marginalised communities, has always been peripheral to the virtuosity of classical and contemporary art. Their potential to comment on aspects and life-worlds beyond the local, the ritual, and the sensorial still awaits serious theoretical consideration. However, here the fundamental aspect of human experience of a global pandemic that Vinay tries to capture is more than just the experience of the virus, but also how we know about the virus; what are the sources of our knowledge about the virus. Vinay's imagination of *life during Covid-19* is testimony to more than just how knowledge of the pandemic world is produced through circulation of images. It also shows us that the division of the world into geographies/polities that actively create knowledge and those that passively receive knowledge is disturbed by the way the local is able to reflect upon and re-present that knowledge. But more importantly, the visual vocabulary that is used to reflect and represent is borrowed from cultural practices of marginalised communities who, as mentioned previously, have been using these images to tell their own stories of assertion and knowledge creation. *Covid-19 Stories* then at its heart is about how diverse traditions of reclaiming one's being-ness and human-ness from diverse geographies and communities can help us reimagine our knowledge and experience of the world.

14

SURVEILLANCE TO SOUSVEILLANCE

Watching the Watchers
June 2020

Sushrija Sakshi Upadhyaya

Introduction: Era of Mass-Surveillance

Surveillance can be defined as monitoring that is undertaken by legal, social, or personal entities in a position of authority. Surveillance suggests an omniscient authority with a 'god's eye view' watching from above (Mann 2016). The concept of surveillance can be recognised in an individual, e.g. 1984's Big Brother by George Orwell or as a social-economic-political class, clan, militia, or group that utilises the information accumulated through surveillance to maintain its power over others (Orwell 1949). This idea of surveillance can be traced back to Michel Foucault, who in 1975 reviewed the ideas of Jeremy Bentham to understand social control in modern societal structures (Foucault 1975). Bentham, in his study, explored the composition of an invented architectural figure in prisons and called it the Panopticon. The structure of the Panopticon was such that the guard could keep an eye on the prison inmates without being seen. Herein, the guard could be on duty or not but either way, the prisoners would always sense being watched. This uncertainty and ambiguity of their situation were deemed to keep them in check (Bentham 1838). The reverberations of Bentham's 1791 Panopticon can be consistently felt in the modern society. Foucault, in 1977, further noted that in a techno-political society, the awareness of being watched forces us to self-police and discipline ourselves as if we were invariably under observation. Our power-driven modern society is deluged with devices capable of tracking and monitoring our private data while feeding them to various government and private authorities. Thus, just like the prisoners in Bentham's Panopticon, citizens in a surveillant state can never be sure whether they are being watched or not (Lyon 2006).

The modern world with technology is making a fast transition into a 'mass surveillance society', which can be defined as the monitoring of a

DOI: 10.4324/9781003320524-18

substantial proportion of a population by pervasive technologies, typically through government agencies, corporations, and even cybercriminals (Campbell and Carlson 2002). It is crucial here to observe that in today's world the distinction between state and non-state actors is more theoretical than ever before. The technology that makes mass surveillance possible gets developed through collaboration between the government and private corporations. Our cell phone carriers, social media accounts, and personalised search engines operate as gigantic information reservoirs for the government.

Many of the private entities reportedly hand over the intimate data of their users to make profits (Franks 2017). Surveillance today has spun into a global industry that subsists of several companies that develop and sell surveillance technology to numerous government agencies across the world. This is further used for spying and policing purposes in the form of a wide range of advanced systems to identify, track, and monitor individual citizens and their private lives. This lucrative business is exceptionally secretive, and its overall value is unknown to the world (Privacy International 2018).

Surveillance – Technology and the Pandemic

Authoritarian as well as democratic governments across the globe have either deployed or are actively inclined towards the utilisation of technology for surveillance to track and monitor their citizens in the face of Covid-19. The data is collected in real time through technologies adopted for contact tracing through movement tracking smartphone apps, wrist bands, CCTV footages, credit card transactions, location data, and recording conversations between people. The pandemic seems to have provided the governments with a green light for drawing unusual steps. The trend has been driven by China and South Korea, which already had an active surveillance operation in place (Wright 2020). The Aarogya Setu app in India and telecom-generated data in Israel went on to gather delicate information prompting intense criticism from privacy and legal advocates across the world. SoftMining's app in Italy got knocked off with malicious code capable of opening backdoors into personal devices while Pakistan deployed secret surveillance technology with Inter-Service Intelligence (ISI) to track coronavirus patients. Austria and Switzerland's DP-3T and TraceTogether application of Singapore, on the other hand, are designed collaboratively by researchers to preserve user privacy. In this spirit, Google and Apple have declared a joint effort to facilitate the adoption of Bluetooth technology to aid governments and healthcare agencies reduce the transmission of the coronavirus (Vynck et al. 2020). Research has specified that a substantive number from the population needs to adopt such contact tracing apps for such systems to be of use, and approximately 60 per cent of the population would need to use any of these apps for the virus to stop its spread (Hinch 2020).

Surveillance – Politics and Policy

State policy towards privacy is a necessary factor regulating the country's socio-political landscape. Till now only a few of the mentioned states have spread out the purpose and process of their data collection along with the definitive time bar. However, unfortunately, even lesser among them have presented precise dates for wiping out any personal data extracted in the process. In this scenario, the government's continuous increasing capability to mine and aggregate data networks to intrude on its citizens is presenting new, dominant, and daunting challenges to individual privacy. There are also concerns generated about the probable usage of these tools after the pandemic. The efficiency of this type of technological solutionism raises suspicion on advances to set up a 'Pandemic Big Brother' like situation. The ongoing crisis is turning the prevalent public-health emergency into a public-order issue with accepted justifications. Yuval Noah Harari (2020) argues that changes in the pre-coronavirus era would have generated years of debate, dissent, and opposition seem to be possible overnight now. There is a potential for heightened surveillance to continue even after the coronavirus pandemic is under control. History warns us that once such infrastructures and competencies are in place, the expanded powers of governments rarely have the political will to roll them back (Harari 2020). It has been indicated that such surveillance technologies have the potential to facilitate increased corruption within the power structures of governments. Surveillance systems under the guise of managing risk or reducing harm can exacerbate a range of problems, including poverty, over-policing, suspicion, as well as exclusion (Mann and Ferenbok 2013). The intrusive tactics of data-hungry powers that occurred rather Orwellian to us just a few months ago are fast developing into the new norms under safety and security policies. Many of these protocols have the capacities to thoroughly modify and revise our socio-economic-political circumstances in the post-pandemic era.

Power and Its Asymmetrical Veillance

In surveillance, the subject of the gaze remains at a disadvantaged point and are often unaware that they are being scrutinised. This makes the placement of power asymmetrical between the 'watched' and the 'watcher'. Surveillers in democracies go on to provide blanket rationalisations and frequently justify surveillant methods in the name of existing societal challenges like national security, crime, fraud, terrorism, and presently the staged plight of the pandemic. The prescribed greater good is not only deceptive but also comes with greater intrusions upon citizen's privacy. An average citizen's intimate data at the hands of government authority can be more powerful than what one can imagine. It can tap and manipulate voting behaviours in a democracy while conveniently disallowing dissent and encroaching on the human rights of citizens. The central and local governments could gather massive amounts of data that can determine political campaigns just like consumers are being tracked for market absorption (Dommett 2019). This creates an illusion of choice. A lot of how these circumstances will re-shape our world will rely on public oversight – our acceptance and resistance in response. Citizen empowerment through modern methods of coordination and innovation can allow the direction of digital platforms towards a more vibrant democratic life. The role of technology and big data can be used to facilitate citizen engagement and improve the monitoring of authorities for public sector accountability.

Exploring Sousveillance

One of the most essential distinctions between free democratic societies and totalitarian regimes is that the 'totalitarian government relies on secrecy for the regime but high surveillance and disclosure for all other groups, whereas in the civic culture of liberal democracy, the position is approximately the reverse' (Walker 1986). The integration of surveillance in a democratic society is attempting to fade its conception in ways not witnessed before. However, technology in the present era also offers citizens enormous opportunities and unprecedented tools to organise and promote a more equal and democratic society. In the modern world, information flows in a multitude of directions, and decentralisation of such technology can allow citizens to be the watchers too. In this trail of thoughts and re-imagination, the idea of sousveillance, which means 'under sight' or 'watching from below' seems interesting with increasing citizen's use of digital technology. In 1998, Steve Mann developed the concept of Sousveillance, about 200 years after the publication of Jeremy Bentham's Panopticon. Mann held that sousveillance would facilitate citizens to rise against the state's 'oversight' and become 'Little Brother' watching the 'Big Brother' from below through handy information technologies. He suggested individual engagement in surveilling government activities for raising informed citizenry. Such a phenomenon will lead to a more balanced state of affairs since everyone including the authorities themselves will be observed (Mann 1998). Sousveillance can be understood as inverse surveillance wherein the monitoring is commenced by individuals who are not in a position of authority. With its spread, citizens could use cheap, portable technologies available to them to oversee and publicise the behaviour of the powerful, which will in return stabilise the equation. Sousveillance seeks to ensure integrity and makes the conception of veillance more balanced in modern societies to avoid its tilt towards totalitarianism.

Sousveillance: Transparency and Accountability of Governments

Sousveillance unveils the future of governance and the values the post-human era can behold. This gives it the competence to confront the various forms of corruption that are intrinsic in a society with the authority's veillance. Such analysis of government surveillance should be vigilant to the role of socio-cultural powers in shaping our societies. Sousveillance requires to be seen as a decentralised force that is self-enacting and exceptionally potent. It not only contributes to the equalisation of power dynamics between the government and the governed but can also widen the possibility of a better community-based operation at the grassroots. Surveillance over the years has operated as a tyrannical reality for the marginalised sections of our society as they have been often rendered powerless to shield themselves from the authority's gaze. This has through ages continuously subjected them to ruthless investigations and regulations.

The true contemporary potential of the privacy revolution cannot be accomplished without taking into account the persistent race, gender, caste, and class inequalities that have hounded the theory and practice of privacy through history. It is important to note that a reform that is strong, systematic and appropriately resistant needs to move beyond *informational privacy stakes* and includes everyday challenges arising from surveillance in all segments of our society. Those who have encountered surveillance with the toughest deprivations of privacy in the acutely oppressive forms have the most profound understanding of its dynamics. It is crucial to emphasise the experiences of this vulnerable section and the violation witnessed by them for learning and further offering ourselves the finest chance of ensuring privacy for all. With the current merging, privacy concerns in the lives of the middle- and upper-class population portray the 'democratisation of surveillance' and hence calls for the 'democratisation of privacy' and its concerns (Franks 2017). It is imaginable to reinstate the panoptic god's eye view of surveillance with captured personal experiences that resonate with the core values of democratic states. Sousveillance can play a crucial role for citizens to seek transparency and accountability from their elected governments. It can be vital in the process of checking the state for its public service obligations. It can also promote denouncement of prevalent abuses through new software and crowdsourced mapping, which could further ensure equitable distribution of resources and justice for all.

Democracy-Friendly Technology

Sousveillance involves the technological competence of citizens to engage in critical political communication and turns to counteract the state's monopoly on the same. Sousveillance can conceivably play a prominent role in unmasking corporate and public official wrongdoings. It can also contribute to potential agencies, which can be adopted to translate public demands into policy reforms. The very prospect that official behaviours might be documented and broadcasted can be unsettling for the powerful, who have for long retained an undeniable top to bottom surveillance against citizens.

The idea is that authorities should learn and accept that transparency is reciprocal. A collective effort of citizens with technology can improve governance and can mitigate the evils of surveillance. Good governance plays an exceptionally imperative role in surveillance societies as otherwise, the government has the authority to administer its will dramatically. It is effective in this background for democratic societies to demand Freedom of Information Acts[1] and hold consistent pressure on law enforcement authorities. However, this often also leads to the state displaying its superior power over its citizens by silencing demanding citizens, journalists, and right to information activists for such laws. As the power struggle on information between authorities and concerned citizens increases, any existing privacy laws might further be impaired to ward off agents and structures which the state harnesses to continue being in its position of power. In such circumstances, techno-driven advocacy through sousveillance is required on all fronts to avoid human rights violations at large.

There are multiple shreds of evidence of sousveillance in our contemporary world, which has empowered every spectator to record and diffuse images and videos from instances observed by them. Mobile phone cameras have been continuously used to capture police brutality, human rights violations, and other government misdeeds from time to time. Although the recording of instances is not a new phenomenon but in the present-day live features and uploading of such recordings on various media platforms allow watchers to immediately share stories with millions of fellow citizens in near to real time. Such collected data can play a critical role in holding the government accountable. To advance, a central destination for accumulating such data can ride real as well as virtual democratic activism a long way. Otherwise, such content might get drowned if published only in the never-ending sea of social media. Uploading recordings online is also considered necessary as the magnificent distribution of it makes it difficult for even the most powerful organisation to take down. One should consider the expansion of more and more sousveillance-friendly technology for higher individual and community agency. Steve Mann sought devices like WearCam and WearComp with sousveillance, which allow a user to watch, record, and broadcast their surroundings. Pervasive and mobile computers that capture and process instances with seamless connectivity provide for extraordinary watching by individuals with personal devices on the ground. The significant use of 'sousveillance-friendly' technology can make way for its constructive metamorphosis in an effective, dynamic, and vibrant political force. Further, the fact that our society has entered the era of augmented and mediated reality, where soon smartphones may become eyeglass-based which can allow overlays to augment and mediate our everyday lives (Mann 2012). Digital Eye Glasses like Google's Project Glass have the potential to transform society and introduce two-sided – surveillance and sousveillance with wearable computing in everyday life.

Conclusion: An Interim Counteragent

David Brin (2000) in 'The Transparent Society', indicated that there is an 'inevitable erosion' of our conventional understanding of privacy and we are therefore predictably heading in either of the two directions i.e. Surveillance or Sousveillance. The hegemonic design of surveillance in our society today does not display an appropriate approach to deal with the challenges that it is plagued with. It is continually displaying features of failed authority in effectively managing the multi-faced crisis of the decade. This situation has presented us with a chance to reflect upon the far-Orwellian course that our societies today are drawing towards a science-fiction dystopia. It is time citizens prepare to act upon the threats that the nexus of large and faceless government agencies tied up with corporations pose towards us. To preserve participatory democracy and to block or at least delay such techno-fascism, it is urgent to acknowledge what is coming while seizing control of it through a steady process of relevant re-imagination. In today's world, along with controlling one's information, it is also required for citizens to concentrate on recognising how such data is being utilised. Due consideration must be devoted to understanding how this personalised data is captured, interpreted, examined, and exposed. It would likewise be advantageous to learn the operation of scientific instruments that raise such data and organise extensive modern discoveries for the advancement of sousveillant systems. This potential of sousveillance must be participated with care, as there's no decree to regulate the usage of such technologies to exclusively resist a surveillant society. This protection from surveillance needs to be pursued with creativity and benevolence to manifest the shared struggles of our times for equality. It should in no way lead to further marginalisation of those who are on the fringes of caste, class, sexuality, gender, and religious hierarchies. Personal technologies can either be operated to create stronger democratic communities virtually and otherwise or to mindless conformity to Instagram stories and Snapchat filters. Citizens can be hanging for the next iOS update, while the governments would extend to inspect more and more components of our routine lives. There are significant choices to be made.

Further, there is a scope of governments and private corporations to develop further corrupt collaborations to curtail the efficacy of sousveillance. Such diminishing citizen autonomy displays an alarming state of affairs and would expect us to collectively fight against such dictatorial and oppressive powers with similar updates. For this, it is relevant to keep track of politics and technology with the potential demonstrations of their combination. At the time, police and spy agencies along with advertising companies use facial recognition and related monitoring technologies way more actively than the average citizen. This provides them with the power to exploit the existing information asymmetrically to their advantage. It is therefore vital that technology rolls out extensively to help citizens and activists find probable solutions for the challenging hegemony in time. It is remarkable to note that here the intention is to neutralise dissent and safeguard the exercise of power by seeking accountability and gaining the consent of the governed. It is important that we push to build legislative frameworks for democratic veillance, or otherwise the ideas of basic civic freedoms would also pose empty. Citizens in this context should also have the legal rights to track their data and observe its use. It is a no-brainer that the abuses would continue to exist by government agencies and private parties but what is noteworthy is that these would then be illegal acts and redressable in the judicial systems. Sousveillant technologies allow making existing errors of veillance visible, unlike surveillant cultures, which oversee in secrecy without the knowledge of the viewed. There is rising discomfort at the possibility that all public acts might be subject to recording, whether from the top or bottom. However, to hold such governing powers accountable that have belligerently mounded manipulations, exploitation, and alliance to employ authoritative technology for mass surveillance – sousveillance undertakes its performance as an interim but important counteragent.

Note

1 Laws on Freedom of Information allow citizens to access data held by their nation's governments. Such information when available in the public domain of democracies for free or at minimal costs avoids secrecy that surrounds government policy development and decision making across the globe. There are constitutional guarantees for the right to information in various countries, but they are usually not supported by legislation.

References

Bentham, J. (1838). *Panopticon, or, The Inspection-house*, Edinburgh: W. Tait.

Brin, D. (2000). *The Transparent Society: Will Technology Force Us to Choose Between Privacy and Freedom?*, Reading, MA: Perseus Books.

Campbell, J.E., and Carlson, M. (2002). 'Online surveillance and the commodification of privacy', *Journal of Broadcasting & Electronic Media*, 46(4), 586–606 [online]. Available at: http://www.tandfonline.com/doi/abs/10.1207/s15506878jobem4604_6#.Ux37Xj9_uSo [Accessed 3 January 2020].

Dommett, K. (2019). 'Data-driven political campaigns in practice: understanding and regulating diverse data-driven campaigns', *Internet Policy Review*, 8(4) [online]. Available at: https://doi.org/10.14763/2019.4.1432 [Accessed 3 January 2020].

Foucault, M. (1975). *Surveiller et punir, Gallimard, Paris*, transl. A. Sheridan, New York: Vintage Books.

Franks, M. (2017). 'Democratic surveillance', *Harvard Journal of Law and Technology*, 30(2) [online]. Available at: https://www.academia.edu/34148858/Democratic_Surveillance [Accessed 4 January 2020].

Harari, Y. (2020). 'Yuval Noah Harari: The world after coronavirus: Free to read', *Financial Times*, 20 March [online]. Available at: https://www.ft.com/content/19d90308-6858-11ea-a3c9-1fe6fedcca75 [Accessed 21 March 2020].

Hinch, R. (2020). *Effective Configurations of a Digital Contact Tracing App: A Report to NHSX*, London: University of Oxford.

Lyon, D. (2006). 'The Search for Surveillance Theories', in D. Lyon (ed.), *Theorising Surveillance: The Panopticon and Beyond*, New York: Routledge.

Mann, S. (1998). '"Reflectionism" and "Diffusionism": New tactics for deconstructing the video surveillance superhighway', *Leonardo*, 31(2), 93 [online]. Available at: doi:10.2307/1576511 [Accessed 10 February 2020].

Mann, S. (2012). 'Eye am a camera: Surveillance and sousveillance in the glassage', *TIME*, 2 November [online]. Available at: https://techland.time.com/2012/11/02/eye-am-a-camera-surveillance-and-sousveillance-in-the-glassage/ [Accessed 10 March 2020].

Mann, S. (2016). 'Surveillance (Oversight), Sousveillance (Undersight), and Meta-veillance (Seeing Sight Itself)', *IEEE Conference on Computer Vision and Pattern Recognition Workshops (CVPRW)* [online]. Available at: doi:10.1109/cvpr.2016.177 [Accessed 12 March 2020].

Mann, S., and Ferenbok, J. (2013). 'New media and the power politics of sousveillance in a surveillance-dominated world', *Surveillance & Society*, 11(1/2), 18–34 [online]. Available at: doi:10.24908/ss.v11i1/2.4456 [Accessed 14 March 2020].

Orwell, G. (1949). *Nineteen Eighty-four*, London: Secker & Warburg.

Privacy International. (2018). 'The global surveillance industry', *Privacy International*, 16 February [online]. Available at: https://privacyinternational.org/explainer/1632/global-surveillance-industry [Accessed 12 March 2020].

Vynck, Gerrit De, et al. (2020). 'How the world is embracing contact-tracing technology to fight coronavirus', *The Print*, 1 May [online]. Available at: theprint.in/tech/how-the-world-is-embracing-contact-tracing-technology-to-fight-coronavirus/412282/ [Accessed 3 May 2020].

Walker, G.D. (1986). *Information as Power: Constitutional Aimplications of the Identity Numbering and ID Card Proposal*, St. Leonards, N.S.W.: Centre for Independent Studies.

Wright, N. (2020). 'Coronavirus and the future of surveillance', *Foreign Affairs*, 6 April [online] Available at: https://www.foreignaffairs.com/articles/2020-04-06/coronavirus-and-future-surveillance [Accessed 10 April 2020].

15

LONG WAY HOME

Aditya Vikram Sengupta

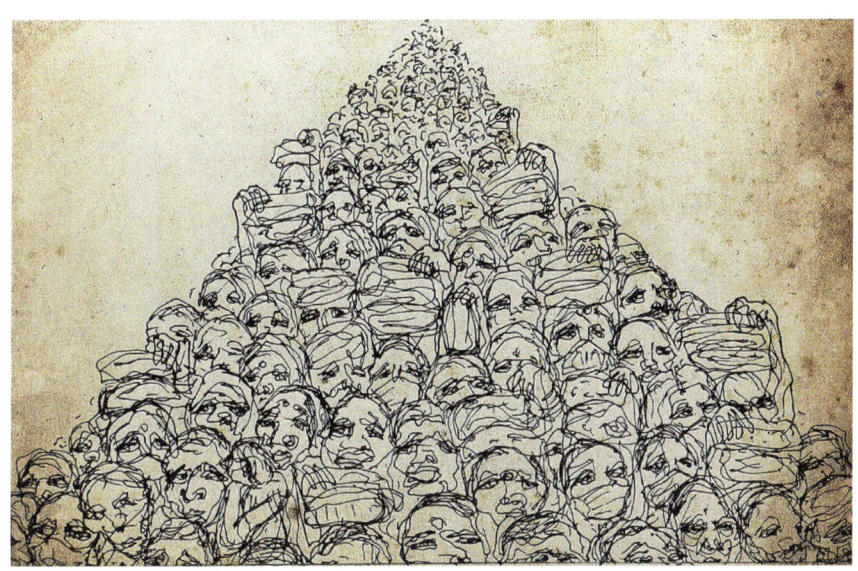

Artwork 15.1 Long Way Home

DOI: 10.4324/9781003320524-19

RELIGION AND GODLESSNESS

16

HANDLING PANDEMIC

How Does a Neo-liberal State 'Manage' the Deeper Malaise?
October–November 2020

Pushpesh Kumar and Debomita Mukherjee

In this chapter, we offer a possible reading of three events that occurred during the Covid-19 pandemic and the lockdown implemented in India – the mass 'reverse migration' of working-class citizens: particularly the rural and urban labour migrants, the Tablighi Jamaat's[1] religious congregation at the Nizamuddin Markaz[2], and the national call for symbolic solidarity through '*thali* banging'[3] and 'lighting lamps'.

The necropolitical approach[4] of the state, where some categories of people are left to die while others are assimilated as citizens (Mbembe cited in Pele 2020), exacerbated by the inabilities and unpreparedness of the state in dealing with the crisis, would have created a crisis of legitimacy for the elected government. This was averted by the media revelation and sudden hypervisibility of the Tablighi Jamaat congregation as a 'state of exception' (Agamben 2005)[5]. Public attention was shifted towards a religious congregation's (apparent) irresponsibility and lack of concern towards the whole nation, the blame of which was subsequently extended to include all Muslims, resulting in violent attacks on them across the country.

The gestures of '*thali* banging' and 'lighting lamp' were meant to show gratitude to the frontline workers and 'drive away Corona'. The lighting of lamps turned into celebrations with fireworks and blowing conch shells in posh urban middle-class households, bearing significant resemblance to 'upper' caste Hindu ritual practices. Ironically, many frontline workers' demands for 'safety gears' and better working conditions did not find similar support in the same body politic. The televisuals of masses of migrant workers walking exhaustively and the chaos in several under-equipped quarantine centres were spectacular with state inaction.

Against this backdrop, this chapter uses media sources – news and social media, and alternative critical spaces – to reflect on these three events and understand the neo-liberal 'management' of a deeper malaise by the Indian

DOI: 10.4324/9781003320524-21

state. Katherine Smits (2014) demonstrates how attachment to a place, traditions, and community are promoted in neo-liberal economic policies that emphasise individualism and 'self-reliance'. Here, the nation is sacralised and solidarity, symbolically reiterated, without addressing the plights of ordinary masses – denying access to food, health facilities, or relief packages for vulnerable segments of the population.

Reverse Migration and Necropolitical Management

The Union Labour and Employment Minister revealed that an estimated 10 million migrants working in various jobs, particularly in the informal sector had attempted to return home during the lockdown (Sharma 2020a) and that no data was available on the number of migrants who had either become unemployed or died of starvation during this time (Nath 2020).

In response to the government's claim of unavailability of information, the Stranded Workers Action Network (SWAN) Report was published, revealing the precarities and vulnerabilities of migrant workers who lost their daily incomes. The report shows that the rate of hunger and distress far exceeded the relief reaching the workers: during the first 21-day lockdown, 50 per cent of these workers had rations left for only a day and many were on the brink of starvation (SWAN 2020). Three weeks into the lockdown, only 4 per cent of the workers had received rations from the government (ibid:10). The helplessness of the workers became evident in situations where, even when some of them got 5 kgs of wheat, they did not have the cash to make it into flour or buy essentials like salt and oil (ibid: 9). To prevent migration of the distressed, the government ordered employers to pay the workers full wages and homeowners not to charge rent. However, the SWAN report (ibid: 15) discloses that 89 per cent of the workers had not been paid by their employers at all. Some, who received rations, were told that their cost would be deducted from their pay (ibid: 15).

Hundred and fourteen people died due to economic distress or hunger, and 168 died on the way using desperate means to return to their native villages to escape starvation and their dwindled access to essential items brought on by the sudden collapse of employment sectors and the lack of effective social protection mechanisms (Sikdar and Mishra 2020). An NDTV report on stranded construction workers at Noida shows a young worker saying, 'We will die of hunger before the virus kills us' (NDTV April 14, 2020). Another complained, 'If the government can facilitate the return of Indians stranded abroad, why can't it arrange for our safe transportation to our native places?' (ibid). Migrants walking home complained (Yadav 2020), 'We are seen as vermin and are left to die'; 'Planes were sent for the rich, but the poor have to walk' (ibid).

The Prime Minister's apology to the migrants was constructed in the language of sacrifice for a bigger cause, 'I apologise for taking these harsh steps that have caused difficulties in your lives, especially the poor people

… But these tough measures were needed to win this battle … Steps taken so far will give India victory over corona.' 'The victory over Corona' is the moral justification used by the state in the face of irredeemable loss and suffering during the crisis. Mbembe refers to them as moral justifications for atrocities inflicted upon the masses for bigger causes or a 'desire for sacrifice' (Pele 2020) instead of taking moral responsibility by the authorities (Alexander 2004). Is the suffering of others also our own? One needs to ask if this expanded circle of 'we' is possible at all within this neo-liberal governance. The trauma and suffering of the migrants indicate that both the government and the new middle-class majority in India largely failed to expand the circle of 'we'.

While the risky labour mobility of migrant workers, close to 300 million in number, helped India's economy, it contributed to minimal poverty reduction and put migrant labourers in the frontline to absorb the shocks of periodic economic crises (Sengupta and Jha 2020). The small savings of informal sector workers does not create a 'buffer' to deal with sudden uncertainties like the pandemic (Sikdar and Mishra 2020). Two critical social protection measures – the right to food (NFSA 2013) and the right to work (MGNREGA 2005) – are place-based and not accessible to the mobile population (Rao et al. 2020). The announcement of 'One Nation, One Ration'[6], ensuring food rations irrespective of place reflects a starting point in the recognition of migrant workers as a legitimate constituency within social protection frameworks (ibid). This, however, came only after the deaths, exhaustion, police violence, hunger, and starvation suffered by the same. Achille Mbembe's work (Pele 2020) demonstrates how increasing masses of individuals are now governed through their direct and indirect exposure to death.

Chomsky and Prasad (2021) discuss the dwindling social responsibility under neo-liberal regimes, reflected in the declining state expenditure on the social sector. The present social sector spending in India has been far from satisfactory (Dogra 2018): the budget for primary education and health has been reduced, and the government has undercut many rights-based Welfare Acts (Ruparelia 2015). The NDA government in India has weakened labour protocols, environmental regulations, and mechanisms of community participation in land acquisitions and forest conservation (ibid). Among these budget cuts, the decreased spending on the health sector, along with historically instituted corrupt practices and mismanagements in public institutions (Harriss-White 2010), directly resulted in the ill-preparedness of the state in dealing with the pandemic with vacant positions in government health centres and hospitals, underpaid doctors and nurses, and lack of Personal Protective Equipment (PPE) kits. Under-funded government hospitals in many states also had serious shortages of hospital beds, Intensive Care Units and ventilators. The health workers, including Accredited Social Health Activists or ASHA workers[7], whose working hours increased with no additional pay, fought the crisis with minimal resources, risking their own safety and that of their family members, simultaneously resisting stigma and harassment from their own communities. Suspected and confirmed Covid-19 deaths in India (Pulla 2020) were also underreported. So, apart from infrastructural lapses, there were questions about medical ethics, including the denial of treatment to many[8] who could have been cured and saved. In a system where overall funding in the social sector is falling and right-based entitlements are undermined, it is difficult to imagine an efficient mechanism to deal with large-scale crises.

Islamophobia, Violent Vilification, and State of Exception

The Tablighi Jamaat meet, held in the early months of 2020 at Markaz Nizamuddin, was a congregation of members of the missionary visiting the mosque from different parts of the country and the world (Bhat 2020). This meeting was like any other year. However, on 13 March 2020, the Delhi government issued an order, disallowing gatherings (of 200 and more) of any kind (Ibid.). Despite the close proximity of the police station to Markaz Nizamuddin, the police made no attempt to enforce these restrictions until lockdown orders were given by the Centre (Ibid.).

During a critical moment in the crisis in early April, mainstream Indian and international news media declared the Tablighi Jamaat congregation as the cause for the spread of the virus in India. There was a sudden amplification of Islamophobia by the media, shifting the public attention from infrastructural lapses and the necropolitical management of the migrant crisis to the new story, which had both an immediate purchase and popular appeal, manifesting in sporadic violence against subaltern classes of Muslims across the country. Some state officials also called the Tablighi Jamaat leadership 'irresponsible'. News headlines read sensational phrases such as 'super spreader' (Irfan, Masih, and Slater 2020), 'Markaz Virus' (quoted in newspapers like India Today), 'planned conspiracy', 'poisonous … hatred towards India' (TRT World 2020) and 'Tablighi Covid Threat' (Republic World 2020), identifying the Muslim missionary and attendees as the chief carriers of this virus, calling them 'anti-nationals' and 'enemies of the nation'. Cartoons and memes showing Muslims to be criminals, and 'Corona Jihad', 'Tablighi Virus' (Naqvi and Bisht 2020), and 'Corona Terrorism' trended in social media with hashtags like #JihadiCoronaVirus, #BanTablighiJamat and *#MasjidoMeinSarkariTaaleLagao* (#ShutThe MosquesWithGovernmentLocks) (Kumar 2020; Rahman and Petersen 2020). Others even warned followers to stay away from Muslims to stay safe.

The television news watching Indian population underwent an anti-Muslim indoctrination leading to widespread violence and discrimination against Muslims in the name of Patriotism (Ibid.). Videos of police brutality on mosque attendees surfaced (in youtube channels of Hindustan Times and others); Muslim vegetable sellers were thrashed and brutalised in

Northern India, the visuals of which circulated on YouTube and other media spaces. In Ahmedabad, a public hospital enforced segregation among patients by allotting separate wards for Hindus and Muslims following state orders (Jha 2020). Residents of Nizammudin *Basti* (colony) lost jobs and found difficulty in procuring new sources of income (Sherwani 2020) and faced ostracisation in hospitals and ration shops, often asked to stand at a distance or refused service altogether (Ibid.). The delayed government response in enforcing airport screenings, travel restrictions, etc., remained outside the arena of public introspection, maintaining Tablighi Jamaat as the epicentre of the pandemic (Mustafa 2020).

The Union Ministry of Health reported that 30 per cent of the existing cases were linked to the congregation (Kumar 2020). Criminal cases were registered against several members of the congregation under various sections of the Indian Penal Code for 'public nuisance', 'malignant act', and 'disobedience to orders issued by public servants', under the Epidemic Diseases Act, 1897, Foreigners Act, 1946, and the Disaster Management Act, 2005 (Wahidi and Thapar 2020). They were overturned by the court stating:

> A political government tries to find the scapegoat when there is pandemic, or calamity and the circumstances show that there is probability that these foreigners were chosen to make them scapegoats…The aforesaid circumstances and the latest figures of infection in India show that such action against present petitioners should not have been taken.
>
> (Cited in Wahidi and Thapar 2020)

Media discourse was an active instrument in creating a momentous rupture in people's imagination of chaos and health infrastructural lapses, and had a widespread appeal among Hindus, while working-class Muslims found themselves in a condition of 'bare life' (Agamben 2005), wherein their most basic legal rights were suspended. They became 'victims of a witch-hunt who are unable to plead their own case' (Bailey 1994). Such lives remain outside the normal juridical system, susceptible to ('legitimate') violence. It resonates with Jean Baudrillard's (1995) idea of how televisuality eclipses the real events. The news provides a vocabulary, an agenda of concern of what dangers we face and from whom (Dorman quoted in Jaramillo 2009), 'manufacturing consent' in the consciousness of the common Indian citizen (read Hindus). Gottschalk and Greenberg (2008) observe how the media's disinterest in a non-violent Muslim perspective fuels the otherness and intolerance suffered by Muslims. It appeared as though the differences between the Jamaat and diverse Muslim groups were erased into forming one collective body, embodying monstrosity. Thus, all Muslims came to embody the criminality attributed to the Jamaat while the perpetrators of violence, armed with moral legitimacy, appeared to enforce the order of the sovereign state and the majority.

A Clarion Call for Appreciation or Normalising the Distress?

By 30 January 2020, India reported its first case of Covid-19, and the Ministry of AYUSH[9] responded by suggesting Ayurvedic, Homeopathic, and Unani treatments, without citing any research findings to back its gratuitous advice (Philipose 2020). As a preventive initiative, Prime Minister Modi (Rajya Sabha TV 2020a) encouraged citizens to participate in a self-restrained lockdown to curb social interactions and gatherings outside homes on March 22. Naming it '*Janta*[10] Curfew,' he suggested a 14-hour stay-at-home lockdown from 7 am to 9 pm to prevent transmission through physical interaction (ibid) and to clap and bang plates (*thalis*) to show support for health workers. Influential personalities called it a 'bold move' and 'masterstroke' (Mannathukkren 2020). The idea of collective '*thali* banging' itself was appropriated from other countries – beginning with singing by Italians in their balconies and picked up by other nations (ibid).

Siddharth Bhatia (2020) discusses Modi's penchant for moral science lectures – the projected image of the Prime Minister as a yogic, selfless, wise elder, whose moral lectures become performative in the challenging times of a crisis, thinning out complaints of substantive socio-economic issues. Such a charismatic leader's invocation to the nation about acknowledging frontline warriors found a wider appeal, even among those who are not die-hard devotees (ibid).

On April 3, Modi directed the citizens to switch off their electric lights at 9 pm on 5 April for 9 minutes, and light candles, *diyas*,[11] or torch lights at their doorsteps or balconies (Rajya Sabha TV 2020b). The ritual aimed to collectively and symbolically fight the darkness of the pandemic and spread the light of hope as a community. This directive was followed by enthusiastic citizens across India, including celebrities and business families, as the internet became flooded with videos and photos of fireworks and celebrations of 'Diwali[12] in April' ending with the blowing of conch shells and the jingling of bells from many apartments. While images of lamp lighting were spectacularised by middle-class urban citizens to reiterate their collective (national) sentiments, there was no concern shown towards the ASHA workers' pan-India protest or other issues raised by frontline workers.

How does the heroisation of healthcare workers[13] (McCormick 2020) resolve the lapses in health infrastructure and provide safety kits to ASHA workers? How do such subaltern frontline workers partake in and make sense of these symbolic gestures in the absence of substantive entitlements? In a context where the secularism of Indian polity is derided, the deployment of religious metaphors and imageries in fighting the pandemic not only sacralises the nation but also enforces the hegemony of the dominant community. It is simultaneously encoded with the real and potential estrangement of those who may not associate with such articulations. These symbolic and ritualised invocations of the majority simply mask the underperformance of the nation either on the infrastructural front or in its unpreparedness to deal with the migrant labour crisis.

In this chapter, we present a synchronous reading of a rather reified understanding of three events during the coronavirus pandemic – the migrant workers' long walk home, the hysteria around the Tablighi Jamaat congregation, and the evocation of affection and national sentiments through *thali* banging and the lighting of *diyas* (lamps), with a critical reflection on the state's power dynamics and governance, which failed to foreground and institute the facilities of social care.

The multiple lockdowns generated a shortage of food and income for millions; the lack of PPEs and other safety provisions put health workers at risk and precarity. Similarly, the unavailability of information and statistics on migrant workers, the undercounting of deaths, and chaos in many health centres were issues of concern in the public domain. At such critical junctures, national sentiments were stirred through the mainstream media's projection of the Tablighi Jamaat congregation as the source of the virus spread, creating an atmosphere of hate and propaganda, leading to sporadic street violence. In such hysteric moments, the discursive power of hate and rumour overpowered critical dialogues on hunger, loss of jobs, unattended patients in public hospitals, lack of PPE for health workers, and the general dismay of citizens. The mass rituals of thali banging and lighting lamps, accompanied by blowing conch shells and ringing of bells simulated the Hindu festival of Diwali, creating a strong bond of community among the masses (read hindu majority). The national majority, charged with hate and anger towards the 'Muslim others' and united through symbolic mobilisation, possibly allowed the neo-liberal state to mask its deeper malaise at a time when it was crippled by its own infrastructural lapses.

The two things suggested in this chapter towards re-imagining state intervention is to increase public expenditure on health. This, along with efficacious management and instituted ethics of care within body politic and the citizenry at large could be a way forward, or one can say a learning towards future crises management. Over the past several years, healthcare in India has been dwindling to new lows (Karan and Selvaraj 2009). Entry of private players in predominant ways, along with poor public health facilities, compel people to look for private outlets pushing millions towards the poverty line (ibid). The understaffed hospitals and abysmal patient bed ratio clearly indicate that India is unequipped to handle a major health crisis like the present pandemic. Therefore, the symbolic, affective, and ritualistic mobilisations of *thali* banging and lamp lighting are woefully inadequate to address the nagging questions of unemployment and livelihood on ground. The hunger and insecurities witnessed among the working class resulting in reverse migration from urban to rural areas during lockdown, and the misery and suffering of long walks are reminders of the collapse of democratic rights in the supposedly largest democracy. What we mean by an expansive vision of 'we' in times of mass miseries, mentioned earlier, is the responsibility of privileged business and capitalist classes and the upwardly mobile middle class to bestow care and concern to the labouring bodies, which build and maintain the mansions and sky rise building and spaces of luxury and consumption in globalising cities. The state, therefore, needs to institute ethics of care, rooted in socialist investment towards institutions catering to the citizens. The 'what' and 'how' of this re-imagining, that is, the root map, can be debated and discussed. However, the learnings from this present scenario suggest that it should include tolerance and respect towards religious and other minorities to prevent phobias and hatred. Last, but not the least, the national Food Security Act 2013 needs a robust implementation.

Notes

1 Tablighi Jamaat is an Islamic missionary movement with a global and transnational participation and is headquartered in Delhi. In March 2020, the Jamaat organised a congregation in India that was attended by pilgrims all over the world.
2 Nizamuddin Markaz is a mosque situated in the Nizamuddin area of South Delhi. It serves as the headquarters of the Tablighi Jamaat movement. The 2020 congregation of the Jamaat was held here.
3 The word 'thali' is the Hindi expression for dishes, particularly made of steel or aluminium. The Prime Minister of India urged the citizens to perform the ritual of thali banging to ward off the virus. Thali banging, maybe seen as a symbolic act, has its root in Hindu worship, wherein idols are worshipped with various sounds of clanging metal instruments.
4 Necropolitics, given by Mbembe (2003, 2019), draws on Foucault's biopolitics and the decolonial approach, explaining 'as the making of spaces and subjectivities in an *in-between* of life and death' (Pele 2020). It is essentially an approach to manage excess populations (within modern capitalism) through their confinement in certain spaces (refugee camps, ghettos, gated communities) and a large-scale exposure to death and elimination (Pele 2020).
5 Agamben situates 'state of exception' as a modern institution, whose imperative in law is to colonise 'life itself'. It is essentially extrajudicial and is invoked in times of national threat, when the 'life of the nation' is at risk, legitimated, and sanctioned through constitutions and international treaties, allowing states to 'suspend the protection of certain basic rights' (Humphreys 2006: 678). In times of public emergency, when state of exception is the rule of law, certain forms of knowledge hold privilege over others, and therefore, are accepted as truth, while others are not. This has a direct effect on the production of knowledge, acquiring certain knowledge while suppressing others (Agamben 2005).
6 One Nation, One Ration Card is an important citizen-centric reform. Its implementation ensures availability of rations to beneficiaries under National Food Securities Act (NFSA) and other welfare schemes across the nation. At the time of lockdowns, however, this provision was unavailable for the workers in big metropolitan cities, which are epicenters of migration. See: https://pib.gov.in/PressReleasePage.aspx?PRID=1704063#:~:text=One%20Nation%20One%20Ration%20Card%20System%20is%20an%20important%20citizen,(FPS)%20across%20the%20countr
7 ASHA Workers are trained female health activists, working as a liaison between communities and the public healthcare system. They are trained to provide healthcare facilities and first aid for minor injuries ailments like fever and diarrhoea.

8 There had been cases where patients were denied access to hospitals on the basis of fear of infection to others. See Yasmeen 2020.
9 The Ministry of AYUSH is a Government of India initiated effort to focus attention on development of Education and Research in Ayurveda, Yoga and Naturopathy, Unani, Siddha and Homoeopathy. It was established in 2014 by the NDA led government (see more https://www.ayush.gov.in/ or https://main. ayush.gov.in/about-us/about-the-ministry)
10 The word 'Janta' refers to the public or citizens in the Hindi language.
11 The word 'Diya' in Hindi language refers to lamps used during Hindu worship and religious festivals. They are small bowl-like structures holding oil and cotton that allows it to stay lit for a long time.
12 See 'Diwali in April: Diyas, candles shine bright as India switches off lights in fight against coronavirus'. https://www.indiatoday.in/india/story/covid-19-narendra-modi-diwali-april-diyas-candles-shine-bright-as-india-switches-off-lightsfight-against-coronavirus-1663641-2020-04-05
13 The frontline health workers such as doctors, nurses, and supportive staffs in the hospitals and healthcare systems were symbolically eulogised through *thali* banging. But these symbolic heroisation during the pandemic did not fully translate into these staffs' access to PPE kits and safety gears, with several of them dying due to infection. At many places, the doctors and nurses were on strike for unpaid salaries and promised compensations for overworking.

References

(2020) '#9baje9minute: Virat Kohli, Rohit Sharma Participate in 'lights off' Exercise as India Unite in Fight against Covid-19', *India Today*, 5 April [online]. Available at: https://www.indiatoday.in/sports/cricket/story/-9baje9minute-pm-modi-initiative-rohit-sharma-sachin-tendulkar-switch-off-lights-fight-against-covid-19-1663633-2020-04-05 [Accessed 4 January 2021].

(2020) 'Modi Seeks 'Forgiveness' of India's Poor over Covid-19 Lockdown', *Aljazeera*, 29 March [online]. Available at: https://www.aljazeera.com/news/2020/3/29/modi-seeks-forgiveness-from-indias-poor-over-covid-19-lockdown [Accessed 14 October 2020].

Agamben, G. (Trans.) Kevin Attell. (2005) *State of Exception*. Chicago: University of Chicago Press.

Alexander, J. C. (2004) 'Toward a Theory of Cultural Trauma' [online]. Available at: https://content.ucpress.edu/title/9780520235953/9780520235953_chapone.pdf [Accessed 29 July 2020].

Bailey, F. G. (1994) *The Witch-Hunt or Triumph of Morality*. Ithaca: Cornell University Press.

Baudrillard, Jean (Trans.) P. Patton. (1995) *The Gulf War Did Not Take Place*. Bloomington: Indiana University Press.

Bhat, M. R. (2020) 'Not a Tableegi Virus: Media Filing Biased Reports to Tarnish Muslim Image', *The Greater Kashmir*, 3 April [online]. Available at: https://www.greaterkashmir.com/news/opinion/not-a-tableegi-virus/ [Accessed 15 October 2020].

Bhatia, S. (2020) 'Modi's Moral Science Lecture for a Nation Facing Crisis', *The Wire*, 20 March [online]. Available at: https://thewire.in/politics/narendra-modi-govt-coronavirus [Accessed 4 January 2021].

Chomsky, N. and Prasad, V. (2021) 'We are Living in an Emergency that Requires Urgent Action', *Tricontinental: Institute for Social Research* [online]. Available at: https://www.thetricontinental.org/newsletterissue/1-noam-chomsky/ [Accessed 8 January 2021].

Dogra, B. (2018) 'Past Trends and Present Needs: Will India's Social Sector Get a Boost in the Budget?', *The Wire*, 29 January [online]. Available at: https://thewire.in/economy/will-indias-social-sector-get-a-boost-budget [Accessed 8 January 2021}

Gottschalk, P. and Greenberg, G. (2008) *Islamophobia: Making Muslims the Enemy*. Lanham: Rowman and Littlefield Publishers.

Harriss-White, B. (2010) *India Working: Essays on Society and Economy*. Cambridge: Cambridge University Press.

Irfan, S., Masih, N., and Slater, J. (2020) 'India Confronts Its First Coronavirus 'superspreader' – a Muslim Missionary Group with More Than 400 Members Infected', *The Washington Post*, 2 April [online]. Available at: https://www.washingtonpost.com/world/asia_pacific/india-coronavirus-tablighi-jamaat-delhi/2020/04/02/abdc5af0-7386-11ea-ad9b-254ec99993bc_story.html [Accessed 15 October 2020].

Jaramillo, D. L. (2009) *Ugly War, Pretty Package: How CNN and Fox News Made the Invasion of Iraq High Concept*. Bloomington: Indiana University Press.

Jha, S. (2020) 'Govt Hospital in Ahmedabad Allegedly Separates Hindu, Muslim Coronavirus Patients; Govt Denies', *Deccan Herald*, 15 April [online]. Available at: https://www.deccanherald.com/national/west/govt-hospital-in-ahmedabad-allegedly-separates-hindu-muslim-coronavirus-patients-govt-denies-825586.html [Accessed 10 October 2020].

Karan, A. K. and Selvaraj, S. (2009) 'Deepening Health Insecurity in India: Evidence from National Sample Surveys since 1980s', *Economic and Political Weekly*, 44 (40) [online]. Available at: https://www.epw.in/journal/2009/40/special-articles/deepening-health-insecurity-india-evidence-national-sample-surveys [Accessed 06 June 2021].

Kumar, B., et al. (2020) 'Challenges in the Delivery of Critical Care in India during the COVID 19 Pandemic', *Journal of Intensive Care Society*, 22(4)1–7.

Kumar, P. (2020) '30 Per cent of Coronavirus Cases Linked to Delhi Mosque Event: Government' *NDTV*, 4 April [online]. Available at: https://www.ndtv.com/india-news/coronavirus-tablighi-jamaat-30-per-cent-of-coronavirus-cases-linked-to-delhi-mosque-event-government-2206163 [Accessed 21 September 2020].

Mannathukkren, N. (2020) 'It's Dangerous to be Taken in by Propaganda in the Time of Corona', *The Wire*, 21 March [online]. Available at: https://thewire.in/politics/coronavirus-india-propaganda [Accessed 15 October 2020].

McCormick, L. (2020) 'Marking Time in Lockdown: Heroization and Ritualization in UK during the Coronavirus Pandemic', *American journal of Cultural Sociology*, 8: 324–351.

Mustafa, F. (2020) 'The Coronavirus spread and the Criminal Liability of the Tablighi Jamaat', *The Wire*, 16 April [online]. Available at: https://thewire.in/communalism/coronavirus-criminal-liability-of-tablighi-jamaat [Accessed 10 October 2020].

Nath, D. (2020) 'Govt. Has No Data of Migrant Workers' Death, Loss of Job', *The Hindu*, 14 September [online]. Available at: https://www.thehindu.com/news/national/govt-has-no-data-of-migrant-workers-death-loss-of-job/article32600637.ece [Accessed 8 December 2020].

Naqvi, S. and Bisht, A. (2020) 'How Tablighi Jamaat Event Became India's Worst Coronavirus Vector', *Aljazeera*, 7 April [online]. Available at: https://www.aljazeera.com/news/2020/4/7/how-tablighi-jamaat-event-became-indias-worst-coronavirus-vector [Accessed 13 December 2020].

NDTV. (2020, April 14). *"We'll Die of Hunger Before Virus Can Kill Us": Migrant Workers*. Available at: https://www.youtube.com/watch?v=95ZtzxiL8l8 [Accessed 11 January 2021].

Pele, A. (2020) 'Achille Mbembe: Necropolitics'. Available at: https://criticallegalthinking. com/2020/03/02/achille-mbembe-necropolitics/ [Accessed 11 November 2020].

Philipose, P. (2020) 'Backstory:The COVID 19 Story Goes Viral', *The Wire*, 28 March [online]. Available at: https://thewire.in/media/backstory-covid-19-viral [Accessed 8 December 2020].

Pulla, P. (2020) 'India Is Under-counting Its COVID 19 Death: This Is How?', *The Wire*, 4 August [online]. Available at: https://science.thewire.in/health/india-mccd-comorbidities-covid-19-deaths-undercounting/ [Accessed 10 October 2020].

Rahman, A. S. and Petersen, E. H. (2020) 'Coronavirus Conspiracy Theories Targeting Muslims Spread in India', *The Guardian*, 13 April [online]. Available at: https://www.theguardian.com/world/2020/apr/13/coronavirus-conspiracy-theories-targeting-muslims-spread-in-india [Accessed 21 September 2020].

Rajya Sabha TV. (2020a) *PM Modi Addresses the Nation on Corona Outbreak*. Available at: https://youtu.be/XPTyktyBj5k [Accessed 21 September 2020].

Rajya Sabha TV. (2020b) *PM Modi's Video Message on COVID-19*. Available at: https://www.youtube.com/watch?v=W5L--1kfLJg&feature=youtu.be [Accessed 21 September 2020].

Rao, N. et al. (2020) 'Destination Matter: Social Policy and Migrant Workers in the Times of COVID 19', *The European Journal of Development Research*, 32: 1639–1661.

Republic World. (2020) *Nationwide Search for Tablighi Jamaat Attendees: The Debate with Arnab Goswami*. Available at: https://www.youtube.com/watch?v=tvP789CbzOU&feature=youtu.be [Accessed 11 January 2021].

Ruparelia, S. (2015) "Minimum Government, Maximum Governance': The Restructuring of Power in Modi's India'. *South Asia: Journal of South Asian Studies*, 38: 755–775.

Sengupta, S. and Jha, M. K. (2020) 'Social Policy, COVID 19 and Impoverished Migrants'. *The International Journal of Community and Social Development*, 2 (2): 1–21.

Sharma, N. (2020a) 'India's Harsh COVID Lockdown Displaced at Least 10 Million Migrants', *Quartz India*, 14 September [online]. Available at: https://qz.com/india/1903018/indias-covid-19-lockdown-displaced-at-least-10-million-migrants/ [Accessed 11 January 2021].

Sharma, C. N. (2020b) 'How Covid-19 Pandemic Exposed India's Chronic Underinvestment in Health Care', *Mint*, 17 August [online]. Available at: https://www.livemint.com/news/india/how-covid-19-pandemic-exposed-india-s-chronic-underinvestment-in-healthcare-11597670943972.html [Accessed 21 September 2021].

Sherwani, Z. (2020) 'How Stigma over COVID Robbed Nizamuddin Locals of Jobs & Dignity', *The Quint*, 24 June [online]. Available at: https://www.thequint.com/videos/fighting-the-coronavirus-tag-delhi-nizamuddin-locals-feel-ostracised [Accessed 11 January 2021].

Sikdar, K. and Mishra, P. (2020) *Reverse Migration During Lockdown. A Snapshot of Public Policies*. Delhi: National Institute of Public Finance.

Smits, K. (2014) 'Neoliberal State and the Uses of Indigenous Culture', *Nationalism and Ethnic Politics*, 20 (1): 43–62.

TRT World. (2020) *India: When Hindu Nationalism Meets Covid-19*. Available at: https://www.youtube.com/watch?v=2DZtMLg-RFE&feature=youtu.be [Accessed 8 December 2020].

Upreti, M. P. (2021) 'Riding on Hope', *The Hindu Business Line*, 4 March [online]. Available at:https://www.thehindubusinessline.com/blink/cover/asha-workers-in-india-await-recognition-and-compensation-for-battling-covid19-on-the-ground/article33988456.ece [Accessed 06 June 2021].

Wahidi, Z. and Thapar, A. (2020) 'Unjust and Unfair: What Three High Courts Said about the Arrests of Tablighi Jamaat Members', *The Scroll*, 24 August [online]. Available at: https://scroll.in/article/971195/unjust-and-unfair-what-three-high-courts-said-about-the-arrests-of-tablighi-jamaat-members [Accessed 11 January 2021].

Yadav, J. (2020) 'I Walked with India's Migrant Labourers: More than Angry, They are Hurt with Modi', *The Print*, 17 May [online]. Available at: https://theprint.in/opinion/pov/i-walked-with-india-migrant-labourers-hurt-with-modi/423643/ [Accessed 15 October 2020].

Yasmeen, A. (2020) 'Coronavirus: So Cause Notice to Nine Hospitals for Denying Treatment', *The Hindu*, 02 July [online]. Available at: https://www.thehindu.com/news/cities/bangalore/coronavirus-show-cause-notice-to-nine-hospitals-for-denying-treatment/article31966184.ece [Accessed 6 June 2021].

17

NO IDEA OF GOD
June 2021

Amitesh Grover

Epiphanies and Exaltations amidst a Pandemic

For all that this pandemic has and will make humanity do, what it has achieved distinctly is this – it has rendered the planet spectacularly godless. I don't think we have come to publicly admit that we are in the midst of an unprecedented wave of atheism. With every rising wave of the pandemic, places of worship shut down and messengers of God went entirely out of business. No prayer, no call to a saviour, no supreme being seemed to answer our desperate cries for relief. Would the creator, if there was one, create a disease that would use the same means of contagion as those that keep us human, namely love, fondness, and fellowship?

You could argue that it is precisely at times of a calamitous phenomenon that people turn to God, any God that will bring in its wake a promise of deliverance. Yet, living amidst this catastrophe – which many claim is natural, while some argue is borne of man's actions – there is enough reason to consider, again, not how God arrives (or leaves), but how profoundly godless our world is. The whole world waits, before temples, mosques, and churches reopen, for a vaccine that will help us defeat the virus and release us from the crushing isolation into which we have been arrested by this disease.

If you come to think about it, the soul's yearning to be touched by God is not unlike the deep craving for a beloved's touch, which we so intensely feel during the physical isolation brought about by the pandemic. Yet, while we will be able to embrace each other again after science defeats the virus (albeit not without paying an unbearable price for it with lives lost), will we ever be able to return to God? Atheism is shocking to some (why wouldn't you believe in God?); it is despairing for others (what keeps you from believing in God?); it is exhilarating for a few (thank you for saying you don't believe in God either). Say what you will, but atheism, like its antagonistic twin theism, has been a part of human history as well. As I wait for vaccines to arrive, and as I continue to access the world remotely, in quarantine, I contemplate about the act of waiting, about the philosophical and

DOI: 10.4324/9781003320524-22

earthly presence of the human alone, and also – more personally – about how I came to be an atheist much before the pandemic arrived.

This act of contemplation is ridden with anxiety. There is growing evidence that humanists and atheists are targeted on the basis of their rejection of a majority religion or their promotion of human rights, democratic values, and critical thinking. A range of tactics is used against humanists, atheists, and non-religious people to shut them into silence, including the criminalisation of blasphemy and apostasy in some parts of the world, the impunity for attacks that certain religious people enjoy in other parts of the world, and the social isolation and discrimination that the atheists have routinely faced from the rest of the society. To speak out and say you're an atheist or humanist can be dangerous in many parts of the world.

Take India as an example. On 20 August 2013, Narendra Dabholkar, a rationalist and anti-superstition campaigner, was assassinated (The Hindu 2013). On 16 February 2015, rationalist Govind Pansare and his wife were attacked by unknown gunmen. He later died from the wounds on 20 February (Deccan Herald 2015). On 30 August 2015, M. M. Kalburgi, a scholar and rationalist, was shot dead at his home. He was known for his criticism of superstition and idol worship (The New Indian Express 2015). Soon afterwards, another rationalist and author, K. S. Bhagwan, received a threatening letter. He had offended religious groups by criticising the Gita (The Hindu 2015). In March 2017, an Indian Muslim youth from Coimbatore, 31-year-old A. Farooq, who became rationalist and atheist, was killed by members of a Muslim radical group (The Indian Express 2017). According to the 2012 WIN-Gallup Global Index of Religion and Atheism report, 81 per cent of Indians were religious, 13 per cent were non-religious, 3 per cent were convinced atheists, and 3 per cent were unsure or did not respond. The three per cent convinced atheists put to the scale in the Indian context translates to approximately 40 million people. Given this astounding number, and the imminent threat they face, how is it that we do not take the predicament of being an atheist any more gravely than we do now?

The Early Days

Fear, ridicule, or misfortune never stopped my Nana (maternal grandfather) from claiming, loudly and boldly, that he is at heart an atheist. Born to a family of Hindu believers, he grew up to be a sceptic of Brahmanism. In my childhood, he often spoke to me about the conflicting dichotomous traditions of Arya Samaj and Snatan Dharam. For most of his life, he aligned himself with the former – a reformist Hindu movement – while my Nani (maternal grandmother) followed the latter, an orthodox and conservative sect. They argued and derided each other's beliefs openly, freely, but always allowed each other the space to practice what they wished to. Nani cooked for his friends when they came visiting home to discuss and debate the tenets of the Arya Samaj, while my Nana arranged for materials and made space in the house for her to host kirtan. She always asked about his friends' well-being, even as she expressed her disapproval for their beliefs; he greeted the priest and friends she invited with respect, appreciated their music, but barely spoke to them.

Nani accepted the epistemic authority of the scriptures: she believed that there is such a thing as ātman (soul), and that if there is a soul, it cannot exist without Ishvara (Supreme Being). Nana, on the other hand, progressively challenged the existence of a soul, or, the omnipresence of a supreme being. In his inimitably provocative ways, he once argued that the performance of last rites and religious death rituals was a sham. "What business does a priest have being there between me and the deceased, instructing me to perform symbolic gestures that don't make any sense!" he quipped at a family member's house, hours before the cremation was about to take place. At another similar occasion, he confessed that he had signed his body off to science, that doctors were free to conduct research on his cadaver, and that the rights of his family to his body would cease to exist after his death. This declaration shocked everyone (no one in the family had done this before) but angered my grandmother the most, to the extent that she didn't speak to him for days. To charm her back and make her smile again, he gently proposed to set aside their irreconcilable difference over spirituality in favour of admitting, instead, to an undeniable, mutually felt truth: "God may or may not exist, but love undoubtedly does."

His views on atheism weren't unique, nor, peculiar. Disbelief in God or Gods is found in several of the Astika (Orthodox) streams of Hindu philosophy. Even before I was curious, or, attentive enough to partake in the philosophical debates, Nana pointed me towards the remarkable, yet little-known, atheistic philosophy of the Carvaka school. The Carvaka school originated around the 6th century BCE as a nāstika (heterodox) school. It is, arguably, the first clear evidence of a materialistic movement in ancient India, in which the teachers and their learners prepared to accept only the phenomenon of pratyakṣa (perception) as valid proof of existence. They rejected all other sources of attestation – sabda (testimony), upamāna (analogy), and anumāna (inference) – as being unreliable. Soul and God were rejected, because they could not be proved by perception. One of the widely accepted principles of Carvaka philosophy was its rejection of any means that sought to establish metaphysical truths. In inferring a truth from a set of observations, one must acknowledge doubt; inferred knowledge is conditional, it claimed.

The Carvakas considered everything to be essentially constituted by one or more of these four elements: earth, water, air, and fire. This system of belief made them close cousins of the followers of the Arya Samaj and also perhaps the reason why Nana gravitated towards its tenets as he read more and more about it later in life. But, he often lamented that his search for the original writings of the Carvaka school took him to a dead end; almost all of the original texts are considered lost. What is not lost is the etymology of the word cārvāka, which is derived from the root carv, 'to chew'. What a poetic metaphor it is: only that what can be seen, touched, and smelt can be chewed; only that which nourishes the body might nourish the soul.

Chewing on a Book

However, while I remember my Nana mentioning the Carvaka philosophy on multiple occasions during my younger days, my adolescence barely allowed me the steadiness I needed to consider the fascinating proposals hidden in there. Much of what I know of this ancient Indian philosophy is something I arrived at much later in life, partly because I preferred the restlessness of fiction, which seemed more in tune with my raging mind, at the time.

In my early 20s, I voluntarily signed up for an undergraduate lecture taking place in the English Literature department on the play *Waiting for Godot*, an astounding play by Samuel Beckett. The lecture was hosted, in a break from the tradition of classroom teaching, under an open sky. It began at noon and lasted till it became dark, quite dark. The professor who delivered the lecture looked no less than a God in a human physique himself – tall, grey, with gentle eyes, sincere mannerism, considered gait, and a distinctive, deep voice.

He opened the book and started without delay, with the keenness of a Sunday priest, who is always enthusiastic to discover in that what he has read a thousand times, something new and freshly illuminating to the mind. He read the dialogues, explained words, played the various parts, and paused every now and then to check if we were keeping up. He progressed from one page to another in the manner of delivering a show to his attendees that day, half a century after the play was written. The lecture gathered a strange kind of sanctity as it proceeded. Everyone realised that it needed to press on uninterrupted. As I got drawn in, I felt the ground on which we sat unguarded becoming thinner – gravity was giving up on us, abandoning its grip on our souls as if to become feeble and weightless like the page we were on.

It is a difficult play to confront, not any less as a student than it is to be its early audience. *Waiting for Godot* is, "a play in which nothing happens, twice." The play's landscape is barren; its universe is forsaken, an environment that eerily evokes the abandonment that pervades our cities under lockdown today. Unlike most plays that contain multiple scenes, this play has only one scene, albeit spread across two acts. In it, two men wait on a country road by a tree. The tree is the only thing that manages to change between the two acts, growing a number of leaves from one act to the next, perhaps to allow for the progression of time but also to cause confusion about how much time might've passed – the script specifies that it is the next day. The characters are of unspecified origin, deal mostly in derisive jokes; the setting's minimal description displays an intent on the part of the writer to present a place that should not be particularised. Nowhere, thus everywhere – a notion often associated with the search for God.

"Not a soul in sight," says one character looking at the audience seated in the auditorium. Another rushes towards the back of the stage, and shouts "There's no way out there." In another moment, he shouts that he's lived his whole life "Here!" but all we see is the barren stage. With sparse action, no plot, and barely any changes, the play is so stripped down, so elemental, that it invites all kinds of social, political, and a/theistic interpretation. Like in the case of anti/theistic texts, the attempts to pin this dramatic text down have not been successful, but my desire to do so is natural, because what we encounter in the writing is a kind of minimalism that reaches for bedrock reality.

The curtain had to be brought down soon after the play started – in one of its first public performances – because the audience got disgruntled, whistled, and hooted derisively. The anti-climax wasn't appreciated at all – Godot never arrives! But, not all early productions got a dismal reception. A particularly significant show took place in Lüttringhausen Prison, near Remscheid in Germany. An inmate somehow obtained permission to stage the play. This was the night of 29 November 1953. He wrote to Beckett in October 1954:

> You will be surprised to be receiving a letter about your play Waiting for Godot, from a prison where so many thieves, forgers, toughs, homos, crazy men, and killers spend this bitch of a life waiting … and waiting … and waiting. Waiting for what? Godot? Perhaps.

It is difficult to say whether the real value of the play is in its performance, or, in its teaching. Less forces us to look for more, and the act of delivering a lecture on the play is nothing short of a sermon, only that this oration opens up speculation in the direction of atheism, agnosticism, and the idea of morality in the absence of God. The lecture lasted seven hours, and left us with a strange fatigue, not unlike that of having run a marathon, only without sweat. At the end, what arrived in Godot's place was godlessness. I remember struggling for words, my mouth melting like flesh exposed to an incinerator, making lips indistinguishable, turning them inside, and making it impossible to utter even a customary goodbye or thank you to the professor. I had grown up with a faint distrust of religion, but even so, I hadn't expected that the final moment of evacuation, of becoming godless, would occur on a perfectly ordinary day sitting on humdrum grass, with not so much a word of warning, amidst a quiet modest middle spring.

Journey back that day felt longer than the lecture had lasted, perhaps because what I had eventually experienced was grief. An odd kind of grief without anchor, without an accompanying personal sentiment, adrift, but grief, nonetheless. I woke up the following morning and latched onto my friend's arm, who at the time was my roommate and was given to piety. I dragged him out in the open, and exclaimed, "God doesn't exist. Oh my god, God doesn't exist!" My gasping squawky cries of relief baffled him. "He said, ok, ok ... ok hmmm" and walked back indoors unimpressed. I wanted to express to him that I had had an intense and profound experience, that godlessness had left me feeling exalted, euphoric, and devastated. I wanted to know if he feels equally overwhelmed when he experiences godliness. But, he didn't turn back. He wouldn't hear any of it. And that was that. We went on to be friends for life despite this fundamental disagreement, and in a sense, it has had echoes of the kind of affection that my grandparents had discovered during a similar contestation years ago – "God may or may not exist, but friendship certainly does."

So, Is the Wait Over?

As far back as 1772, Baron d'Holbach said that all children are born atheists; they have no idea of God. Is then the journey towards Godlessness through shedding, in some part, what was learnt in becoming an adult? Is it a kind of forgetting? Once when an actor needed to prepare himself to play a character in Beckett's play, he began by observing people suffering from dementia. Beckett's characters keep "failing to remember": where they are, how they got there. "Nothing is to be done" is the opening line.

Nana is 93 years old now. In his last stage of life, he cannot talk anymore, barely remembers anything, and looks on into oblivion when he is amidst family. He now occupies his own solitude, unaware of his real surroundings, suspended in a reverie all day as he sits sketching and painting, as if determined that only such things as art, which work through perception, on perception, are the only worthy pursuits of an atheist's life. Has he turned into a Beckettian character who has successfully managed to forget all that he learnt? Like a child who enters the world godless?

Waiting for Godot is the perfect play to read 70 years after it was written, as we sit at home to save humanity by doing nothing. Perhaps, we have all become characters in Beckett's godless universe. If we go on to survive the pandemic (which we will), it will be owed in no small measure to the grit of a growing tribe of atheists who march on to deliver godlessness (in the form of a vaccine to fight Covid-19 this time). As the world moves forward, it will undoubtedly have more and more atheists. We might do better if we keep faith in our ability to evolve to faithlessness in the matter of transcendence. Atheism – or, at least in its more essential form, disavowal – requires more intellectual sinew, more mental courage, than does faith.

Doubt is a matter of conviction and grace. In an interview, the renowned physicist Richard Feynman said:

> I can live with doubt and uncertainty and not knowing. I think it's much more interesting to live not knowing than to have answers which might be wrong. I have approximate answers and possible beliefs and different degrees of certainty about different things but I'm not absolutely sure of anything and the many things I don't

know anything [such as] why we're here … I don't feel frightened by not knowing things.

Of course, in classic sub-continental style, and to return to the faith I keep in fiction, we could look at the whole thing the other way around, instead. It is not us who endure God's neglect, but God who suffers from our rejection. People have forsaken God, because people are, simply, too busy living. Kiran Nagarkar best captures this in the opening page of his book *The Arsonist*:

"If you had to choose between a woman you loved and God, who would you choose?"
The Weaver said, "The woman."
And the mullah asked him, "If you had to choose between a song and God, what would you pick?"
The Weaver said, "The song."
And the priest asked him, "A beautiful sunset or God?"
The Weaver said, "The sunset."
And they asked him how he could blaspheme so.
The Weaver said, "God has eternity on his side, he can always wait. Will the woman, the song, or the sunset wait for me?"

To be God is to be without people for eternity. To be human is to be without God for eternity.

Either way, we are on our own.

References

Deccan Herald. 21 February 2015. 'Rationalist Pansare is dead.' https://www.deccanherald.com/content/461081/rationalist-pansare-dead.html

The Hindu. 20 August 2013. 'Rationalist Dabholkar shot dead.' https://www.thehindu.com/news/national/other-states/rationalist-dabholkar-shot-dead/article5041138.ece

The Hindu. 10 September 2015. 'Writer Bhagwan received threat.' https://www.thehindu.com/news/national/karnataka/writer-bhagwan-receives-threat-letter/article7635331.ece

The Indian Express. 27 March 2017. 'Tamil Nadu youth killed for being an atheist, father says he will become one.' https://indianexpress.com/article/india/tamil-nadu-youth-h-farook-killed-for-being-an-atheist-father-says-he-too-will-become-one-4586999/

The New Indian Express. 31 August 2015. 'Indian Scholar Who Criticized Idol Worship Murdered at Home.' https://www.newindianexpress.com/nation/2015/aug/31/Indian-Scholar-Who-Criticized-Idol-Worship-Murdered-at-Home-807662.html

CREATIVE COMMUNICATIONS

18

THOUGHTS FROM THE NORTH
April 2020

Áshildur Linnet

As an islander, you are always aware that you must rely on yourself. That even though this island is a part of the world, we are oceans apart. This concept has been passed on from one generation to the next for as long as people have been living in Iceland. In the last 20 to 30 years, we, the inhabitants of this northern island, have started to forget that we are not directly connected to the mainland of Europe. Jumping on an aircraft to go wherever we could think of became so easy that for a moment we forgot that we live on an island.

In a blink of an eye, the whole community was forced to rethink our way of life. What we had taken for granted yesterday was a privilege today. Who are we, the people sharing their fate on these cliffs in the Northern Atlantic? And not less important, how do the decisions of others affect our daily lives?

In the first response to the Covid-19 crisis, the focus was all on the health aspects of the pandemic. We were focused and united in protecting the most vulnerable such as the elderly. We had daily press conferences, where the Civil Protection and the Directorate of Health gave information and insights on how we were all doing. How many had been infected, how many were on ventilators, where in the country, and what to do if you thought you might be infected. This was broadcasted live on national television and radio. The conversation that followed was like going back in time when everyone watched the same television program offered on the only station available. We were all in this together, or were we?

Did the information and the spirit of solidarity that spread so fast through the community reach everyone? What about the people who did not speak Icelandic? What about those who never watch or listen to the stations of the national broadcasting services? Were they included or somehow left out, unaware of the solidarity among those who understood the official message?

How the information flow was handled was very impressive, but it also demonstrated that we forgot a part of our society. We have always been prepared for emergencies, but they had more to do with natural hazards like avalanches and earthquakes – emergencies that involved evacuating

DOI: 10.4324/9781003320524-24

geographically defined areas. These were situations where all the people were housed in one or two emergency shelters. The information that needed to be communicated was developed based on who was there and which form of communication would be most appropriate for their understanding. This time it was different and the way we communicate, the way information spreads, is different from when the last pandemic hit in 1918 or the other emergencies we have dealt with in Iceland.

The number of refugees and immigrants in Iceland has been steadily rising in the past two decades.[1] After the financial crisis in 2008, the reconstruction of the economy was dominantly focused on tourism. It was a success, and we had a tourism boom. Between 2010 and 2019, the number of tourists visiting annually went from 488 thousand to 2 million.[2] With a population of 318 thousand in 2010,[3] you can easily calculate that receiving these 2 million guests was not possible without outside help in terms of labour. The number of immigrants rose fast and by the end of 2019, they were 14.1 per cent of the inhabitants. In areas where the tourism growth was most evident, for instance around Keflavík International Airport, it rose to 27 per cent of the population as 98.7 per cent of all visitors to the country came through the international airport. The largest immigrant group is Polish, comprising 38.1 per cent of all immigrants in the country. No other nationality comes close to the number of Polish immigrants as the second-largest immigrant group comes from Lithuania (5.7%) and the third largest from the Philippines (3.9%).

When international air traffic was suddenly turned off and people were not busy at work, we started realising how little we know about this important part of our society, the immigrants. That the ways we communicate, pass on and look for information might not be familiar to the new arrivals in Iceland. All of us had been too busy with work or completely oblivious to raise these issues. The immigrants were like the migrant birds, coming for a short time to work but had stayed on and were not planning to leave. The pandemic and its economic recession, mainly in tourism, had reminded us that we are on an island. The islanders and the immigrants were not just here during the good times, they would be staying together during the bad times as well. The immigrants were also on the island, and we forgot that they are people, a part of society, not just migrant labour. We were all coexisting or at least pretending to, as the wheels of tourism kept spinning, making our economy flourish and bringing the world a step closer with affordable flight fares.

In general, Icelanders are seen to have a rather positive attitude when it comes to immigration issues. Up to this day, no national party that bases its ideology and debate on xenophobia has been elected for parliament or local governance. Studies also show that most people do not have a problem with the number of immigrants in the country. Not surprisingly, young people are more positive about immigration than the older generations. About 64 per cent believe that immigrants enrich cultural life, and 74 per cent of

Icelanders believe that immigrants have a good or very good impact on the economy.[4] These statistics struck me and prompted me to question what gets in the way of this view when we are faced with a social task such as protecting ourselves and our community from Covid-19. Our acceptance of immigrants stemmed from our perception of them as labour, rather than equal participants in our society. This was evidenced in the communication strategies adopted when the Covid-19 pandemic began to spread.

It proved challenging to create the right channels to communicate with the immigrant communities, and most of the resources were at the beginning only available for Icelandic speakers. It took a great deal of effort from some dedicated women from immigrant communities to make sure the official information of the civil defence and the health authorities was available in multiple languages. It was gratifying to be an observer, in my role as a migration expert, to see how this came about. Through my professional role in the Red Cross, I was able to ensure that the main languages of the beneficiaries were included. Finally, in the end of March 2020, the official information was available in nine foreign languages. The information provided on the official Covid-19 web page of the civil defence[5] was only a part of the information flow and the challenge was to inform people about this trustworthy source of information. Access to information was plenty, the sources not all trustworthy. Translation was only one step on the access to information that we needed to take during the outbreak of the pandemic.

In Iceland, elementary schools and kindergartens were kept open, but the daily routine for most children changed with limited hours of schooling each day. For most kindergarten children, it meant one day at home, one day at school. For the elementary schools, attendance was not compulsory, and parents were welcome to keep the children at home as long as they attended to school work in cooperation with the teacher. Anecdotal information suggests that in most schools the attendance was more than 50 per cent. If we look into the first numbers from the schools, it seems that attendance among immigrant children was much lower than among the locals. That leads us again to the question of access to information and if the official message and the evaluation of both health risks to children, the importance of having a daily routine, and the encouragement by the public health authorities to send children to school did not reach the immigrants. The non-Icelandic-speaking part of the community was left out in the information flow, and as a result their reaction was different. They possibly did not feel the solidarity and trust the general public had in the advice of the Civil Defence and Directorate of Health.

Where information comes from might be a factor here. What role did different responses from nations, for example, your host nation and your home country, play? Why did the Italians and the Danes close their schools while children in Iceland were expected to go to school? All of this was explained in detail to the Icelandic-speaking community but perhaps not others. As the situation lasted for several weeks, children of immigrants missed out on participation in the community, which is very important for their future. Even though Icelandic is a language spoken by few, it is the official language, the language of the education system, healthcare, social life, and all public services. To gain and maintain language skills is instrumental for the future of immigrant children. It is also crucial for Iceland to build cultural connections that will allow for more active participation of all migrants in the country. Their language skills and cultural understanding is an important key to be able to actively communicate, inform, and deliver information to migrants. They are a part of our community regardless of how long they intend to stay.

One of the tasks my colleagues and I, at Red Cross, took on was to tailor our regular services to meet both requirements made by the public health authorities and the needs of the people we work with. It was not simple, and we had to be both flexible and creative. An important part of delivering information was asking people how they prefer to get the information we manage. In no way am I suggesting that our information flow was perfect, it was probably far from it. What we do know is that it was appreciated by our beneficiaries. We were, on numerous occasions, informed by them that the information was helpful, reassuring, and met their needs. We understand that information is aid and is a part of empowering communities to deal with challenges. In a pandemic where you can protect yourself with behavioural change, the information on how you do that is a key factor.

One of the more creative tasks we took on, in cooperation with community volunteers, was creating videos that explained the key message of the public health authorities and directed people to safe sources of information. We had to analyse the official message, get that into a script for our videos, find someone to shoot the video, find people to do voice-overs, edit, act, and all the things you need to make a simple video message. You might ask yourself why several migration experts take on the role of making videos? You could say that the endless optimism embedded in the workplace and the belief in finding active, talented, and knowledgeable volunteers made this possible. Possibly a dash of the Icelandic mentality that it will all sort itself out was a part of it.[6]

The active communication route before Covid-19 was sending messages to our beneficiaries through text messages – a preferred way of the target group, to receive relevant information regarding our services. We knew it worked and we suspected that sending a link to a video could be more effective to get the key message to people instead of texting a link to a web page. If we believe that people remember 10 per cent of what they read, it was worth the effort to produce videos to get to the 50 per cent of what they remember if they both hear and see the message. With the ultimate goal of setting the target even higher to 90 per cent of what they do remember.[7] The Covid-19 response was in huge part about changing behaviours. About spreading awareness so that people would be able to protect themselves and stop the spread of the infection. The videos became a reality and the team, the volunteers, and the audience were all able to learn something in the process. Not only about the coronavirus and how to protect oneself but also about cooperation and the ability to work together as members of the community. We got filmmakers and musicians on board. People generously provided the use of a studio without charge. Volunteers acted and did voice-overs even though they had never done anything like this before. The videos were posted in six different languages providing a marginalised group of immigrants with important information.[8]

In July 2020, on this island in the Northern Atlantic, we were opening our borders. We managed to get the Covid-19 infections down to two or three people. The situation around the pandemic was getting relaxed and people were back to an almost normal way of living. The restrictions on gatherings were lifted in some parts, summer had arrived, and for a moment it felt surreal that only weeks before we had been battling this unpredictable virus. The authorities were testing people at the borders, and we had faith that this would be a safe way. Then it hit – one infection causing multiple infections and around 300 people quarantined. The pandemic was far from over.

While the world continues to grapple with the impact of the pandemic, it brought forth to us the importance of access to information. If we want to build an inclusive society, it is important to increase access to information and remember that 'new' people in a 'new' country need extra support in familiarising themselves with the local ways of getting information. We cannot exclude people from access to information that is crucial for their survival and well-being. Information is power and in the matter of Covid-19, it is a lifesaving power. In addition to the process of re-imagining methods of communication, we must device creative and innovative methodologies that are sensitive to the diverse cultural and linguistic backgrounds of the immigrant populations.

Notes

1 Legislation in Iceland does not distinguish between immigrants based on their permits. Any person who has a valid permit to stay is considered an immigrant in the data presented by Statistics Iceland.
2 Icelandic Tourist Board, 2020, *Heildarfjöldi erlendra ferðamanna*, see: https://www.ferdamalastofa.is/is/tolur-og-utgafur/fjoldi-ferdamanna/heildarfjoldi-erlendra-ferdamanna [Accessed 30 April 2020].
3 All numbers regarding population and number of immigrants used are from the same source of Statistics Iceland available on the web page www.hagstofa.is [Accessed 30 April 2020].
4 Félagsvísindastofnun Háskóla Íslands, 2019, Könnun á viðhorfum almennings til innflytjenda og fjölmenningarsamfélagsins. On: https://www.stjornarradid.is/library/04-Raduneytin/Felagsmalaraduneytid/Vi%C3%B0horf_%20til_innflytjenda_september_2019.pdf [Accessed 30 April 2020].
5 All information of the Civil defence regarding the pandemic is published on www.covid.is

6 In Icelandic, the phrase is 'Þetta reddast', meaning it will all be ok in the end or sort itself out. Many immigrants find this mentality at the same time very irritating and fascinating as it includes a belief that you can somehow pull off all kinds of things without any planning. The mentality might be a small population syndrome if you could say so. If things had to be sorted out the experts might not necessarily be at hand so those who were there would figure it out and solve the problem with a group effort.

7 Not to emphasise the percentage, the idea of Dale's Cone of Experience is that how much information we remember depends on the method used. Reading is considered less effective than hearing and seeing the information. By doing we are considered to remember the most. See various information on Dale's Cone of Experience: https://www.qscience.com/docserver/fulltext/qproc/2015/4/qproc.2015.elc2014.6.pdf?expires=1591381323&id=id&accname=guest&checksum=00C77A8E733DC9B10771CC022064AD4C

8 The English video is available at: https://www.youtube.com/watch?v=NM7F0IWyslI, other languages were Arabic, Farsi, Russian, Spanish and French.

References

Davis, B. and Summers, M. (2015). 'Applying Dale's Cone of Experience to increase learning and retention: A study of student learning in a foundational leadership course', *QScience Proceedings*, 2015(4), p. 6.

Félagsvísindastofnun Háskóla Íslands. (2019). 'Könnun á viðhorfum almennings til innflytjenda og fjölmenningarsamfélagsins' [online]. Available at: https://www.stjornarradid.is/library/04-Raduneytin/Felagsmalaraduneytid/Vi%C3%B0horf_%20til_innflytjenda_september_2019.pdf [Accessed 29 April 2020].

Icelandic Tourist Board. (2020). 'Total Number of Foreign Tourists', *Icelandic Tourist Board* [online]. Available at: https://www.ferdamalastofa.is/is/tolur-og-utgafur/fjoldi-ferdamanna/heildarfjoldi-erlendra-ferdamanna [Accessed 30 April 2020].

Information on COVID-19 and vaccination in Iceland [online]. Available at: https://www.covid.is/ [Accessed 29 April 2020].

Red Cross. (2020). 'Information for asylum seekers in Iceland – Covid19', online video, YouTube, https://www.youtube.com/watch?v=NM7F0IWyslI [Accessed 28 April 2020].

Statistics Iceland. n.d. [online]. Available at: https://statice.is/about-statistics-iceland/ [Accessed 25 April 2020].

19

JUST WAFTING BY…

Gitanjali Joshua

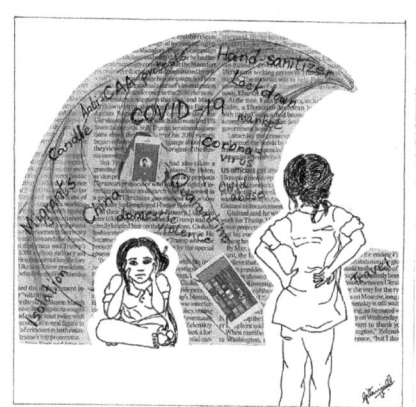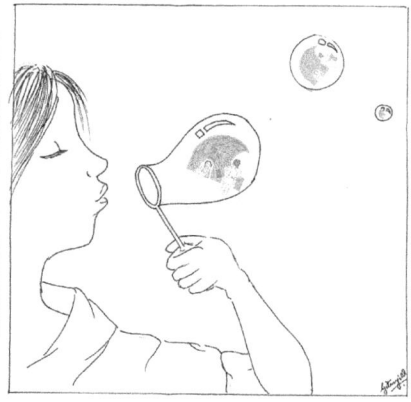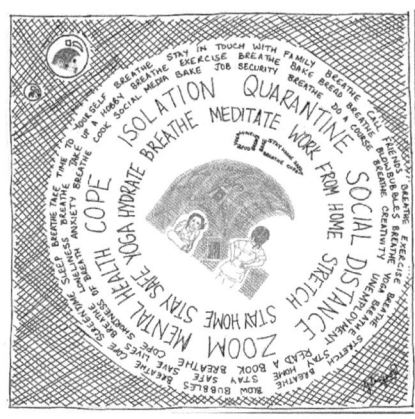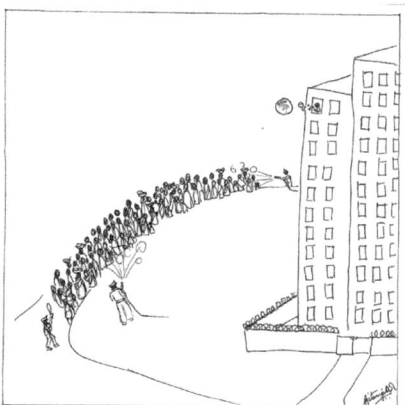

Artwork 19.1 Just Wafting by… (Panel 1).

DOI: 10.4324/9781003320524-25

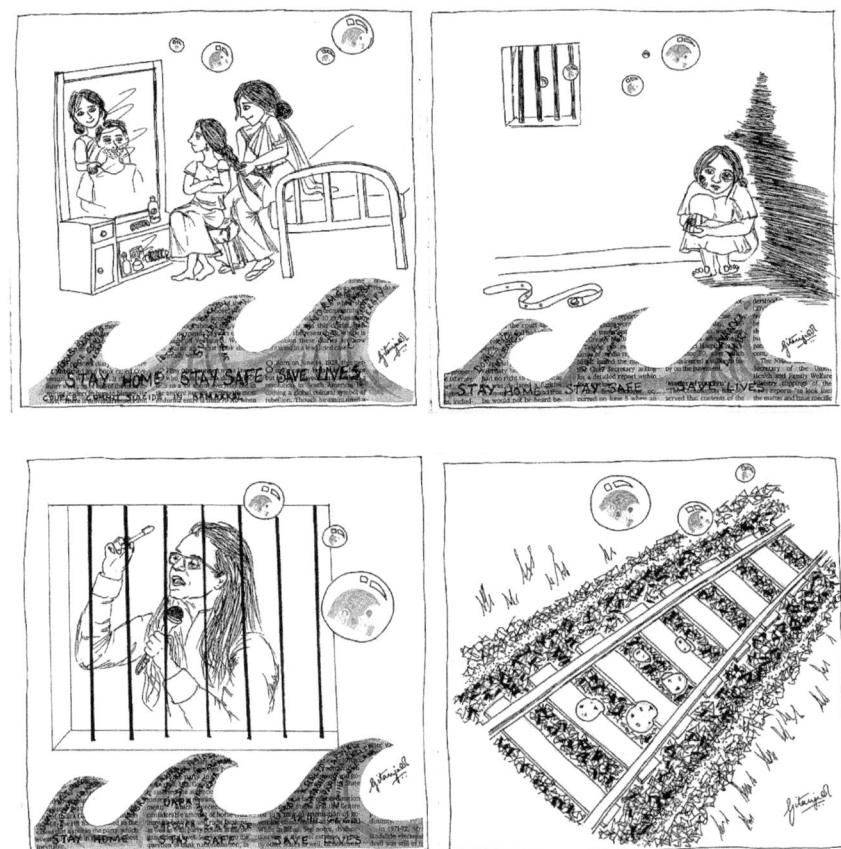

Artwork 19.2 Just Wafting by… (Panel 2).

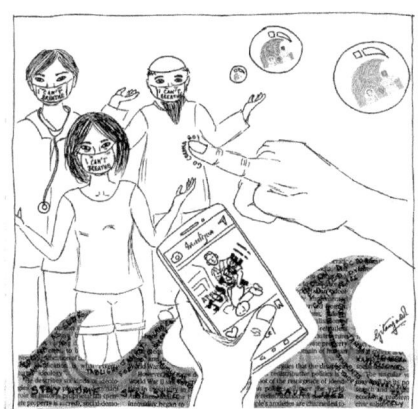
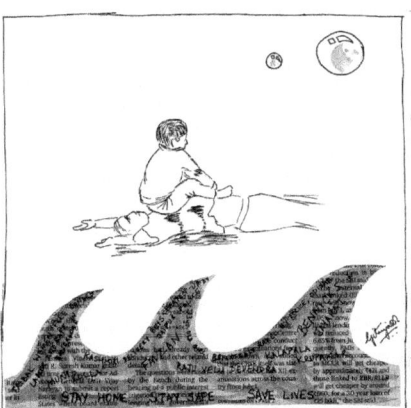
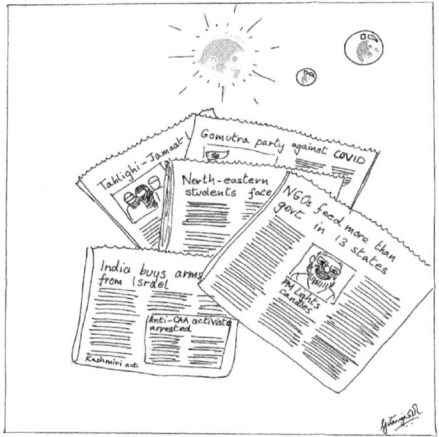

Artwork 19.3 Just Wafting by… (Panel 3).

20

RE-IMAGINING INDIGENOUS KNOWLEDGE IN POST-COVID-19 SOCIAL WORK IN UGANDA

April 2020

*Sharlotte Tusasiirwe, Laban Kashaija Musinguzi,
and Boaz Kukundakwe*

Introduction

The first case of Covid-19 in Uganda was confirmed on 21 March 2020. Like most countries in the world, Uganda introduced a series of strict lockdown measures to stem the spread of the pandemic. While some of the measures such as the closure of schools and places of worship, restrictions on movements in addition to general recommendations such as hand washing, social distancing, and staying at home helped to slow the spread of Covid-19, these measures did not completely stop the spread of the virus. Uganda had a recorded cumulative total of 36,407 cases and 290 confirmed deaths by 8 January 2021 (MoH 2021). The justification for the strict lockdown measures included saving people's lives and preventing a total collapse of the healthcare system. Information reported in the Ugandan media, however, suggests that the measures have created untold suffering, including escalation of gender-based violence, loss of livelihoods, mental distress, child abuse, and loss of lives due to other non-Covid diseases (Musisi 2020; Sali 2020; Twinomujuni 2020; Waiswa 2020). While the evidence shows that Covid-19 is a public health crisis of significant magnitude, it is also clear that Covid-19 is as social as it is biomedical. For example, some of the Covid-19 control measures, such as social distancing and regular hand washing, are all more social in nature than biomedical interventions. Besides, most of the effects of the Covid-19 response measures are largely social in nature than biomedical. For example, reports suggest that prolonged lockdown, restrictions on movements have resulted in increased cases of domestic violence, child abuse, and mental and emotional stress, among others (Musinguzi et al. 2021). Some of the other social effects reported in the media include increased cases of teenage pregnancies and child marriages (ibid).

DOI: 10.4324/9781003320524-26

It has been reported that over 2,372 girls became pregnant during lockdown while 128 girls were married off in the Ugandan districts of Kitgum, Ngora, Kyegegwa, Kasese, and Lyantonde (Daily Monitor 2020).

In response to Covid-19, several actors including social workers have, through art, music, dance, drama, and Indigenous practices, devised various means and ways to cope, educate, and manage Covid-19. In this chapter, we draw from two examples of Indigenous knowledge and practices called Ryemo Gemo among the people of Acholi in Northern Uganda and the artwork from a local artist drawn in the middle of the pandemic (January–April 2020) when everything had come to a standstill due to the strict lockdown measures imposed by the government. Through art and Indigenous knowledge and practice, we seek to demonstrate how local people are (re) shaping, re-imagining, and reconceptualising the intersections of emergency thinking, illness, wellbeing, and Indigenous knowledge in Uganda. Strong and culturally relevant post-Covid-19 social work in Uganda lies in utilising these often-neglected Indigenous knowledge, practices, and art.

Coronavirus Pandemic in Uganda: Through the Lens of an Artist

Art can be a powerful visual communication tool. Contemporary artists in Uganda have, since the pandemic, created art that responds in many ways to the Covid-19 pandemic. Among the artists using Art to respond to the pandemic is Cliff Kibuuka, whose recent exhibition at Umoja art gallery titled UGA-CENTRIC was conceived out of the pandemic (Muwanguzi 2020). Reflecting on what happened during the lockdown when everything came to a standstill, some of Kibuuka's paintings such as the "Home Sweet Home Series (Covid-19)" 2020 (Muwanguzi 2020) communicate a message of hope, as opposed to the gloom that people were accustomed to seeing on television sets and listening to on radio about Covid-19. Therefore through art, artists can relay local realities and enable people to understand what is at stake. As Nabulime and McEwan (2011) observe, art has the "capacity to move beyond the spaces of galleries" into the social. In this section, we will explore three artwork pieces developed by one of the authors, Boaz Kukundakwe, as part of his work as an artist. They document the story about Covid-19, the feelings, emotions, its impact, and how governments and communities have responded to it. The use of Boaz's Art pieces is therefore illustrative of what local artists have been able to do in Uganda to express what the Covid-19 pandemic means using visual communication.

In Artwork 20.1, the artist uses the analogy of the eagle to represent the monster-like coronavirus attacking and killing people worldwide. Coronavirus is like the eagle with its sharp talons, which attacks and devours the chicken and its chicks. The face of the virus is tough, with wide eyes. It is ugly, salivating, and ready to attack whoever is exposed to the virus. However, the virus is in chains, with a padlock, representing the different strategies used by

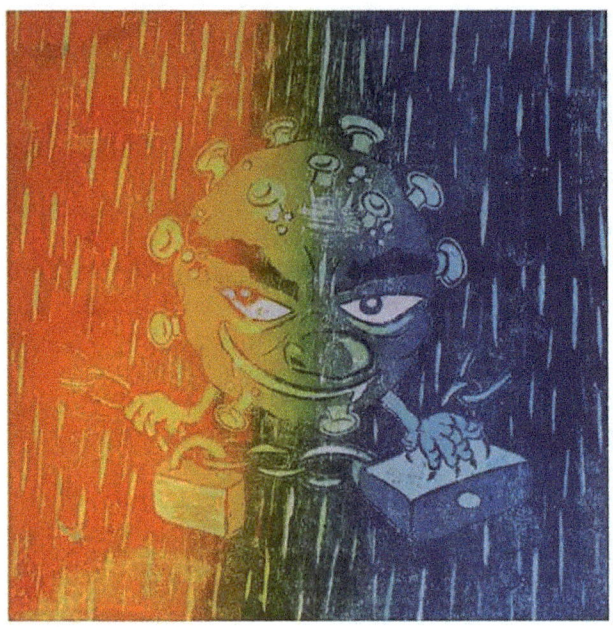

2/4 'Lockdown' woodcut print. Booz K, '20

Artwork 20.1 Lockdown!

countries like Uganda to contain the virus including lockdown, quarantine or self-isolation, and closure of borders. These strategies have resulted in positive and negative impacts represented by the different sides of the art piece in different colours. The piece sends a clear warning to the public to practice measures put in place by the government of Uganda through the Ministry of Health to avoid the spread of the virus. While the virus is depicted as that which can fly, it is also depicted as containable. Artwork 20.2 titled Together in Adversity articulates the impact of the virus and the strategies adopted.

Artwork 20.2 represents the furious and scary coronavirus on the right, which is vividly posing a great threat to the figures in the centre, who seem to come together by an 'invisible force'. Close to the virus is the savings box. The savings box represents a popular economic empowerment program known as village savings and loan association (VSLAs) in several African countries (Musinguzi 2016). VSLAs are popular because of their potential to increase financial access and livelihood improvement for the poor (ibid). Therefore, the savings box placed next to the virus in artwork 20.2 depicts the economic impact of the pandemic on the livelihoods and incomes of people. With the sudden loss of employment and closure of businesses for the self-employed, people have been forced to rely on their savings. With the extended lockdown in Uganda that has gone for over three months, the limited savings for some have been depleted, leaving individuals and families, especially in urban areas like Kampala, struggling to provide the basics

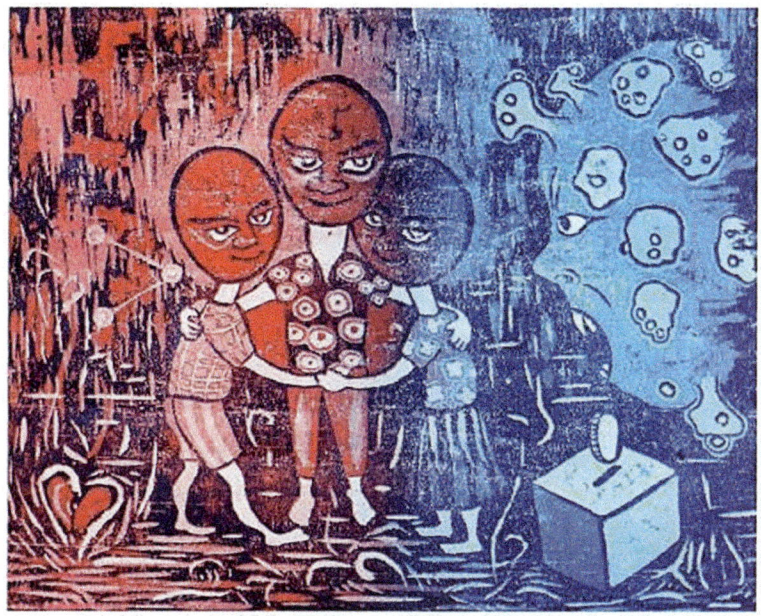

2/4 "Lessons for Humanity" Woodcut Print Betz K. '20

Artwork 20.2 Together in Adversity!

for themselves and their families. Nuwagaba (2020) argues the pandemic has seen the low-income population struggle to pay rent, cover utility bills, and even afford food. There are also cases of people who live by the day translated in the local language as *Zenkola Zendya* (hand-to-mouth), who have been impacted severely by the lockdown and stay-at-home restrictions. This category of people includes taxi operators, market food vendors, and motorcycle taxi operators (locally known as bodaboda riders) casual labourers, including people who earn a livelihood through carrying heavy loads for people in town and markets, among others.

Consequently, the pandemic has also sparked conversations in the community about the importance of saving for future emergencies but with the majority struggling to survive by the day, the possibility of such saving remains a dream for many. In Artwork 20.2, people have been drawn close to each other to represent the time families are spending with each other during the lockdown. Children have been sent home from schools, their parents are not working or working from home, and therefore for some families this has meant time spent bonding and building relationships. For other families, however, spending time together amidst livelihood anxieties caused by the lockdown has resulted in increased anxieties, and cases of domestic violence have escalated (Musisi 2020).

Families and communities have not been just passive victims of the pandemic. As Artwork 20.3 below illustrates, individuals and communities

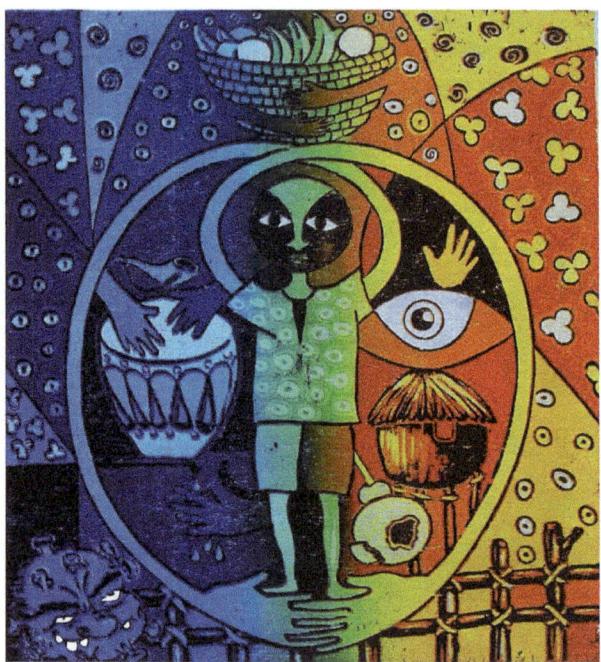

1/4 "Crisis in my eyes" Woodcut Print, Boaz Kukundakwe '20

Artwork 20.3 Crisis in My Eyes!

have not only drawn on their Indigenous knowledge, philosophies, and practices to spread a message about the pandemic and how to prevent it but to also support each other in the communities. Most notably, local communities have drawn on their Ubuntu values of compassion, sharing, and caring to support those struggling (Nussbaum 2003; Mugumbate and Nyanguru 2013; Tusasiirwe 2020). As we will discuss later, communities have also drawn on their Indigenous practices like Ryemo Gemo to work together to alert the community about the pandemic (Awany 2020).

Artwork 20.3 presents a person in the centre appearing seemingly helpless and enclosed by the hands on which he/she is supported. The hands of the human figure join each other in a way that suggests the Ubuntu collective way of being, the unity, and cooperation needed to endure the pandemic (Tusasiirwe 2020). In most parts of Uganda, placing hands over the head depicts an overwhelming situation to the extent of almost giving up. However, in this art piece, the hands are providing support. It is on the hands that the person is standing. When information about Covid-19 became more available, people were told to regularly wash their hands and not touch anybody with unwashed hands. This art piece shows that taking care of your hands becomes a protection against Covid-19. Therefore instead of giving up by wrapping hands over your heads, the artists here show how hands can be

170

supportive or protective against Covid-19 if they are washed regularly. The hands also represent the Ubuntu value of mutual help, which is needed more than ever before given the challenges posed by the pandemic, in particular the sudden death of people and the loss of livelihood, among others. These challenges require putting in practice the *Runyankole/Rukiiga* proverb of *Agetereine nigo gata iguufa*, which literally means that through concerted efforts of people working together impossible issues like this pandemic can be overcome. We draw on a case example of a concerted effort by communities in Northern Uganda, who have drawn on their Indigenous practice of Ryemo Gemo to alert communities to work in solidarity against the pandemic.

Indigenous Practice of Ryemo Gemo and Covid-19 Response

At the beginning of the Covid-19 measures in Uganda, the Acholi and Luo communities in Northern Uganda drew from an Indigenous practice 'Ryemo Gemo' to sensitise and mobilise communities. Ryemo Gemo is a practice based on a long-held belief system, which means noise making (Mao 2020). It is a ritual done when there is an illness in the community that is categorised as a killer pandemic (Gemo). On 31 March 2020, Acholi people in northern Uganda banged jerrycans, containers, saucepans, and drums, making a tremendous noise to drive out the coronavirus from the community (Awany 2020). As Mao (2020) explains:

> When Gemo (evil spirit, pandemic) is identified, the family is supposed to do at least the following; isolate the patient in a house at least 100m from all other houses, with no visitors allowed; a patient is cared for by a survivor of the disease or an elderly woman or man; two long poles of elephant grass are erected at the door to identify a house with a patient and notify those approaching; movement is restricted, people stay within their household; no food from outsiders is allowed; pregnant women and children are given strict instructions to avoid contact with patients; household members are encouraged to live harmoniously with each other, avoid harsh words or conflicts within the family; sexual relations are to be avoided; dancing is not allowed; smoked meat may not be eaten, save for fresh cattle meat; a survivor is expected to remain in isolation for one full lunar cycle before moving freely in the village, and; a person who dies of Gemo is buried by a Gemo survivor or a person who has taken care of several sick persons and not become ill; the burial takes place at the edge of the village.
>
> (Paragraph 2)

There is also a spiritual aspect to this practice where before daybreak, participants of Ryemo Gemo in the community bang any object that can bring out a loud sound and chant *wang ceng ote ci ote* (may the rising sunset with this epidemic) (Mao 2020). Similar practices have existed in other parts of Uganda. For example, the practice of banging, making a loud noise to alert, awaken, communicate, and heal the community can also be related to the drumming of a specific drum called "*Gwanga Mujje*," among the Baganda of central Uganda. According to Wamala (2014), the drumbeat *gwanga mujje*, communicates doom. The drumming serves as a critical call communicating togetherness against and during calamities such as Covid-19. Just like Ryemo Gemo, the *gwanga mujje* drum beat is used to transmit a signal against a catastrophe that calls for coming together. As Wamala (2014) observes, through such practices, communities were mobilised and rallied against HIV and AIDS. The drumbeat was used to create awareness about a terrible catastrophe that everyone needed to band together, and the Ugandan government succeeded in informing the country that HIV and AIDS were destructive forces (Wamala 2014). Also, as was noted in the case of Ebola, historically, such rituals have been instrumental in the face of epidemics (Hewlett and Amola 2003; Kinsman 2012). In all, practices like Ryemo Gemo and Gwanga mujje are used to chase away a disease associated with bad spirits but are also a tool used to raise awareness of the bad elements of the disease and as a tool for community mobilisation. These are locally grown responses that resonate with the context and are clearly understandable to the local communities practising them.

However, such Indigenous practices are often dismissed, both by biomedical practitioners in the Uganda Ministry of Health, policymakers, and sometimes religious leaders, calling it witchcraft that is ineffective in combating such calamities. For example, in the case of Ebola, Kinsman (2012) reports how the famous Roman Catholic clergy had visited the affected villages telling people "to ignore such witchcraft." In the case of Covid-19, President Museveni of Uganda during his address to the nation criticised the Acholi people for not respecting public health directives to contain the virus (Awany 2020) and sent one of the Ministers to talk to Lawirwodi (paramount chief) of Acholi, Rwot David Onen Achana, and ask him to ban the practice (Mao 2020). Response from communities tends to be misinterpreted, ignored, and marginalised, as the focus is mostly placed on top-down responses from government, international organisations like the World Health Organisation (WHO), and scientific experts, among others. Post-Covid-19 needs to teach us that pandemics like coronavirus are as social as they are medical, and recognition and integration of local communities' responses and knowledge may help in managing them in much better participatory and non-colonising ways.

Although Indigenous practices are under attack and reducing in their performance, with the coronavirus pandemic, we have seen reclamation of such practices, including artists coming up with music and songs, using traditional instruments and Indigenous languages to mobilise communities about the pandemic. It is through such practices that people recognise the seriousness of the message and are able to internalise it.

Music and Covid-19 Response in Uganda

There has been a surge in music and songs developed by Ugandan musicians to communicate messages about the pandemic, its symptoms, and how to prevent its spread, among others. Most notable are songs developed by popular musicians like *Corona Virus Alert* by BobiWine and Nubian Li[1], *Corona distance* by Bebe Cool[2], Katonda Yekka Ku Corona[3] (God is the only answer for Covid-19) by Pastor Frank Kyeyune, and one by Dickens Ahabwe[4] about Covid-19 played in one of the local dialects called Runyankore using the traditional music instruments known as Enanga. These songs did not only spread a message about the virus, they also demonstrated the importance and significance of Indigenous languages in the communities. A mixture of languages including Luganda, Lusoga, and Runyankore are used to widen the audience who may be excluded from guidelines using only English, for example, the communications from WHO and also some of the addresses from Uganda's Ministry of Health, which predominantly use English. The downside, however, is that while some songs are rich in contextual information, use of local languages and metaphors is deeply embedded in local experiences; some of the concepts used even though translated in local languages appear to reinforce or communicate the WHO and Uganda's Ministry of Health (MoH) messages. While some of the concepts like social distance appear alien to some people, musicians tend to use them to fit within the framework that has been constructed by biomedical knowledge within the precincts of western hegemony.

Western Enlightenment, Colonisation, and Indigenous Knowledge and Practices: Social Work Reflections

When communities participated in Ryemo Gemo, several critics attacked the communities, and their representatives like Members of Parliament, to explain the demonic practice their communities were engaging in. Indeed as Mao (2020) argues, the critics of Ryemo Gemo are those embodying "the neo-colonial mentality of the culturally alienated African petty bourgeoisie – the intellectuals and political leaders of Africa" (Paragraph 5). Although the global social work definition acknowledges that social work is underpinned by theories of humanities and Indigenous knowledge, there has been neglect of these very areas in social work in Uganda and globally. "Part of the legacy of colonialism is that Western theories and knowledges have been exclusively valorised, and indigenous knowledges have been devalued, discounted, and hegemonised by Western theories and knowledge" (IFSW 2020, knowledge section). Indeed, as authors of this chapter, we have had conversations about Indigenous knowledges, practices, and languages, and we have stated that this is everyday knowledge that resonates with people's everyday practices but remains marginalised in responses to pandemics, where the focus is mostly put on top-down responses from government, international organisations like WHO and UN, or scientific experts. The voices, knowledge, and experiences of local communities are ignored and at worst demonised and dismissed as primitive ways of responding to the pandemic. The way that international organisations like WHO disseminate their messages or at least how it is received by some of the elite or governments in the Global South is as if the messages are universal and are cast in stone. Little if any effort is made to engage with the local community to come up with local understanding or local approaches and practices that communities are most familiar with. Studies (Gilmore et al. 2020) have shown how lack of involvement of communities stifled effective response to COVID-19 in several countries. As the world grapples with Covid-19, it is important to start to rethink these processes.

The explanation for the valorisation of western approaches and knowledges while Indigenous knowledges and practices are devalued is the legacy of colonisation and the ideology of the colonised who have come to believe that their ways of being and doing are 'primitive' 'backward' 'demonic'(words used by the coloniser).

Concluding Remarks

In this chapter, we have highlighted the role of creative arts and Indigenous practices in mobilising communities and communicating critical messages during the pandemic. Music and song remain an important part of the lives of the communities we work with in Uganda. Communities love music, dance, songs, and other creative forms of expression. Through songs, people learn, tell stories, show love, sorrow, heal, laugh, mourn, uplift, and pass secret messages to each other (Wenje et al. 2011). As Wamala (2014) notes, the use of the *gwanga mujje* drumbeat is not only deeply rooted in local communication culture, communities also recognise the seriousness of the messages with little persuasion. The visibility of the role of music, song, Indigenous languages, and instruments demonstrates their significance in the communities.

Therefore, in re-imagining post-covid-social work, social work educators need to find ways to support their students to develop skills in creative and performative arts since these are channels accessible to the communities. For example, the Department of Social Work at Makerere University has been working with students to develop small but relevant skits on Covid-19 response. These skits have been shared on social media platforms, such as Facebook and Twitter. In the spirit of interdisciplinary learning and teaching, it is also possible for the Department of Social Work to partner with the Department of Music, Dance, Drama, and Art at Makerere University and beyond to allow students to learn skills to develop creative art skills along with social work skills. Songs could be used in an emancipatory way to raise issues impacting communities and to find ways to address them. In most of these songs, it is individual artists who have developed songs; where they have worked with others, it has been a collaboration with other artists. Given the collective way of being among Ugandan communities, a more community participatory approach, where community members are engaged in the development of the songs and other creative arts may be a more community engagement approach that social workers can facilitate. Communities can be facilitated to draw on their talents and strengths such as Indigenous language to advocate for change. The use of songs and other oratory skills to facilitate change is not new in Uganda and other African countries, which are predominantly oral societies. The role of creative arts as a behavioural change communication tool in addressing the HIV/AIDS pandemic in Uganda has been documented. In particular, the role of songs by Ugandan artists like Philly Lutaya, who admitted publicly to having HIV/AIDS and began singing songs to raise awareness about the disease and how to prevent it (Bastien 2009).

The use of Indigenous modes of communication like dancing and singing has been explored (Wenje et al. 2011; Wamala 2014). Bastien (2009) explores why songs developed by local artists in Tanzania were effective in spreading awareness about HIV/AIDS and its prevention: the songs were rich in contextual information, used local language and local metaphors, and were deeply embedded in local experiences. In re-imagining the use of songs and creative arts in a more contextually relevant way, the need to engage the communities targeted to come up with messages to be included in songs that reflect the daily life realities in the communities might be one way to effectively utilise this familiar and culturally appropriate communication channel.

As social workers (Twikirize and Spitzer 2019; Tusasiirwe 2020) have argued, Indigenous knowledge and practices although critical in our communities are yet to survive the onslaught of oppression, hegemony, and arrogance of former colonisers and African elites. Indeed, as seen in the critics of Indigenous practices such as Ryemo Gemo discussed earlier, we can allude that some of the African elites remain representatives of colonisers, and therefore, to reclaim the value of Indigenous knowledge and practices, decolonisation of the mind and our leaders must take place. As we have seen, the struggle for decolonisation is more evident in the current pandemic. For example, while some music and songs produced by local Ugandan artists depict a lot of local experiences, it is not difficult to see the struggle they face to completely shade off the influence of western hegemony in the form of WHO and Uganda's Ministry of Health messages about Covid-19. This hegemonic power is hidden in the name of providing the so-called standard message to all communities, which push artists to "conformity" with the "standard messaging." Artists have also been "forced" to use concepts such as social distancing, which makes one question the reflection the songs have about the dream of social distancing in the crowded slums in Kampala, which comprise an audience of such songs. Reference to the use of sanitiser for hand hygiene is even stranger, especially for the biggest part of the audience who may have never heard or seen or could even afford sanitisers. However, as we noted above with Ryemo Gemo, where the practice was denounced as demonic, in the wake of Covid-19, such contradictions also appear to present opportunities to revamp the debate about indigenisation and decolonisation. We view decolonisation in this context to mean that the colonisers and colonised begin to question and challenge the dominance and imposition of western enlightenment worldviews and ways of being and doing while devaluing and marginalising Indigenous knowledges and practices.

A decolonised response to a pandemic puts at the centre local or Indigenous people's knowledge, practices, and worldviews. It works in collaborative and dialogical ways with the local communities, where their knowledge is not demonised, as foreign knowledge becomes imposed as the only right way of responding to the pandemic. Decolonisation includes disrupting the colonial thinking among the critics of Indigenous knowledge that Indigenous knowledge and practices are inferior. The pandemic is a challenge to social work to rethink its neglect of the creative and performative arts, in particular, music and songs, which remain as channels accessible and culturally appropriate to our communities. For social workers in Uganda, Covid-19 should be seen as an opportunity to disrupt the legacy of colonialism that devalues locally available knowledge and practices and enhance interdisciplinary learning and teaching..

Notes

1 https://www.youtube.com/watch?v=PUHrck2g7Ic.
2 https://www.youtube.com/watch?v=DOmAncrXRvM.
3 https://www.youtube.com/watch?v=HXwvhpjqc0o.
4 https://www.youtube.com/watch?v=tdc5GxMixhM.

References

Awany, J. (2020). 'Traditional and community engagement is crucial for fighting epidemics like COVID-19', *LSE Firoz Lalji Centre for Africa*, 19 May [online]. Available at: https://blogs.lse.ac.uk/africaatlse/2020/05/19/uganda-community-engagement-and-traditional-practices-are-crucial-for-fighting-epidemics-like-covid-19/ [Accessed 24 May 2020].

Bastien, S. (2009). 'Reflecting and shaping the discourse: the role of music in AIDS communication in Tanzania', *Social Science Medicine*, 68(7), 1357–1360. https://doi.org/10.1016/j.socscimed.2009.01.030

Daily Monitor. (2020). '2,300 school girls conceive, 128 married off during lockdown', *Daily Monitor* [online]. Available at: https://www.monitor.co.ug/uganda/news/national/2-300-school-girls-conceive-128-married-off-during-lockdown-1909280

Gilmore, B., Ndejjo, R., Tchetchia, A., De Claro, V., Mago, E., Lopes, C., and Bhattacharyya, S. (2020). 'Community engagement for COVID-19 prevention and control: a rapid evidence synthesis', *BMJ Global Health*, 5(10), e003188.

Hewlett, B. S., and Amola, R. P. (2003) 'Cultural contexts of Ebola in northern Uganda', *Emerging Infectious Diseases*, 9(10), 1242.

Kinsman, J. (2012). '"A time of fear": local, national, and international responses to a large Ebola outbreak in Uganda', *Globalization and Health*, 8(1), 15.

Mao, N. (2020). 'What would Okot p'Bitek tell Museveni about 'gemo'? (Part II)', *The New Vision* [online]. Available at: https://www.monitor.co.ug/OpEd/Commentary/What-would-Okot-p-Bitek-tell-Museveni-about--gemo--/689364-5522082-4eqi9/index.html [Accessed 3 May 2020].

MoH. (2021). 'Coronavirus (Pandemic), COVID-19' [online] Available at: https://www.health.go.ug/covid/ [Accessed 8 January 2021].

Mugumbate, J., and Nyanguru, A. (2013). 'Exploring African philosophy: the value of ubuntu in social work', *African Journal of Social Work*, 3(1), 82–100.

Musinguzi, L. K. (2016). 'The role of social networks in savings groups: insights from village savings and loan associations in Luwero, Uganda', *Community Development Journal*, 51(4), 499–516.

Musinguzi, L. K., Ssempebwa, J., Ssempebwa, C., Kibirige, J., and Lukungu, B. (2021). The Situation of and Impact of COVID-19 on School Going Girls and Young Women in Uganda. Forum for African Women Educationalists (FAWE) Uganda Chapter.

Musisi, S. (2020). 'COVID-9 and Mental Health in Uganda: How COVID- 19 and the response of the Uganda Government may affect mental health' [online]. Available at: https://www.jasprogramme.ug/publication/covid-19-and-mental-health-in-uganda-how-covid-19-and-the-response-of-the-uganda-government-may-affect-mental-health [Accessed 24 July 2020].

Muwanguzi, D (2020). 'COVID-19 Art', *The Independent News Paper*, 22 October [online]. Available at: https://www.independent.co.ug/covid-19-art/ [Accessed 1 January 2021].

Nabulime, L., and McEwan, C. (2011). 'Art as social practice: transforming lives using sculpture in HIV/AIDS awareness and prevention in Uganda', *Cultural Geographies*, 18(3), 275–296. https://doi.org/10.1177/1474474010377548

Nussbaum, B. (2003). 'African culture and Ubuntu', *Perspectives*, 17(1), 1–12.

Nuwagaba, A. (2020). 'Understanding the impact of Coronavirus', *The New Vision* [online]. Available at: https://www.newvision.co.ug/new_vision/news/1519193/understanding-impact-coronavirus

Sali, S. (2020). 'Covid 19 and Gender: Examining the gender dynamics of Uganda's national response' [online]. Available at: https://www.jasprogramme.ug/publication/covid-19-and-gender-examining-the-gender-dynamics-of-uganda-s-national-response [Accessed 24 July 2020].

Tusasiirwe, S. (2020). 'Decolonising Social Work through learning from experiences of older women and social policy makers in Uganda', in S. Tascon and J. Ife (Eds.), *Disrupting Whiteness in Social Work*. New York: Routledge.

Twikirize, M. J., and Spitzer, H. (2019). Indigenous and innovative social work practice: evidence from East Africa. In M. J. Twikirize and H. Spitzer (Eds.), *Social Work Practice in Africa: Indigenous and Innovative Approaches*. Fountain publishers.

Twinomujuni, B. (2020). 'Covid 19 and the Right to Health in Uganda: Analysis of the National response and its implications for the realization of the right to health' [online]. Available at: https://www.jasprogramme.ug/publication/covid-19-and-the-right-to-health-in-uganda-analysis-of-the-national-response-and-its-implications-for-the-realization-of-the-the-right-to-health [Accessed 24 July 2020].

Waiswa, P. (2020). 'Sexual Reproductive Health and Covid 19 in Uganda: Avoiding the pitfalls of unintended consequences for maternal newborn, child, adolescent and nutritional health in the national response' [online]. Available at: https://www.jasprogramme.ug/publication/sexual-reproductive-health-and-covid-19-in-uganda-avoiding-the-pitfalls-of-unintended-consequences [Accessed 24 July 2020].

Wamala, C. V. (2014). 'Theater, gender, and development: merging traditional and new media to address communication challenges in Uganda', *Signs: Journal of Women in Culture and Society*, 39(4), 866–874.

Wenje, P., Erick, N., and Muhoma, C. (2011). 'Wende Luo (Luo Songs) as an intervention tool in the fight against HIV/AIDS among the Luo of Western Kenya', *Journal of AIDS and HIV Research*, 3(8), 151–160.

21

THE EARTH AND COVID-19

April 2020

Anil Vangad

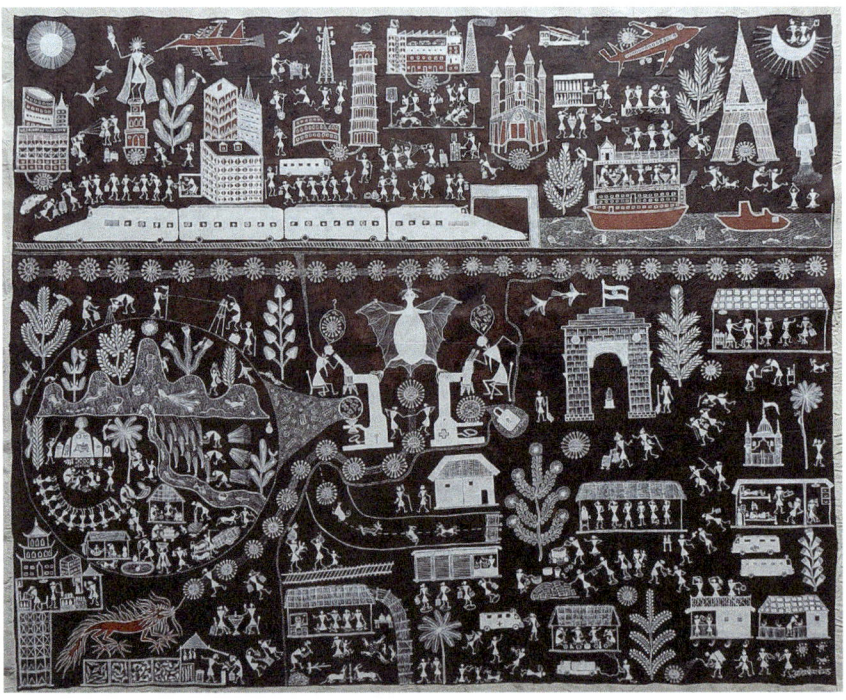

Artwork 21.1 The Earth and Covid-19.

The encircled space at the bottom left corner depicts life before the advent of 'science', when we lived in the midst of mountains, trees, and plants. We depended on farming, worshipped gods, and led simple lives. Gradually, as I have portrayed outside the circle on the top, symbols of 'development' in the form of technological innovations, such as engineering instruments, used to measure land, started appearing. Land became a commodity to be

DOI: 10.4324/9781003320524-27

bought and sold. Above that is the microscope – an unmistakable symbol of 'science'. We increased our knowledge about land and other resources and began exploiting them. I have depicted 'developed' countries such as the United States, Italy, France, and Germany by depicting the share market, train, airplane, tall buildings, rushed pace of life, and so on. We did not anticipate that all this 'development' would lead us to a crisis like Covid-19. In the bottom left corner, I have depicted Wuhan city and its wet market, from where coronavirus seems to have emerged, eventually spreading to the entire world. However, the circle on the left that depicts rural life and the life of yore remained protected from the illness to a large extent. On the right, I have shown how the lockdown wreaked havoc for migrant workers, as they had to walk for miles without any means of transport. I have also depicted how fellow humans offered food to the migrants. The biggest irony in all of this is that coronavirus has forced us to adopt the lifestyle we followed in the past, when we lived in less crowded spaces, ate healthy, home-cooked food, and did not need much to survive.

The text was narrated by the artist in Hindi to Dr. Sandali Thakur who then transcribed and translated it.

QUESTIONING THE 'NORMAL'
AND THE NORMATIVE

22

TO DO IS TO BE?

May–June 2020

Rusham Sharma

In a situation that has left all of us with an atrocious amalgamation of fear and uncertainty looming large in our minds, we are forced to live the present as a period where we are 'doing' to not feel nothingness. 'Present' here, on a very personal note, refers to a period of transition that I am merely 'passing', and 'doing' is distracting myself to retain the satisfactory notion of straightening my spine on the bed. Most importantly, 'nothingness', quite ironically, refers to the erasure of the numbness and hopelessness from my mind. The way we spend this *present* to feel said *nothingness* is inevitably contingent on our mental health and personal backgrounds that are overwhelmed by the stark national socio-economic division operating messily in different spectra altogether.

Each wave of the Covid pandemic in India has struck us with different versions of grief, heartbreak, and wretchedness – collectively rendering us 'powerless'. This grief will soon be documented in WHO reports and national and international surveys with retrospective perspectives of where we went wrong as a people. But as I cope with the anguish of the second wave of Covid-19 in India, I retrospect over a few unresolved thoughts – What could the people of our country have done to alleviate the hopeless anguish of others, as a community? What purpose did this said 'nothingness' serve?

I had been too busy attempting to evoke the aforementioned 'nothingness' inside of me – to actively wash away the wave of ambiguity I used to wake up with, to eat away the wave of ambiguity with breakfast, coerced into doing, coerced into being. My feeling of helplessness was met with the individualistic response of feeling of use, feeling powerful by doing work, by being. I suppose that many of us adopted such individualistic/subjective mechanisms to cope with this unprecedented crisis.

Retrospection is a valuable exercise; it ignites re-imagination. However, I found myself labouring my energy into looking for the cause that led to my individualistic, often denial-inducing, and helpless state of evoking nothingness, prioritising productivity over our collective welfare. Our material conditions and adherence to institutions of authority have unfortunately

DOI: 10.4324/9781003320524-29

driven us towards consumerism, productivity, and hatred towards those who defy or question institutions of power. Why are conventional parameters of productivity determining our worth and response mechanisms to grief on such a global level?

We have been conditioned to believe that life has brought along with itself an instruction manual of 'doing' and 'being' to comprehend where these terms intersect, and how much; how *'doing'* and *'being'* conveniently turns into *'doing and being'* with a coerced ignorance of how it affects lives. We were never given the power to imagine a social order to lead us to the awareness that we have the power to re-imagine it. This exposes a broken system – of our assumed interpretation of community and its welfare, inter-personal relationships, individuals, and the state. No retrospection begins without an examination of the personal. The personal slowly descends to further diagnosis of its relationship with the community and the state.

As an 18-year-old teenager who spends her day in her room attending online classes, a lot of affirmative effort goes into grabbing my rollercoaster moods and taming them to be a merry-go-round of doing work to feel a sense of worth. In a global system that profiteers by overestimating the value of the amount of work done (and undermining the value of labour that goes into), guilt and numbness become a perfect accompaniment to the days left unproductive. I feel powerless with a constant search for the needful mechanisms to do and to keep doing, which can go from sleeping in jeans disconcertingly to getting up out of bed soon after to considerably more destructive ways. The worse thing is that they work. They work by allowing me to feel that my day has structure and time is bound. Being 'normal' has become falling prey to a system that has exploitation as one of its dire consequences.

To tailor my life around this system, I hold myself accountable for functioning as a broken individual who, hence, forms a broken system. I permit myself a disproportionate responsibility of 'fixing myself' that I also inherently link to social morality. This thought makes me think of the same-ness with which my (private) school has been operating in terms of pedagogy and overall environment.

I say same-ness as they fixate on the already-concrete facade of normalcy that people are being forced to co-opt as a 'lifestyle'. Phrases that incorporate the idea of interpreting this pandemic as a *'blessing-in-disguise'* or the *'new normal'* not only take away the seriousness of this situation but snatch the liberty of conceptualising education as a tool of freedom and liberty from those who are engaged in it. It penalises those who fear the future of education by touting them off as unprepared and incapable of the competition that 'awaits' them in life. Listening and questioning are de-legitimised as necessary tools not only to seek learning but to become responsible citizens of a country. I, for one, am always flooded with messages from teachers for updates on the hours of studying I do, on the co-curricular activities I have been doing, on the marks I am expecting in upcoming exams, and on how productive I have been. Consequently, I lose track of the books to be read; experiences to be had; ideas to be explored; and concepts of solidarity and love that I must fail at, process, learn and unlearn, all at the same time. I feel that the system leaves me as a traumatised person attempting to unravel her wasted (non) experiences of adapting to a broken world.

Somewhere along the nothingness of the pandemic, I questioned, just for the sake of general wonderment: What makes the notion of productivity so powerfully cruel that our re-imagination is capable of being curbed? The evolution of this thought led to a rather obvious conclusion – it is not broken individuals that make a broken system full of incompetence. It is, however, a broken system that manufactures broken individuals. This realisation can prove to be a successful factor in comprehending our brokenness, our anger at our unproductive selves, and our compulsion in filling the nothingness of our day with work. Maybe this realisation is a necessary (perhaps successful) effort in trying to pick up our broken pieces and keeping them handy. Maybe a collective realisation among communities or organisations would pump us to arrange such broken pieces of ourselves into life.

When capitalist structures work hard, we lose sight of the obvious, structural nature of this 'brokenness' and link it to us being 'bad individuals' who are lazy, incompetent, disobedient, and defiant. For the sake of humour, I may just say that exploiting us to the level that we feel 'failed' might be the sole thing capitalists work hard at and claim no credit for. We are tamed into believing that people are not positioned according to the structural nature of inequalities in terms of class, caste, gender, etc., but only in terms of 'hard work'. With this over-dependence on 'hard work', we numb ourselves to the complexity of capitalist social systems and dehumanise ourselves by self-blame and categorise our method of work into 'good/bad'. Of course, I am not calling for the absolute giving up of work. I want the option for us, as a people, to be able to avail ourselves the right to rest, grieve, and pause at times of a global pandemic (and otherwise).

Is it too dreamy a vision to have to be able to freely access the broken systems of this world that, in turn, break us? All the 'modern democracies' take pride in claiming to be modelled on a system of simultaneous critique of their actions, exercisable feedback mechanism, and a competent justice delivery system. What we do not hear about are the devious tactics played so cunningly by the capitalist governments that fear us into forgetting, into accepting death, into accepting survival as life. This fear plays out in micro-forms such as the guilt of being unproductive or major forms like the prioritisation of restoring economic gains over living conditions of marginalised people.

It is not us. The global system is broken – by wars that go unnoticed, injustice, imperialist operations, globalisation. Organising ourselves by incorporating ethics of political love and care can turn this upside down.

Is it too unrealistic to dream of a world where we ask strangers, workers, and neighbours how they are doing and pause to hear their answers? Is it permissible to let these Covid-caused deaths be processed, to let this grief bind us, to cry? A world where we read the number of Covid deaths as statistics is already dystopian. As a community, a 'productive' start of our days could be to re-orient our perception that questions our actions – both collective and individual.

We ought to re-envision our community as one that allows us to cope and process instead of accompanying our grief with a repressed fear. We ought to re-imagine a new way of living by never forgetting the course of this pandemic, through retrospection of what our 'normal' has been.

23

THE MYTH OF MAJORITY

Re-imagining Minorities
July 2020

Soumita Basu

Equality is not and should not be based upon what the majority wants; majoritarianism is actually the enemy of equality. However, even the terms 'minority' and 'majority' are ill-defined and used inappropriately to derail conversations on inclusion. Ideally, any discussion on inclusion should not even have a mention of 'majority' and 'minority'. It should be about following the principle of 'no one should be left behind' and carving a potential for good quality of life for all, without anyone having to navigate the 'hindering biases of others'. Yet, experiences of being marginalised are rampant and probably increasing. The ordeal of people with disabilities is only an example of this systematic marginalisation. The global pandemic has highlighted our biases, stereotypes, and tendencies to be discriminatory in our actions, and insensitive in our ideas. The problem often stems from our lack of practice in inclusive thinking in our everyday lives.

Let us understand how marginalisation plays out in reality, using the example of people with disabilities. People with disabilities are usually referred to as a marginalised community. If we go by the official figures, around 3 per cent of the population in India has one or more of the 21 types of disabilities recognised by the Government of India. Many have been advocating for years that there be a proper census of people with disabilities. They are grossly under-documented. First, only people with disability certificates with over 40 per cent disability are counted. Many people who may have a more severe disability are not taken into account, as they may not have registered themselves for a government disability certificate. There are more than 180 million people in India who suffer from arthritis, a recognised disability in India. That itself is nearly 13 per cent of the Indian population.

Second, many painful and crippling conditions like Fibromyalgia,[1] which happens to be the second-most common condition affecting bones and muscles (WebMD), are not recognised by the Indian government as a disability. Urine incontinence, which often restricts a person's outdoor life, is not

DOI: 10.4324/9781003320524-30

considered a disability in India. It affects one in every three women. Most mental health conditions are not considered at all. DALYs[2] is a tool used to understand disease burden and, according to the World Health Organization (WHO), depression-related disorders constitute the second-leading cause of disability in the world. According to a recent *Lancet* article (India State-Level Disease Burden Initiative Mental Disorders Collaborators 2020), one in seven Indians suffers from mental illness.

The Spectrum of Ability and Disability

The World Health Organization (WHO) defines disability using three dimensions: impairment of physical or mental functioning, activity limitation, and participation restriction in normal daily activities – social, professional, or recreational. It is clear from the previous paragraph that a large percentage of the population lives with some or the other disability. At this point, it is imperative to note that disability is not 'black' or 'white'; it is a spectrum. For example, many people wear spectacles due to visual impairment. Not all of them experience total blindness but fall somewhere on the visual disability spectrum depending on the degree of impairment of their eye lens. Similarly, while some suffer from mild depression, others experience a more severe form of it. While some limp because of gnawing knee pain, others have to use a wheelchair because of complete impairment of the lower limbs. It is a common experience of wheelchair users to be looked upon with suspicion if they get up and take a few steps. Many wheelchair users can take a few steps or stand for a few seconds. Just like we do not walk from one end of the country to another and take a vehicle, such wheelchair users cannot walk beyond a few steps and need a mobility aid.

Can we re-imagine ability and disability to say that they are relative? Many rheumatologists and physical therapists with experience in treating patients from South Asia and North Europe consider the average neck and waist mobility of South Asians to be more than that of North Europeans, for example. Another haunting image of normalised 'ability' is that of women in rural India walking an average of 5 kilometres to fetch drinking water. Many well-nourished urban women (or men) in India would not be able to do the same without rigorous training. Ability is a perception. The same woman who walks for kilometres carrying three pitchers full of water for her family is perceived by the society as physically weak. She is often deemed unfit for athletic activities. Carrying pitchers of water, no matter how physically strenuous, is always seen as an act of nurturing the household. And that, of course, is solely a woman's job! The physically strong woman is made to sound like a myth, even as women outlive men in almost all stages (Saini 2020). Shaili Chopra (2020) opines that in popular perception, being strong is being unfeminine. No matter how many kilograms of flour a woman kneads into a dough with her strong wrist, in an arm-wrestling match against a man, she will always be deemed an underdog. Re-imagining notions of ability and disability will help in breaking mental barriers.

If we use WHO's definition of disability, we will see that most people around us live with visible or invisible disabilities. They fall somewhere on the spectrum and are not fully able-bodied (physically or mentally). We will notice many who do not identify themselves as someone living with disabilities. They have normalised their 'disability' and accepted their limitations and restrictions as they are not located at the high end of the disability spectrum. The very extreme of the spectrum are peopled by those with severe disabilities, then there are many with moderate disabilities, then those with mild disabilities, and then again, a few non-disabled or 'fully able-bodied' people.

Look hard at the 'fully able-bodied' people. You will find only a few, very few of them. Now let us imagine them in bright red costumes, while others in grey. This makes them draw and capture all the attention, as the focus light is projected on the space they inhabit. All others do not take our fancy anymore. They are called the minorities. The largest part of the population becomes 'marginalised'.

The ones capturing all our attention are usually fully able-bodied men, mostly young able-bodied men. If participation restriction can be a measure, women often have been disabled by society. They bear the burden of this perceived 'weakness'. The young able-bodied men seem to be at the helm of power. It is this group that holds all decision-making power, implements the decisions in the name of the majority, and normalises traits that only a few enjoy.

Most of the designs around us – clothes, houses, cities – all favour non-disable-bodied young men. All the norms in our communities – in our kitchens, our offices, our schools – have been formulated keeping the experiences of the non-disable-bodied young men as the frame of reference. The architectural designs of our built environment and the practices within them are reflective of this limited perspective. Think of office timings that do not account time for caregiving, norms for personal days at work that overlooks the need for leave during menstrual cycle, pockets in clothes having a gender bias in terms of numbers and functionality, or even lack of adequate lighting on streets and in public toilets. This is no surprise, given that women occupy less than 10 per cent of positions in the top management of the best architecture firms in the world (Terraza et al. 2020). As if everything seems to be made *by* non-disabled young men, *for* non-disable-bodied young men. Participation for all others becomes restricted. Ability, then, can be best defined as a person's position in society, in terms of proximity to power and capacity to draw attention.

Take one of the necessities of life – clothing. Even today, women's clothing with pockets are more an exception than the norm. Men's ensemble always has a pocket, often multiple. Pockets add ease while going about everyday activities. Women's formal clothes, especially Western formals, are far more restrictive in movement and ease than men's formals. All clothes are designed for able-bodied people, celebrating a particular body type – the hourglass shape for women and the well-chiselled straight figure for men. After years of demanding plus-sized clothes, there are a few brands offering them now. Yet, it seems as if little imagination has gone into their design. Most of the plus-sized clothes for women look like merely larger replicas of designs made for petite hourglass-shaped bodies. So many times we have seen a man with a well-grown belly being embarrassed, as his shirt gets pulled around the button closure, displaying the insides! This is a design problem that has very simple solutions, only if adapted around his body shape. Can't someone like him conquer our imagination to be the focus of design?

Frozen shoulder is a very common problem. People struggle to get into the regular clothes available in the market. Dressing up becomes a painful activity. This struggle with dressing up, often giving up one's privacy only to fit into a piece of clothing, is common across people with various physical conditions. Most people with any kind of locomotor or neuromotor impairment (arthritis and shaking fingers are very common examples) take an average of four times longer[3] to dress up than the completely non-disable-bodied counterpart. And these clothes are often oversized to make them a little easier to wear. But then, it becomes difficult to keep them on! Now re-imagine clothes that fit you, instead of you struggling to fit in.

When I started my inclusive clothing brand, Zyenika,[4] many asked me if it was possible to design clothes adapted to people's physical challenges. This, when we have made fabrics of cotton, silk, bamboo, and even charcoal! This, 50 years after we stepped onto the moon for the first time! Why is our imagination so limited? Why do we hesitate to think about a vast majority of our society, who might not be holding positions of power and privilege but are very much part of this world? Zyenika has designed a range of elegant and trendy clothes that are easy and quick to wear, without any pain. I was my first muse and designed clothes adapted to my own severe disabilities. Being thoughtful is all it takes. Creativity usually follows easily; human ingenuity takes a bow.

Being inclusive mandates that we see the needs of everyone. Any blindness-friendly infrastructure like contrasting colours and brighter lights helps people across the spectrum, even if they do not identify as a person with disability. A tactile surface enhances the experience for everyone, including an able-bodied person, not only that of a fully blind person. While the experience of someone totally blind or with severe visual impairment is significantly improved with accessible infrastructure, it is an enhancement for everyone. Now imagine that you have brightened up your infrastructure completely. There may be those who are photosensitive, and a completely bright infrastructure might exclude their participation. Offering them photosensitive glasses might be an easy solution to that. Can we imagine a space where everyone's needs are met? The first step is to *know* everyone's needs. And it mandates that everyone's participation and voice is included. Accessibility is the opposite of uniformity.

Covid-19 and the Invisibility of People with Disabilities

Covid-19 is said to be a great equaliser. Is it really? Has it been able to break the shackles of our imagination and make it more open to difference and diversity? Has it been able to make us re-imagine 'minorities'? Or is it yet another ride, where we are travelling with our eyes wide shut? Possibly, what the pandemic has done is to shake the bubble a bit and magnify the existing inequalities. Yet, it does not seem to have extended our imaginations.

It is universally accepted knowledge that persons with disabilities are more vulnerable to coronavirus than others (MSF 2020), yet no policies have taken their vulnerability into account. Most quarantine centres in India are inaccessible and have a dormitory-style common bathroom, completely unusable for those with disabilities, as has been complained by many on Facebook. Persons with disabilities who need constant physical assistance would not be able to quarantine alone. These issues have been completely overlooked. While physical distancing norms were being prescribed, possible alternatives for those physically dependent on others were not thought about. Many need caregivers for carrying out their daily activities. How can physical distancing be maintained for them? When the lockdown was suddenly announced in March 2020, many people dependent on caregivers – because of disabilities or old age – were left stranded. There were reports of many stuck in their beds, developing bedsores, and of families struggling to meet their basic needs (Malhotra 2020). After concerted advocacy by disability rights activists, the Department of Disability Affairs stepped in, and the government announced special passes for the caregivers. However, by then the lockdown had already been implemented and getting the pass in that situation was extremely difficult for many, if not impossible. Even with a special pass for travel during strict lockdowns, many caregivers could not reach, as public transport was unavailable or Resident Welfare Associations of the residential complexes did not allow them entry. Policies for people with disabilities are either non-existent or an afterthought in India. The cost of knee-jerk reactionary policies in a pandemic situation is human lives.

Getting medical care for any ailment apart from those infected by Covid-19 seemed like an uphill task. This became particularly difficult for those with chronic illnesses. While their health deteriorated and they suffered, their situation was often not considered a 'medical emergency' for the hospitals to take cognisance, as was evidenced by conversations with many people turned away during the pandemic. 'Medical emergency' is a term applied solely to conditions that may be fatal in a span of 72 hours. Deterioration of health to the point of losing the quality of life is not considered medical emergency. People with Thalassemia needing regular blood transfusion found it difficult to navigate to a safe place for the transfusion. Those with spinal cord injuries and chronic pain, survivors of cerebral attacks, those needing physiotherapists, those under post-operative care, and those with kidney disorders requiring regular dialysis stayed in the margins of our imagination during the pandemic. Anoo Bhuyan (2020) reported in IndiaSpend that even though the Government of India issued guidelines about maintaining access to maternal and child health services, dialysis services, blood transfusion, and tuberculosis treatment, people suffering from chronic and non-Covid-19 illnesses around the country have been struggling for healthcare. Regressive conditions regressed faster due to absent medical care or lack of access to the same for non-Covid-19 patients.

Dr. Anubha Mahajan is the founder of the organisation Chronic Pain India, which also has a strong peer support group. She herself needs to be hospitalised every month for the administration of medicines to manage her condition of Complex Regional Pain Syndrome (CPRS). During the lockdown, she fainted a few times due to severe pain. She started to lose mobility in some of her limbs and her speech began to get garbled, as she was not able to access her regular treatment, which included physiotherapy. When she hired a private nurse at home for part of her treatment, her healthcare cost tripled to INR 1.5 lakhs (about 2000 USD) a month. Access to several regular medicines like Hydroxychloroquine (often used to manage autoimmune conditions) and the anti-epilepsy drug Vigabatrin became difficult. Either they were not available at all due to shortage and a focus on exports, or they were being sold in the black market at ten times the cost. For example, one strip of 10 Vigabatrin tablets that normally costs around INR 450 (about 6 USD) was selling at INR 3,500 (about 47 USD) by April 2020 (Bhuyan, 2020).

If your first reaction is that we could not have done better, think again. Volunteers have proved to be the lifeline for people with disabilities as well as senior citizens. Being a more vulnerable group in the context of spread of infection, people with disabilities and senior citizens could not step out for their daily essentials. Volunteers readily brought medicines and groceries for them; a few even got cooked food. An all-India network of volunteers came together via social media platforms such as Facebook and fetched Vigabatrin for a child in Bangalore from parents in Chennai, who shared their son's strip of medicines. Anubha organised online physiotherapy sessions at affordable prices. While it may not be the best substitute for in-person sessions, it proved to be beneficial for many with aggravating pain and other conditions. Such alternatives could have been proposed and enacted by the government. It just needed thoughtful action.

The lack of inclusive thinking was stark in all notifications by the Indian government. No television announcements, including the Prime Minister's live press announcements during the pandemic, were accessible to the deaf community. The only live sign language interpreter for Prime Minister

Narendra Modi's speech on May 12 was so incompetent that the National Association of the Deaf declared that the PM's message was incomprehensible. It has been reported that many deaf people stepped out during the lockdown, as they were unaware of it. Similarly, none of the notifications was accessible to those with visual impairment. The All-India Confederation of the Blind complained that the mandatory *Aarogya Setu* app was completely inaccessible. As digital India grows, it grows without in-built accessibility measures mandated by the Rights of Persons with Disabilities Act (RPWD), 2016.

Amidst the chaos of the pandemic, the government had proposed to dilute the Rights of Persons with Disabilities (RPWD) Act of 2016, by decriminalising minor offences and encouraging out-of-court settlement for many offences against people with disabilities. This proposal arrived on the pretext of 'increasing ease of doing business' (Jurist 2020). Disability rights activist Shampa Sengupta reacted to this on a Facebook post,

> But if penalty clauses are diluted, how will a person with disability demand justice if someone intentionally insults them in a public place? I have personally seen the faces of many disabled people from rural Bengal light up when I read out this clause of the Disabilities Act to them. The majority of them have never heard about the United Nations, but for them, this one clause is a reason to believe that they too can live a life with dignity and urged us to 'ask the Government which business house is finding it difficult to work here because of disability law'.

Not only the RPWD but the Right to Education Act is also being blatantly flouted. School education has been completely shifted online. There have been many reports (Kundu 2020; Mani 2020; Sunil 2020) narrating how children from poorer sections of society are not able to access online education due to lack of access to internet or digital devices. People with disabilities are also excluded from online education for a variety of reasons. Apart from affordability, the websites and apps are not accessible to the blind. There are no systems in place for people who need scribes. While the finance minister mentioned accessibility issues for the blind and deaf in a recent presentation on education, there was complete oversight for students with intellectual disabilities (ANI 2020).

The shift towards a more digital platform for work has been a welcome change for many. Social media has been constantly ringing with posts from people with disabilities about this change. While they were happy with the movement, they also called out the hypocrisy of ableism, as they have been denied such accommodations for years on the pretext that it would be too disruptive. Though this crisis has opened up opportunities for people with disabilities that did not exist earlier due to the resistance of an 'able-bodied' society, an accessible work environment is still a challenge. The pandemic has not been able to make paradigm shifts towards inclusion yet. Online video calls or meetings have become an integral part of 'work from home', and it is not very mindful of people with disabilities. Online presentations are not accessible to the blind. Being on live video might be difficult for people with mobility issues and chronic pain.

It is possible to be mindful of specific needs of people with disabilities and integrate them in our everyday life and work ethic. Rising Flame, an organisation working on disability rights, recently conducted an online writing workshop for a group of women with multiple disabilities. This meant having a live sign language interpreter and a live transcriber, giving the option to participants to talk or type, ensuring every slide or typed communication was read out, and giving all participants the choice of keeping their videos on or not. What stops others from investing in such resources to be more inclusive? Is it the perceived 'value' of the person being included that discourages such investment?

Conclusion

People with disabilities have discussed the merits of euthanasia in closed Facebook groups. Why can they not be made to feel more valued? There are reports from across the globe that doctors are trying to decide who gets to live in the situation where life-saving equipment like ventilator is in shortage. A news report by NPR (2020) from Houston points to the rationing plans by state health officials that exclude some people with significant disabilities from ventilators and other treatment. Prejudices against the community of people with disabilities tend to undervalue them and rip them off their human dignity, a basic human right to life. Can all that life has to offer be assigned a tangible value? Is a person's worth restricted only to their role in the production line? And what if the production line is missing out on talent only because it has closed its doors to some people? What if the production line gained more by placing a ramp instead of a staircase? But really, aren't most things that are cherished fall outside the categories of profit and loss? The very idea of productivity is still entrenched in the perceptions seeded by post-industrialisation thinking, which privileges the number of units produced in a given hour over everything else. It leaves out quality, innovation, creativity, and of course compassion, completely out of the definition of productivity.

We need to re-imagine our world and transform our worldview of the majority. We need to re-imagine a world where it does not matter if one is a minority because there is no such thing. In reality, we are a community of many, many minorities. The idea of the majority is a myth. To re-imagine this, we need kindness and compassion. By definition, certain communities who are pushed to the margins are called 'marginalised communities'. Take a moment, make a note: they are *pushed* to the margins; they don't belong there!

Notes

1 Fibromyalgia is a disorder characterised by widespread musculoskeletal pain accompanied by fatigue, sleep, memory, and mood issues. Available at: https://www.mayoclinic.org/diseases-conditions/fibromyalgia/symptoms-causes/syc-20354780, [Accessed 15 July 2020].
2 Disability Adjusted Life Years.
3 See https://disabilitycreditconsultants.ca/dressing-impairment/
4 See https://zyenika.com/

References

ANI. (2020) 'Visually challenged students, NGOs hail FM Sitharaman's announcements on development of special e-content', *ANI News*, 17 May [online]. Available at: https://www.aninews.in/news/national/general-news/visually-challenged-students-ngos-hail-fm-sitharamans-announcements-on-development-of-special-e-content20200517152613/ [Accessed 5 May 2020].

Bhuyan, A. (2020) 'How healthcare became unaffordable for non-COVID patients during the pandemic', *India Spend*, 19 June [online]. Available at: https://www.indiaspend.com/how-healthcare-became-unaffordable-for-non-covid-patients-during-the-pandemic/ [Accessed 23 June 2020].

Chopra, S. (2020) 'If we think women are physically weak, Haley Shapley breaks the 'rules", *SheThePeople*, 22 April [online]. Available at: https://www.shethepeople.tv/books/if-we-think-women-are-physically-weak-haley-shapley-breaks-the-rules/ [Accessed 12 July 2020].

India State-Level Disease Burden Initiative Mental Disorders Collaborators. (2020) 'The burden of mental disorders across the states of India: The Global Burden of Disease Study 1990–2017', *Lancet Psychiatry*, 7th edn., pp. 148–161.

Kundu, P. (2020) 'Indian education can't go online – only 8% of homes with young members have computer with net link', *Scroll*, 5 May [online]. Available at: https://scroll.in/article/960939/indian-education-cant-go-online-only-8-of-homes-with-school-children-have-computer-with-net-link [Accessed 15 July 2020].

Malhotra, N. (2020) 'Disabled Indians can't be afterthought in Covid. Disability secys needed in all ministries', *The Print*, 25 May [online]. Available at: https://theprint.in/opinion/indias-disabled-cant-be-afterthought-in-covid-crisis/428162/ [Accessed 31 July 2020].

Mani, G. (2020) 'Online classes: Poor students in Delhi struggle due to lack of internet connections', *New Indian Express*, 18 May [online]. Available at: https://www.newindianexpress.com/cities/delhi/2020/may/18/online-classes-poor-students-in-delhi-struggle-due-to-lack-of-internet-connections-2144781.html [Accessed 18 July 2020].

MSF. (2020) 'Inclusion in the time of pandemic: Tools and resources to support an inclusive preparation and response to the COVID-19 emergency', *Medecins Sans Frontieres* [online]. Available at: https://disabilityinclusion.msf.org/COVID-19.html [Accessed 18 July 2020].

Saini, A. (2020) 'The weaker sex? Science that shows women are stronger than men', *The Guardian*, 11 June [online]. Available at: https://www.theguardian.com/world/2017/jun/11/the-weaker-sex-science-that-shows-women-are-stronger-than-men [Accessed 3 July 2020].

Sunil, S. (2020) 'How India's poor students are falling through the gaps as schools go digital', *The Print*, 24 July [online]. Available at: https://theprint.in/india/education/how-indias-poor-students-are-falling-through-the-gaps-as-schools-go-digital/467173/ [Accessed 24 July 2020].

Terraza, H. et al. (2020) *Handbook for Gender-Inclusive Urban Planning and Design*. Washington, DC: World Bank. Available at: https://openknowledge.worldbank.org/handle/10986/33197. License: CC BY 3.0 IGO.

24

COVID-19 AND THE INTERSECTIONAL CONSEQUENCES FOR WOMEN WITH DISABILITIES

Experiences from Sri Lanka
May 2020

*Niro Kandasamy, Binendri Perera,
and Karen Soldatic*

Introduction

On 30 January 2020, the World Health Organization (WHO) declared the outbreak of the novel coronavirus (Covid-19), a Public Health Emergency of International Concern, and shortly afterwards, on 11 March declared the outbreak a pandemic. The WHO has continued to state that the pandemic can be controlled through decisive public health responses. As Covid-19 spreads across the world, researchers are beginning to document the consequences on people's lives politically, socially, and culturally (Jalali et al. 2020). Importantly, governments are being urged to ensure that the public health responses are inclusive of vulnerable communities, including people with disabilities; those living in poverty, women, racialised communities; and those without adequate employment or access to welfare supports (Berger et al. 2020). It is well documented that government control measures are varied in response to preventing the spread of Covid-19 (Satkunanathan 2020). In fact, governments within the Global North and the Global South have shown little consistency in their approach, especially with the shift to the second wave of community transmission of the virus.

In this chapter, we contribute to the growing body of scholarly work that seeks to identify and document the particular experiences of persons with disability, by tracing and explaining the social and cultural impacts of Covid-19 on ethnic minority women with disabilities in rural and former conflict areas of Sri Lanka. At the initial time of writing in late June 2020, there are 1,951 confirmed cases and 11 deaths in Sri Lanka.[1] In what

DOI: 10.4324/9781003320524-31

follows, we expand on the material and social implications of Covid-19 government restrictions in Sri Lanka and provide two case studies of women with disabilities to demonstrate its effects on ethno-religious minority communities. This includes a Tamil woman living with congenital and war-acquired disabilities and a Muslim woman living with a physical impairment. To understand the effects of the public health response, however, we first turn to the nature of political unrest in Sri Lanka that continues to leave minority groups in a position of vulnerability, fear, and uncertainty.

The President of Sri Lanka, Gotabaya Rajapaksa, has stated that the public health crisis caused by the Covid-19 pandemic is unforeseen within the constitution and that there is no other option but to hold the election as soon as possible.[2] The President has been responding to the public health emergency without democratic Parliamentary oversight (Peris 2020). The President imposed an island-wide curfew under the Quarantine Ordinance,[3] and those caught violating the said curfew are being arrested (Chuang 2020). The inevitable result has been a 'doubling of the chaos' by mixing the public health crisis with a constitutional crisis, which undermines the political rights of marginalised communities, who are also highly vulnerable to the worst outcomes of Covid-19, specifically, persons with disabilities and those living with chronic health conditions and illness.

The armed forces have been deployed to track and apprehend individuals testing positive to Covid-19 with minimal protective gear, which has also resulted in a wave of infections within the Sri Lanka Navy (Economynext 2020). These actions depict an ableist approach to the handling of public health measures. Persons with disabilities in Sri Lanka generally face discrimination due to institutional, infrastructural, and attitudinal barriers, which actively deny or undermine the fundamental rights of persons with disabilities (Jiffry and Perera 2018). The militarised national response ignores the necessity for implementing stringent public health protective strategies and reinforces the marginalisation of persons with disabilities, as it places them at greater risk of susceptibility to the virus through the disregard of vital public health protocols with Sri Lankan government's militarised response. The lived experiences of persons with disabilities during Covid-19 continue to remind us of the implications of the state's lack of commitment to actioning socio-legal development and commitment to international law, such as the Sri Lankan Government's ratification of the United Nations Convention on the Rights of Persons Living with Disability (Perera, Kandasamy and Soldatic 2020).

Persons with Disabilities and the Ongoing Denial of Rights and Justice

In 2011, the Department of Census and Statistics recorded that 8.7 per cent (1,617,924 persons) of the total population of Sri Lanka are persons with disabilities, however, the proportion is likely to be higher (DOJF 2017).

There are a range of external factors that have caused physical, sensory, and/or psychosocial impairment (commonly referred to as mental illness) among the population: the three-decade-long armed conflict, uncleared landmines, and natural disasters such as the 2004 Tsunami, poverty, and malnutrition. Our earlier work on the social and cultural impacts of these factors indicates that people with disabilities in Sri Lanka face numerous barriers to their survival and realisation of the political right to participation in society due to stigma, discrimination, and poor implementation of disability policy (Samararatne and Soldatic 2015). The outbreak of the coronavirus pandemic has exacerbated these challenges for persons with disabilities, resulting in their further marginalisation and exclusion from society. As we have identified elsewhere (see Perera, Kandasamy and Soldatic 2020), persons with disabilities face specific challenges during the Covid-19 pandemic militarised curfew, such as a lack of access to essential services, aggravated impacts on economic security due to the inability to engage in work (formal and informal paid employment), discriminatory distribution of government aid packages, ongoing access to education, in addition to public information that is accessible to different communicative strategies of different impairment groups, such as persons who are blind, those who belong to the deaf community, and those who have mobility impairments. Persons with disabilities face a higher risk of poverty and exclusion that can undermine government public health protections aimed at reducing the effects of the Covid-19 pandemic, thus requiring additional and more targeted forms of assistance. These necessary adjustments to ensure that persons with disabilities can fully afford their rights and protections during Covid-19 have not been implemented.

For example, the curfew and resulting limitations on the freedom of movement compelled people to rely on the delivery of essential services to their homes. Moreover, access to medicine through online orders, delivery restrictions faced by rural communities, and long waitlists during the curfew have also aggravated consequences for persons with disabilities, who require prescribed medicine and pharmaceutical products (Ubeyratne 2020). These particular and unique needs to date have not received government attention, hence persons with disabilities have to either place themselves at risk of the virus through attending external medical appointments or endure without these necessary interventions, often to secondary health effects. Also, the government's latest mechanism of allowing persons to go out on different days of the week based on the last digit of their National Identity Card Number overlooks the fact that the majority of persons with disabilities require mobility assistance and support due to inaccessible infrastructure and built environments (News Sri Lanka 2020).

To illustrate the impact of the Sri Lanka Government on the everyday lives of persons with disabilities, the next section of the chapter presents two short case studies of women with disabilities from ethno-religious minority communities who are disproportionately affected by Covid-19.

The case study approach is used to illustrate the heterogeneous effects of Covid-19 and public health responses, by providing insights into the lived experiences of women with disabilities and their actions, strategies, and feelings compelled by the ableist, exclusionary measures. As Mazumdar and Geis (2001: 265) remind us, 'the characteristics, experiences, hopes, and needs of persons with various sorts of abilities and disabilities will not be identical'. These insights are critical to any research that seeks to examine the effects of Covid-19 on persons with disabilities: it is only through careful in-depth analyses, such as the case study approach, that a complete picture can be obtained. The preliminary insights presented next underline the value of this approach. The two case studies are based on women with physical impairments; Nisha has a mobility impairment, and Harini has a physical and sensory impairment. A pseudonym has been used for Harini's name. Nisha explicitly stated that she wished for her first name to be used.

The interviews with Nisha and Harini were collected in May 2020 just as Sri Lanka was implementing a range of Covid-19 restrictions. Our decision to interview the two women was partly shaped by our long-standing connections with them through a larger project that examined their gendered-disability advocacy work in Sri Lanka. The chapter is based on rapid case study interview responses of the two women with disabilities from diverse ethno-religious backgrounds [Tamil and Muslim] and document analysis of newspaper articles and official government statements that were collected during the first few months of the Covid-19 pandemic in Sri Lanka. Investigating the impacts of the unfolding pandemic in the context of militaristic government responses provides the opportunity not only to elucidate individual experiences but also to better understand how government restrictions were affecting women in distinct ways. Because no research was available on this subject in the context of Sri Lanka, we adapted qualitative methods of interviewing to describe the effects of Covid-19 on the two women whose experiences follow. Both of the women reside outside the main urban centre, Colombo, in smaller peri-urban areas with lesser access to resources and services.

Nisha

Nisha, a Muslim woman, is an advocate for the rights of persons with disabilities and President of one of the local Disabled People's Organization (DPO). She is financially independent and runs her own business in the town where she lives. While the Covid-19 curfew has compelled her to remain at her home for months, she opened her business as soon as the curfew was relaxed. She knows that the income from the business is crucial for her to maintain economic security and independence as a woman who is supporting her family and to actively continue her disability advocacy work, which is unpaid. She states that she is following the government's guidelines on doing business during the Covid-19 threat to ensure the health and safety of both herself and her customers.

Nisha arranged for a trishaw to come to the town, to bring her to her place of business in the mornings and take her back home in the afternoons. Persons with mobility impairments have always faced difficulties in accessing public transport in Sri Lanka because the buses have long been unwilling to accommodate their needs or purchase disability-accessible standards and public bus stock. Nisha, therefore, has to solely rely on private arrangements during this period because public transport mechanisms have not operated at all during the pandemic curfew. She had to plan her working hours based on the number of hours the trishaw driver was prepared to remain in the town to wait for her. Nisha states that:

> The time period I can open my shop every day depends on the working hours and trips that the trishaw driver – whom she refers to as a younger brother – would have. Some days I have to close the shop very early. Since the customers get familiarized with my watch only when it is consistently open this is bad for my business. But what else can I do?

While the Covid-19 outbreak affected able-bodied citizens' freedom of movement and freedom to work generally, persons with disabilities faced heightened challenges in moving amidst restrictions and in returning to work. The Sri Lankan government's response to the pandemic has not taken these unique circumstances into account and as a result, this has heightened the economic insecurity of many persons with disabilities already in positions of extreme economic precarity.

Mobility, however, is much broader than economic security. It also impacts access to basic essential goods and services and maintaining critical support in relation to a doctor, pharmaceutical, and general health services. For Nisha, as a result, this has meant reliance on her friends to buy essential items during the Covid-19 curfew, as she could not stand in the queues to enter stores or move swiftly at the temporal rate required to move through the aisles, which are often wheelchair inaccessible, to buy basic necessities within short periods allowed for people to do their shopping. She explains that:

> the shops are crowded when the curfew lifts and there is a lot of jostling. I cannot move to their speed, run around, and get my work done. So, I can only wait in the trishaw while a friend buys my necessities for me as well.

While persons with disabilities were highlighted as a vulnerable category during the Covid-19 period, there were no mechanisms put in place to accommodate and facilitate disabled people to obtain their basic needs.

The Sri Lankan Government's ableist assumptions about individual mobility, bodily movement, and the collective flow of consumer products through central markets and shopping centres always assumed that persons with disabilities were dependent upon others – that is, that family members and informal networks would be willing to take up these responsibilities for family members living with disability.

Nisha's main concern is not herself but the difficulties faced as persons with disabilities collectively, who are forced to rely on the 'goodwill' of others and the types of long-term dependencies this may create. For example, Nisha narrates that she is aware through her advocacy work that there have been numerous instances where persons with disabilities could not access the medicine they needed because pharmacies would not deliver outside a certain radius. She also relates to the difficulties persons with disabilities faced in placing online orders/phone call orders due to their disability and not having access to technology or digital literacy. Nisha notes that many persons with disabilities have been denied access to education and that their access to social and economic opportunities in general diminished, which have been aggravated with the restrictions resulting from the Covid-19 outbreak.

Harini

As outlined through Nisha's experiences above, the public health responses can exacerbate the gendered-disability impacts of Covid-19, while showing individual and collective forms of mobilisation and resistance that emerge in these spaces of exclusion. Similarly, Harini, a Tamil woman, is affected by the government's inadequate responses to persons with disabilities who are living in rural areas with the means and basic necessities to ensure their survival during the pandemic. Harini, who was employed as a shop assistant, was forced to return to her village when the government announced the island-wide restrictions. Persons with disabilities are included in government income payments if they register for the payment. However, this payment is the same as the current disability income payment and, therefore, does not provide additional assistance nor the coverage of income loss persons with disability earn on top of their government monthly disability support payment. Furthermore, the process of registering and receiving the payment is, in itself, inaccessible due to the Covid-19 disruptions in public administration and the associated mobility issues that arise, as outlined above, in attempting to register for the payment.

At the time of writing this chapter, Harini was yet to receive the government's single cash payment of SLR 5,000 (USD 25.00) for persons who are earning a low income affected by Covid-19, despite registering at multiple locations. Like Nisha, Harini refers to the difficulties faced by her peers in accessing the aid packages that are routinely given to persons with disabilities by the Department of Social Services due to inaccessible and exclusionary information communication and coordination shortcomings. Harini explained that she had contacted several government officials to secure financial payments, however, she was unsuccessful at all her attempts. At the time of undertaking this research, Harini had not received government welfare payments since the lockdown period began several weeks earlier. Consequently, Harini relies on her family to support her financially. However, due to the loss of income in the household, Harini's family has been forced to use the home garden as their main source of food and they live without other food staples such as milk powder and eggs. Harini's family has supported her socially and emotionally during the social isolation; she feels energised by the strong family networks that are helping her overcome the distress caused by the loss of income and her feelings of economic insecurity.

The family lives in a rural village where the grocery delivery vans that drive through their village sell food at a higher cost. Moreover, the lack of access to public transport has made it difficult to travel to the town to purchase food items at cheaper, regular market prices. Harini states that fewer buses are operating and due to the strict curfew hours, there are greater risks associated with going to the supermarket and general market that are more susceptible to transmission, as it creates high levels of restricted mobility (The Morning 2020; Gunawardhana 2020). The lack of public transport coupled with the loss of income has forced Harini to reconsider attending her upcoming medical appointments as well. Thus, Harini finds herself at home most days with very little access to the outside world; however, she remains hopeful that she will return to work one day.

Conclusion

There is no doubt that the effects of the Covid-19 pandemic will become clearer as information is gathered about the short-term effects, as this chapter shows, and the longer-term effects on women with disabilities in the Global South. The two short case studies presented in this chapter, about Nisha and Harini, begin to highlight the importance of understanding the intersectional consequences of Covid-19 on women with disabilities. The evidence begins to chart a complex map of the ways persons with disabilities have been forced to negotiate their basic and social needs to survive. In response to the vulnerability facing persons with disabilities across Sri Lanka, Nisha, and other disability community leaders have taken the initiative to engage in collective actions to link the official support mechanisms with persons with disabilities. Nisha speaks with pride about the solidarity and resilience that her disabled community and their advocacy and networks have demonstrated during this emergency period. It is in these moments of rapid collective mobilisation that closer attention is required, not only for witnessing the ongoing failures of the state but for recognising the productive agency of persons with disabilities in redefining their lives during a localised and global crisis.

Re-imagining policy responses to support women with disabilities requires a multifaceted approach to address their needs that have gone unaddressed even before the Covid-19 emergency. Policy makers must give priority to basic demands, such as mainstream disability supports to ensure that all sectors address disability needs, recognise the distinct experiences of women from diverse ethnic backgrounds alongside identifying their daily activity restrictions and associated levels of required support, provide women information in their respective languages so that they can access welfare services, and ensure the inclusion of disability in national agendas that respond to the pandemic. To adopt and implement these responses, however, policy makers must develop grounded knowledge of gendered-disability experiences that foregrounds the lived experiences of the women, thereby avoiding misunderstandings and stereotypes that can undermine disability-inclusive policy responses.

Notes

1 By early January 2021, this number had increased to 6,897.
2 At the time of writing this chapter, the parliamentary election was set for 5 August 2020.
3 While the legality of these regulations was questioned, the Magistrate Court of Gampaha upheld them this week in the case B1108/20 (11.05.2020).

References

Berger, Z.D., Evans, N.G., Phelan, A.L., and Silverman, R.D. (2020). 'Covid-19: control measures must be equitable and inclusive', *thebmj* [online]. Available at: doi: 10.1136/bmj.m1141.

Chuang, N. (2020). 'Here in Sri Lanka 22000 have been arrested for breaking curfew and police are rewarded for their vigilance', *The Telegraph*, 15 April [online]. Available at: https://www.telegraph.co.uk/travel/destinations/asia/sri-lanka/articles/a-postcard-from-sri-lanka/ [Accessed 16 April 2020].

Disability Organizations Joint Front. (2017). 'UN Universal Periodic Review – Sri Lanka 2017. Third Cycle, 28th Session 2017'. Submission for the Review of the situation of persons with disabilities in Sri Lanka. Available at: https://www.ohchr.org/Documents/Issues/Disability/RightAccessJusticeArticle13/CSO/DisabilityOrganizationsJointFrontSrilanka.pdf [Accessed 27 March 2020].

Economynext. (2020). 'Sri Lanka scrambles after Navy Coronavirus cluster than fanned out in curfew, Covid-19 count 619', *Economynext*, 29 April [online]. Available at: https://economynext.com/sri-lanka-scrambles-after-navy-coronavirus-cluster-that-fanned-out-in-curfew-covid-19-count-619-68940/ [Accessed 1 May 2020].

Gunawardhana, T. E. (2020). 'The queuing calamities', *Life Online*, 28 March [online]. Available at: http://www.life.lk/article/latest_stories/The-queuing-calamities/1/19179 [Accessed 8 April 2020].

Jalali, M., Shahabi, S., Lankarani, K.B., Kamali, M., and Mojgani, P. (2020). 'COVID-19 and disabled people: perspectives from Iran', *Disability & Society* [online]. Available at: doi: 10.1080/09687599.2020.1754165.

Jiffry, A. and Perera, B. (2018). 'Status of persons with disabilities in Sri Lanka. Sri Lanka: State of Human Rights 2017', *Law & Society Trust*, 99–136.

Mazumdar, S. and Geis, G. (2001). 'Case study method for research on disability', in S. N. Barnartt and B. M. Altman (eds.), *Exploring Theories and Expanding Methodologies: Where We Are and Where We Need to Go*, 255–275. New York: Emerald Group Publishing.

News Sri Lanka. (2020). 'Permission to go out for essential requirements based on last digit of the ID Card', *Government Official News Portal*, 26 April [online]. Available at: https://www.news.lk/news/political-current-affairs/item/30036-permission-to-go-out-for-essential-requirements-based-on-last-digit-of-id-card [Accessed 29 April 2020].

Perera, B., Kandasamy, N., and Soldatic, K. (2020). 'Sri Lanka's response to COVID-19: militaristic enforcement and its effects on disability', in N. Georgeou (ed.), *State Responses to COVID-19: A Global Snapshot*. Penrith: Western Sydney University.

Peris, H. (2020). 'Nominations close and elections postponed amid Covid-19', *Groundviews*, 24 April [online]. Available at: https://groundviews.org/2020/03/24/nominations-close-and-elections-postponed-amid-covid-19/ [Accessed 30 April 2020].

Samararatne, D. (2012). *Critical reflections on recognising and enforcing disability rights within the Sri Lankan legal framework*, Annual Research Symposium, University of Colombo. Available at: http://archive.cmb.ac.lk:8080/research/bitstream/70130/3375/1/AnnualResearchSymposium2012Universityof Colombo.176-178.pdf [Accessed 8 May 2020].

Samararatne, D. and Soldatic, K. (2015). 'Inclusions and exclusions in law: experiences of women with disability in rural and war-affected areas in Sri Lanka', *Disability & Society* 30(5), 759–772 [online]. Available at: doi: 10.1080/09687599.2015.1021760.

Satkunanathan, A. (2020). 'Justice in the time of a pandemic', *Groundviews*, 29 March [online]. Available at: https://groundviews.org/2020/03/29/justice-in-the-time-of-a-pandemic/ [Accessed 18 May 2020].

The Morning. (2020). 'Pictures: supermarket, ATM queues following the lifting of curfew', *The Morning*, 23 March [online]. Available at: http://www.themorning.lk/pictures-supermarket-atm-queues-following-the-lifting-of-curfew/ [Accessed 29 April 2020].

Ubeyratne, R. (2020). 'Surviving COVID-19: Lankans share their stories', *Pulse*, 3 April [online]. Available at: http://www.pulse.lk/everythingelse/surviving-covid-19-lankans-share-their-stories/ [Accessed 10 April 2020].

EDUCATION

25

THE PRIVATE LIBERAL ARTS UNIVERSITY AND THE PANDEMIC

Some Reflections
March–June 2020

Ridhima Sharma

This is the story of many stories set in a private Liberal Arts University in India. Like any other story, this one is also marked by a time-place specificity, by its here and now. This 'here and now' is historically informed by various factors, some of which are shaped by the move towards privatisation of higher education in India, the proliferation of private liberal arts universities in the country, and the various notions that a liberal arts education comes attached with. I am one of its minor characters, situated in what I view as a 'come and go' relationship with the university, in my capacity as a visiting faculty. Like all other stories then, this one is also a partial, situated, and contextual one shaped by my, the storyteller's, socio-economic location as well as position vis-à-vis the institution.

Those involved in a similar engagement with a university may be familiar with the dynamic of such a relationship. Contract-based, subject to change based on the courses that may or may not be taught the next semester, reliant on a session-to-session payment are common features of this relationship with the university. The payment plays a sizeable role, especially for those who are unable to/do not wish to/are not in the place to teach full-time, for a variety of reasons and are reliant on this 'fee' as their source of livelihood. What also plays a considerable role in this choice, especially for younger research scholars still in the early stages of their career, is the opportunity to engage with students, be able to teach and find its many meanings, joys, and challenges.

In what follows, I describe various facets of the university that I am located in, in an attempt to make sense of how it has been impacted by the pandemic that seems to have shaken the world as we knew it. In doing so,

DOI: 10.4324/9781003320524-33

I am as invested in the university and the space that it was, before the pandemic struck, as I am in the project of interrogating the shifts as a result of the pandemic. If we are being called upon to 're-imagine a new order' in the wake of the pandemic, it is significant to first take stock of the 'old', with all its inadequacies and fault lines. Unsurprisingly then, this moment is marked by an ethico-political charge for those committed to the process of re-thinking the order of things. Writing this chapter is an exercise in this (re)thinking and examining the political and ethical stakes of the university as a space committed to socio-political transformation in the current moment and in the aftermath of the Covid-19 pandemic.

Understanding the University's Texture: Choice, Merit, and the Business of Benign Protectionism

I start the larger story with two vignettes: one as I experienced it and the other as narrated to me by a student. More than a year ago, just days after I had joined the university as a Visiting Faculty, I was told by a senior colleague over a cup of tea,

> This is very different from a public university. You will be expected to be on your toes because the students are really smart and well-read. They are vocal, they ask questions. Teachers can get away with so much in a public university but that would just not happen here!

What confused me then as a bizarre cautionary note to give to a new entrant soon exposed itself as a belief held widely by many at the university – the notion of the university in question as not just built on 'merit' but one that claimed a distinct status from a public university. Having come from a public university that took pride in its rigour and training (and thus had its entrapments of merit), this was telling. As I got familiar with the space, I could not help but wonder if this construction, this manner of declaration of merit, was tied closely with the glaring absence of caste-based reservations in the university.

The second episode revolves around a student's first-hand experience of/ with the university campus when she came to take a 'campus tour' with her family, much before she had applied to the university as a prospective student. As I was to learn later, anyone could 'book a tour' at any point in time (they could be as young as 14!) and be familiarised with its aesthetically appealing campus, 'smart' classrooms, inviting canteens, and a meticulously curated image as an 'open-minded', student-centric, liberal university via an especially appointed 'tour guide' for the job. The student pointed out that she was confused about what to pursue right after school and liberal arts seemed like a good choice, which would provide her with a fair degree of exposure to a variety of disciplines and eventually help her pick an area of specialisation. From my conversations with students, this indeed emerged as the most popular reason for opting for a Liberal Arts degree – choice. As another student said,

> I was baffled at the choices available. These choices were not just limited to the subjects we could study and the combinations we could study them in, but the food we could eat, the activities – sports, cultural events, special kinds of academic projects and peer mentorship programmes that we could have access to. I was over-joyed at the prospect of studying both music and finance. It seemed like a lot of worlds would be open to us!

I open with these two vignettes because they gesture towards what I believe are the two central planks that structure the ethos of the private Liberal Arts university in question – merit and choice. In a special arrangement where academically 'meritorious' students offer services to the university (for instance, as research assistants) in return for scholarships granted to them, one of the roles that a scholarship awardee can take on is that of the guide who provides tours to potential students and their families – the same tour that they would have undertaken before they joined the university. The strategic use of certified meritocracy to bolster the university's claims of offering choice is a specific kind of move that speaks to familiar concerns around the privatisation of education and the neo-liberal forms of governmentality in educational institutions. Those invested in the future of education have been warning us about these for years now. I claim that these two, seemingly innocuous episodes constitute the microcosm of a private liberal arts university. They offer us a glimpse into the material and symbolic practices that shape its space. Let us take the example of what is known as the 'academic fair', an event that I have never experienced but was described to me by colleagues and students. After taking a diverse set of courses in the first year, the students are required to opt for their major and minor specialisations second year onwards. To facilitate this choice, the university organises the academic fair, where various teachers from all disciplines set up stalls in an attempt to 'sell' courses to the students. As part of the event, the students are familiarised with the course outline, structure, and evaluation components, etc., which then become important criteria for their decision-making.

This language of buying and selling education as a service, where teachers and students–parents are enjoined as service providers and consumers has been a significant source of concern for those invested in the future of education. This is the concern, the mortification even, that scholars like Pathak (2019) have described when they look at advertisements of private universities in newsletters of private airlines and marvel at their complete lack of 'hesitation in selling their courses as a product with immense value for the corporate sector'.[1] Pathak (2019) writes:

> The collaboration with 'foreign universities', the 'high ranking' as declared by some agency or the other, the 'international' faculty and, above all, the lure of 'placement and package' – the narratives of these ads suggest that the meaning of education has changed drastically. It seems the emergent middle class – guided by a mix of technocratic rationality and market-driven desires – is willing to buy this sort of education.

While the much-needed unease with the privatisation of education has a long history, I think the current moment of the pandemic has urged or should urge us to refine and push our critique in a manner that takes cognisance of first, our place in the project of the commodification of education, without eulogising the public university and second, the nature of what is being touted as the 'future of education in India'. If liberal education has often been posed as the solution to the 'engineering mindset' (Pathak 2019; Pant 2007), there needs to be a discussion on the character of institutionalised liberal education in India and its self-fashioning as the din of the elite.

In 'An Historical Review of Liberal Education', Hoerner (1970) refers to the haziness of the origin of liberal education, largely on account of a lack of clarity on what exactly constitutes liberal education. Hoerner cites Woodring's definition as perhaps the most useful one – 'It is the education that liberates men from the bondage of ignorance, prejudice, and provincialism. It enables us to see the world whole and to see ourselves in perspective' (Hoerner 1970: 3). He posits that liberal education is notionally at least 2,000 years old, with the imagined subject of some of the ancient philosophers being the 'free man'. The 'free men' then, he adds, were also the leisure class 'trained exclusively in the liberal arts without any utilitarian tinge … trained in the reflexive pursuit of the good life' (1970: 4). The very moment of the inauguration of liberal education, as nebulous as the term may be, has therefore been haunted by the question 'who can afford to do liberal arts?'. This already presents an interesting problem where the pursuit of perspective can be afforded by class privilege. This helps us situate the place of 'merit' and 'choice' in the contemporary institutionalisation of liberal arts.

While this issue is not unique to a liberal arts university, I contend that it is the combination of neo-liberal forces that push for privatisation of education on the one hand and the self-fashioning of liberal arts universities on the other-both inextricably intertwined, that allows for notions of choice and merit to flourish in specific ways. The neo-liberal agenda of profit-making by offering 'more choices' acquires the shape of the 'campus tour' or the 'academic fair' when disciplines have to sell themselves to consumers as the most lucrative, most interesting, and most rewarding choice. A part of this 'selling' includes the need to appeal to various constituencies, of which parents are the most significant. Perhaps, more significant in many ways than the students are the parents who provide the enormous amount of material resources needed for the students to acquire the university experience. It is no wonder then that the university pitches itself to the parents as its primary audience – they are given special attention during the campus tours, informed periodically (every 15 days) about the students' attendance, and kept in the loop in the event of any misdemeanour on behalf of the student. On the issue of excessive parental involvement, a colleague mentioned to me,

> As a teacher, I am uncomfortable with marking parents on every email. I do feel that students are adults and all communication should not have to be routed through their parents. Yet, the university functions in a manner that mandates parental involvement. Since they are the ones paying the exorbitant fee, we have to be accountable to them especially in cases of disciplinary action against the students or say, a change in their scholarship status.

He explained further that a part of the university's appeal to parents is its disciplinary mechanisms that keep students 'in check'. What is seen as surveillance by students is exactly what is sold by the university to the parents as its USP, as its great investment in the lives of the students. This surveillance which often masquerades as benign protectionism manifests in the form of curfew hours, 'raids' of hostel rooms, stringent checks of classrooms, especially post-sunset to check for 'inappropriate' activities, which include public display of affection. In the event of a disciplinary breach, the nature of punishment is graded – starting from being grounded on campus to being suspended or even rusticated.

Anyone occupying an institutional role in a university is likely to be familiar with the negotiations that teachers, students, and various other actors make with punitive norms and processes. What is noteworthy here, however, is the double bind that consistently operates –the presentation of the university as one committed to a 'liberal' ethos in terms of the choices it offers as well as its regulation of the bodies of various actors, notably students. This was stated lucidly by one of the students when she pointed out,

> The university has something for both students and their parents. This university appeals to the sense of propriety and safety, of parents who are reluctant to send their children abroad or even to far-off cities within India. It can give them the correct impression that their children will not be allowed to go awry, while also convincing the students, at least in the beginning, that they will have the choice to lead the kind of lives they will build for themselves. Most of us are happy to grab the chance because we get to stay away from home while also keeping our parents happy.

This sums up how the university can place itself delicately but firmly on the twin branches of discipline and freedom to choose.

And Then There Was the Pandemic...

It is against this context that one must situate the Covid-19 pandemic and its impact on the university. We are in the midst of a moment where universities in India and across the world are being held accountable for leaving students in the lurch whether it is by shutting down hostels, rendering their immigration status vulnerable, or proposing to hold exams during the pandemic.[2]

On 14 March 2020, in the wake of WHO's declaration of the spread of coronavirus as a pandemic, the state and union government issued directives to the Universities. After much speculation on the future course of action by the University's administrative authorities, the students received official communication on the temporary closure of the university. All activity on campus was suspended. In the two days that students had, they packed their belongings amidst understandable chaos and confusion and made the necessary arrangements. Students were advised to leave for their respective homes. Transport facilities to the railway station, bus stand, and airport were provided. Some students were picked up from campus by their parents. It was also recognised that all students, especially those from other countries, would not be able to go home and were allowed to stay on campus with provision for housing, dining, and other essential services. They were instructed to take the required precautionary measures. To that end, a health advisory was issued especially to students who chose to stay on campus.

Students were also informed about the university's determination to maintain 'continuity in instruction' and migrate classes online so that the remaining month's course work could be completed. While students were urged to take care of themselves, they were reminded that the moment must not be seen as a vacation and rather an opportunity to engage with online classes 'in the comfort of their homes' and 'the company of their loved ones'. Meanwhile, a 'Tech Task Force' was set up to devise and oversee the modalities of online teaching. Teachers were informed of the decision to hold a quickly organised but detailed online seminar on conducting online classes.

Murmurs about a difficult, unprecedented decision had already started doing the rounds a few days before these announcements. A week before the announcement on temporary closure, I had walked into a class of anxious, speculating students, many of whom wished to go home. The air was thick with tension, uncertainty, and confusion. In another class, a member of the students' council had been put in a tight spot by her classmates, demanding from her an explanation on why the university was still operating when the Covid-19 situation seemed to be going out of hand at the national and state levels. The council representative explained that the university was in a tough spot, confronted with an unprecedented situation, and was struggling to perform the tightrope walk between ensuring students' safety and maintaining continuity in the university's activities.

One of the (unofficial) refrains of the university around this time was its emphasis on its location (which was removed from the main city) and its status as a residential campus with a minimal influx of people from outside. This, therefore, became a significant moment to ascertain whom the university regarded as those on/from the outside. I mention this because a few of us as visiting faculty remember being struck by the fact that at a time when there were conflicting and frequently changing opinions on the necessity of masks for prevention, it was only the security guards, canteen workers, and *safai karmacharis* (cleaning staff and workers) who were asked to wear masks. The visiting faculty and non-residential and regular staff were not asked to do so, despite coming from locations outside the campus. This was also the period when in the name of the need for hygiene, the *safai karmacharis* could be seen doing more cleaning shifts than usual without additional payment.

As visiting faculty who was not on campus on 14 March 2020, when the university was in the thick of much churning and was attempting to do the best it knew, there was a nervous energy in the air. There was uncertainty and chaos, but there was also the sense of venturing into something not fully known. This was to be the first tryst of most teachers and students with online learning. Everyone was given four days to reach their homes, settle, and prepare for the upcoming online classes. Teachers were instructed to redesign their course structure, deadlines, and evaluation components, in keeping with the shift to online teaching and learning. It was reiterated to visiting faculty like myself that all terms of our contract (which included the number of teaching sessions, etc.) were to remain unchanged, except the shift from offline to online medium.

Thus began the story of experiments with online learning. The site of learning had changed from the site of the 'smart classroom' to the 'smartphone' (or well, laptop). From discussions among teachers and emails sent to us, it became known that initial awkwardness, technical glitches, and struggles to ensure participation co-existed with instances of increased peer support and demonstration of commendable adaptability by both teachers and students in almost all classes. While most teachers recognised the anxieties brought forth by the moment and readily devised new ways to teach and evaluate, the students demonstrated the will to learn in an environment different from the one they were used to. Far from their friends and the manner of community support they had been used to, the students were now in their homes with perhaps greater safety but also greater challenges for everyone involved to negotiate their learning in the spaces of their homes.

The mode was new and certainly involved reconfiguration in practices and modes of teaching and learning for everyone involved. The administrative staff was working overtime to oversee the scheduling and technical workings of the online classes. The teachers were restructuring various aspects of their courses while also learning the modes of teaching online. The students were grappling with all these changes and the rude shock of their university, as they knew it, coming to a halt. However, the fact that most of the actors came from reasonably cushioned backgrounds as far as their class-caste location and access to material resources is concerned made the online transition far easier than it could have been in a university that houses students and teachers from diverse and different locations. Almost all actors involved had access to devices and an internet connection.

And yet, there were challenges that one would not necessarily imagine in an elite university. For example, one of the students recalled how her friend who lived in a relatively remote, hilly area had to especially procure a WiFi connection on account of this transition and had to severely struggle with issues of a slow and patchy connection.

> For such students who kept getting booted in and out of sessions, the classroom experience was just bad. You start feeling like a burden on the class if you have to constantly keep asking questions because you missed parts of what was said, or you have to keep explaining the state of the internet connection.

Some students thus wondered if they could have been given more time to make the necessary arrangements. The fact that a private university does not feel the need to consider these questions of the unequal distribution of resources and their access only reiterates its self-image as one that harbours students from certain backgrounds. Even after the completion of the remaining course online and despite emails from students regarding difficulties of access, these were seen as individual grievances and aberrations in the larger order of things and no larger institutional response was deemed necessary.

Meanwhile, another story was in the making. The workers at the university who engaged in various kinds of manual labour, including cleaning and construction were in the midst of a storm. Rendered vulnerable and even more precarious, many of the workers wished to return to their homes, much like the students. Some of them did. A few months later, many of us learnt from students that the workers who chose to leave had not been paid for months by the university. After a series of interactions between some concerned students and the authorities, the students reported that there has been no concrete action from the university. It is significant to note here that much like everything else, students' parents were involved in these conversations too. It was after many emails sent by several students' parents to the authorities that the university assured them that they were taking the necessary steps to address workers' issues but the steps did not quite follow. A few students stated that many of the leading student voices on the issue subscribed to a politics that believed in holding institutions accountable rather than seeking the help of what they viewed as NGO-ised networks/

ways of working. However, with no other options in sight, some of them came together to set up a 'distress fund' to collect monetary resources for the workers' financial distress, medical emergencies, and other vulnerabilities from students and concerned members of the civil society.

These issues, notwithstanding, the story of online migration at the university was constructed as one of triumph, one where the university successfully rose to the occasion and ensured that everything that needed to be done was done in a timely and efficient manner. At the time of writing this chapter (around June 2020), while the university is currently preparing itself for the upcoming semester, it is determined once again to defeat the virus in what is being seen nationwide as a 'battle'.

As must be evident already, the many stories of the private liberal arts university, the one I am engaged with and others, in general, are complex and layered. Though steeped in privilege and deriving power and legitimacy from modes of neo-liberal governmentality, they allow for possibilities of fostering meaningful relationships and acquiring perspectives that have the potential to think against the status quo. A student narrated,

> I had commerce in the 12th grade. I was convinced that I wanted to study Economics or Business. Had it not been for the liberal arts training at the university, I would have never been exposed to disciplines like Sociology and Cultural Studies. And I would have never specialized in them. Not only were these completely unknown to me, but my parents were also opposed to the idea of me pursuing humanities and social sciences. The model here is such that it makes it possible to negotiate these things with parents. Once you have entered the university and spent your first year here, having come up with the decision for majors in the second year, the parents can't say or do much. Had it not been for this place, my life trajectory would have been different, I would have been a different person completely unaware of how gender and caste play out in our lives.

It cannot be denied that the space can offer possibilities for critical thinking and a certain amount of political action in interstitial pockets, despite the absence of a culture of collective mobilisation on campus.

A colleague also pointed out a facet of the transactional teacher–student relationship, that those committed to the ethos of public education would be critical of. In his view, such a relationship that frames the university and looks at its teachers like service providers is a respite from the *gurukul* (residential school) like *parampara* (tradition), a feudal culture of revering the teacher that elevates him to a pedestal. In a transactional approach where students and teachers were graded by each other, he felt that there are possibilities of democratisation of a classroom because it limits the possibilities of abuse of power by the teacher.

Concluding Thoughts

I argue that with all its possibilities and limits, the space of the private liberal arts university is confronted with several foundational questions about its fundamental rubric and ethos at the current moment. The kernel of these questions always existed but the virus has exacerbated the existing faultlines and posed an urgent need to ask as well as attend to some compelling questions. First, what does 'choice' mean in a context where students build networks in classrooms with only those like them, whether they are built offline or online? Is 'choice' reduced to an empty signifier when not confronted with a meaningful difference? Another way perhaps of asking the same question is to ask what choices are available to those whose work and labour is central to making the story of the university during the pandemic a 'success' story. What constitutes 'success' and 'efficiency' if the labour in the construction of said success and efficiency is devalued? If we wish to maintain our obsession with barometers of merit and success even during the pandemic, one way to do it with integrity is to value, notionally and monetarily, the labour which makes it possible. This labour itself is placed in a graded hierarchy of value – from the *karmacharis* to the administrative staff to the teachers (couched as service providers) and students (enjoined as consumers). For those of us located as actors in the university, in whatever capacity, these concerns point to the issue of what kinds of negotiations and resistances are possible in spaces of this nature, where political action is not imagined beyond the idiom of charity. In that sense then, what I began as a story of a private liberal arts university is also a series of questions posed to those like us, located within and dependent upon these universities who see value in teaching and engaging with them but need to rethink the terms of this engagement. The pandemic, I hope, can urge us to do that.

Notes

1 See https://thewire.in/education/youngsters-are-you-ready-to-rethink-education
2 See https://timesofindia.indiatimes.com/city/delhi/students-left-in-the-lurch-after-jnu-du-jamia-close-hostels/articleshow/74739641.cms and https://www.newindianexpress.com/states/andhra-pradesh/2020/mar/19/closure-of-us-varsities-leaves-students-in-lurch-2118676.html

References

Hoerner, J. (1970) *An Historical Review of Liberal Education*. Coral Gables, Florida, USA: University of Miami.

Pant, H. (2007) 'In Defence of Liberal Education', *India International Centre Quarterly*, 34 (3/4):168–177.

Pathak, Avijit. (2019) 'Youngsters: Are You Ready to Rethink Education?', *The Wire*, [Accessed 26 June 2020] [online].

26

RE-IMAGINING EDUCATION IN THE POST-COVID-19 WORLD

December 2020

Vaishali Diwakar

> It was my mistake to enrol all my three daughters in a private English medium school unlike all other children in my basti (slum). This online education is a huge burden on my resources. I thought English education in a private school would give better opportunities to my daughters and they would not have to work as a domestic worker like me. But now I repent and feel we should not dream of a better future for our kids.

These are the words of despair of the domestic worker working in my home – a single mother of three daughters, 6, 9, and 11 years old, respectively. All three go to a private school. During the pandemic, they were attending lectures from one mobile phone and struggled with digital technologies and online submissions. They would make frantic calls to the teachers to understand these new apps and technologies, and were almost always on the verge of crying, scared of the humiliation by teachers in the next day's online class. There was helplessness, fear, and vulnerability in my domestic worker's eyes. She feared she was losing the dream of giving a better life to her daughters. All this along with my own challenges of teaching in an online class forced me to think of this reality from a sociological lens.

Covid-19 has created exceptional circumstances across the globe. Many aspects of our everyday lives went through major transformations. These transformations have been observed and experienced across class, caste, gender, religion, ethnicities, and economies. It has radically changed how we look at many conventional notions of survival along with our basic survival practices at the very micro-level. The lockdown periods redefined the essential and non-essential categories of goods and services needed for human survival. As an educator, this redefining of essential and non-essential made me rethink many aspects of education that are generally taken for granted. It raised, for me, many questions about the future of education not just in the Indian context but also globally. The fast-changing Indian education

DOI: 10.4324/9781003320524-34

system shares some of the concerns of the global education system and at the same time demands a closer and fresh look at the Indian context with its own specificities.

In March 2020, suddenly there arose a need for partial automation of the education system to cope with the changes emerging as a result of the pandemic. When the nationwide lockdown was declared in March, the entire attention was diverted to getting access to food supplies, healthcare, creating awareness among the masses about Covid-19, and migrant labourers and their return to their villages. While there is no doubt that these were pressing demands and needed urgent attention, the education system was also dramatically disrupted without getting any time to wind down the semester systematically. In India, schools had less than 24 hours to figure out how to respond to the closure notice. By the end of March 2020, 320 million students in India lost access to education for an indefinite period (Kavita Anand 2020).

It seemed as though the entire world was divided into essential and non-essential during the lockdown, and without any label as such, education came under non-essential. Teachers had to find their own ways to complete the remaining syllabus and update assessment sheets and were struggling to do justice to their responsibilities even when nobody was sure when the school/colleges would reopen and when things would resume to 'normal' in all respects. As an insider – a teacher in a college – while witnessing these changes and playing the role of an educator, I was constantly engaging with issues within the education system and particularly the higher education system, that was presented with these unusual circumstances. This chapter focuses on these issues, concerns, and experiences of teaching and learning during the pandemic.

Methodology

After three to four months of online classes, in July/August 2020, I carried out a survey to understand the challenges faced by teachers and students while adapting to the changes in the education system. I collected data from 55 university or college teachers and 75 students on their experiences and the issues faced during online teaching and learning. Due to the strict lockdown, the data was collected through an online questionnaire consisting of multiple-choice as well as open-ended questions. The data also includes informal discussions with teachers and students from my college as well as other universities and colleges. The online questionnaire was shared with students and faculty across streams from conventional disciplines of Arts, Commerce, Science, Humanities to professional disciplines of Engineering, Food and Nutrition, Medicine, Management, and interdisciplinary fields like Film Studies and Women's Studies. I used the snowball method of sampling to reach teachers and students from Pune, Mumbai, Guwahati, Latur, Manipal, Ahmednagar, and Wardha. Among teachers, 68.5 per cent of the teachers were teaching undergraduate courses, 46.3 per cent were engaged in postgraduate teaching, 22.2 per cent were teaching junior college, and 4 per cent were teaching professional courses. Contextual analysis of the open-ended questions was done within the broader framework of interpretivism and critical realism. The quantitative data was used to make simple correlations.

Why Bourdieu Matters: Reproducing Inequality

From March to December 2020, over ten months, the education system saw certain irreversible changes as far as teaching and learning pedagogies and evaluation practices are concerned. Education, in India, is considered a prerequisite for a better life and better opportunities. Therefore, education was considered a fundamental right in the Indian Constitution, especially after the Right to Education Bill was passed in 2009. This Act makes education a fundamental right of every child between the ages of 6 and 14 and specifies minimum norms in elementary schools. It requires all private schools to reserve 25 per cent of seats for children of the above-mentioned age group. The Right to Education aimed at ensuring the right to education for every child.

However, given the unprecedented circumstances of Covid-19 and the consequent lockdown, to access this fundamental right to education, additional pre-requisites were required. To be part of the online education system, one was required to have a smartphone/laptop, an internet network with good bandwidth, the technical knowhow about online interactive platforms, and access to the Learning Management System (LMS) like Moodle[1] to attend lectures and to be part of the evaluation system. In India, a large section of students faced challenges to fulfil these requisites and remained outside the education system.

During the pandemic, many people, especially those in the working class, lost their source of livelihood. This had a ripple effect in terms of parents' compromised ability to pay fees for their child's education and provide new basics such as the internet and smart devices. This resulted in a lack of access to education for many, especially female students. In various informal discussions in the classroom and during mentoring sessions, many college students expressed that the experience of being part of the education system now includes many new awkward experiences such as constant reminders for paying fee instalments, not being able to attend the final year examination because of low bandwidth, constantly getting prompted to switch on the videos to make sure they are physically and mentally present and students continuously apologising for their inability to have better network connectivity.[2] The sudden switch to online education has deepened the existing socio-economic hierarchies and made access to education harder for those on the margins of these hierarchies.

Over the last 20 years of my service as a teacher in a reputed college, I have witnessed the marginalisation and difficulties faced by students from a working-class background or first-generation learners. With the 'new now',[3] one can see the shifts in the usual lifestyle parameters like the brand of clothes and shoes students wear, money spent in the canteen, stationery used for assignments, brand of mobile phones, contents of the lunch box, and medium of commuting as the bases of inequality among the student community. A new hierarchical order is in the making.

A popular thought among the general public and academicians has been that digital technologies act as equalisers and since students are not attending school or college, it will help to get rid of comparisons and thus reduce the hierarchy (Sarkar et al. 2017; Black et al. 2019). However, today we see the focus of hierarchy shifting from purely lifestyle parameters as mentioned above to one's very existence as a digital native. Student's access to education is now defined in terms of their access to digital technology. Pierre Bourdieu (1990) has elaborated on how the education system reproduces inequality. He emphasises various kinds of capital, viz. economic (money or wealth), cultural (gained through family and education), social (social networking), and symbolic (status and social honour). According to him, differential cultural/social/symbolic capitals explain differences in educational achievements. As far as the contemporary education system is concerned, there is a need to add 'digital capital' (access to digital technology) to the list of Bourdieu's types of capital to understand the layers of inequality created by it.

Bourdieu (1990) argues that children from privileged classes gain knowledge from families and family practices such as household conversations on various topics, visits to museums, and art-related events. Later when these children go to schools, this embodied cultural capital is mistaken for intelligence. They convert their cultural capital into good grades and educational achievements and after completion of education, they further reconvert their cultural capital back into economic privilege. During the pandemic, 'digital capital' is playing the same role in perpetuating inequality in terms of access to education. According to Bourdieu (1990), the process of fit and fitting takes place throughout the life course but is most concentrated in early socialisation. Bourdieu uses the term 'cultural arbitrary' to explain how certain things are made to seem universally significant because they are important to dominant people and institutions. These practices are inscribed in our 'habitus[4]' and are supported by societal values and existing discourses in the concerned social field. This also results in what Bourdieu calls 'symbolic violence'.[5] In the context of reproduction of inequality in the field of education, he further adds that symbolic violence of cultural arbitrary is based on pedagogic action – whether that be family education, institutionalised education or the diffuse education[6] of the peer group and every day. Today, students with digital access can be thought of as owners of 'embodied digital capital' who can grab the best opportunities to build their futures. It may seem premature to say that the same digital capital can be reconverted into economic capital, but it is a reality we see it unfold in the digital classroom every day. During the pandemic, can we say that digital capital plays a far more significant differentiating role than cultural capital? The data collected for this project throws light on this question.

Online Education: What Does the Data Say?

According to Hindol Sengupta (2020), the Covid-19 crisis marks a point of transition in the field of education as far as the adoption of online teaching and learning platforms is concerned. Education is one of the key sectors which will witness this transition in a big way. Before the Covid-19 crisis, notes a KPMG and Google study, the online education market in India was set to grow to $1.96 billion, with 9.6 million users by 2021, from $247 million and 1.6 million users in 2016 (Sengupta 2020). Based on this estimation and the situation created by the pandemic, in April 2020, it is predicted that the nature of education is ripe for change in India and interest in online education will soar in India as it has elsewhere (Sengupta 2020). However, in India, this has a special resonance due to its peculiar class composition.

A majority of teachers who participated in the survey expressed anxiety regarding the drastically changing education system. Both teachers and students communicated a fear of coping with the online teaching–learning challenges. About 88 per cent of teachers felt that online education will create inequality and a digital divide among the students. Teachers perceived online teaching as a temporary substitute in these unusual circumstances. They indicated that online teaching and learning cannot be the norm because the ground reality for the majority of students from marginal sections is seriously challenging the continuation of education in such circumstances. They were concerned about students facing discrimination due to and on the digital online platforms.

As far as the positives of online teaching are concerned, many teachers reported being able to use more innovative audio-visual methods to reach out to students. Some teachers also expressed that online education provides flexibility and time to learn at one's own pace, allows people to ensure health and safety during the pandemic by letting them stay indoors, takes away the stress of travelling to school/college/university and lets people work from the comfort of their homes. These were seen as worthwhile opportunities. Interactive activities via quizzes and apps were seen as the advantages of online teaching.

However, the negatives regarding online teaching are numerous and notable and need more attention and analysis. Around 40 per cent of teachers reported the 'facelessness' of the classroom and the anxiety of losing connection with students. A significant number of teachers, as well as students, were concerned about the challenges due to inadequate infrastructure: lack of continuous electricity supply, expensive technological devices-phones, laptops, uninterrupted data/internet connection and resources to access the same. Around 75 per cent of students surveyed expressed that they faced issues with internet connectivity.

The absence of personal interaction with students, especially with those who need additional support in their studies, was also at the centre of some teachers' apprehensions. Teachers also agreed that teaching often lapses into a monologue, a top-down delivery, and thus becomes very monotonous. In the conventional education system, teachers and students are not formally trained in online teaching-learning methods. Creating e-content for the subjects needs specialised training. These new teaching methods were haphazardly and hurriedly imposed on both students and teachers, and everyone struggled and learned these methods mostly on their own. Gradually, some teachers began to add innovative content and made online learning interesting and interactive but for most of them, it is still a monotonous and insipid method. Teachers observed that digital learning also adversely affected peer learning, vibrant discussions, fieldwork, and classroom debates. Teachers organised virtual visits and used break-out rooms for discussion, but they also mentioned that these activities are more effective and interesting if conducted in person. According to 60 per cent of teachers, classroom teaching–learning facilitates discussions, learning, and unlearning in a healthier environment than online classes.

While commenting on the issues impacting students, teachers mentioned that some students spoke about problems, such as reduced attention span, frequent headaches due to constantly looking at small screens, and extra efforts required for sustaining interest during the online lectures. Loss of human connection in terms of immediate feedback, encouragement, appreciation, and motivation was a source of major disquiet.

As far as the equality between students is concerned, the majority of teachers said that online teaching will not bring equality among students. Though inequality is created and persists in offline classroom interactions as well, some teachers predicted that unequal internet access and the cost and accessibility of 'smart' devices will further deepen the inequalities and create new hierarchies. According to Mr Kasinath from IT for Change, if online education is going to be the way forward, then 90 per cent of the children in India will not be a part of it (Interview in *Hindu*, 18 December 2020).

Moreover, as Professor Nayar points out, "learning" in its totality is *not* about books and classrooms alone. More broadly, learning also involves the negotiation of identities, social interaction and "coming-of-age" responsibility and decision-making abilities. Peer-work, peer-pressure, bullying, but also solidarity, relationships, developing and sharing coping mechanisms, and support work are a part of "learning" – for which the campus is the site' (Nayar 2020: 2).

Why Gender Matters?

A few teachers expressed concern about the space and privacy issues within the home, especially for female students and also the responsibility of household work they shoulder. In my teaching career of over

20 years, I have observed that many female students who are first-generation learners look at college hours as a respite from abusive homes, domestic violence, the drudgery of housework, sibling care, and in some cases managing entire households. The physical space of college usually provides a spatial and temporal zone, where one can leave these odds behind, behave one's age, and enjoy mundane yet important activities, such as visiting libraries, doing assignments together, 'bunking' classes, and hanging out with friends in the canteen. It has been observed in many conversations with students in pre-pandemic times that sometimes, just leaving home for six to seven hours gives them a sense of 'normalcy' and relief. Many female students have mentioned that coming to college and spending a few hours outside the family gives a lot of confidence and assurance that there is a way to find reprieve from their situations, a sense of freedom from their stressful family lives however temporary it may be. When seen from a female student's point of view, online education has snatched probably the only space they had to get rid of their limiting, abusive surroundings.

In the online survey, 26 per cent of the students admitted that they used to look at classroom space as an escape from the drudgery and unpleasantness of the household. Some of the female students said that chaos at home is a serious issue for them. They were not able to concentrate on their studies due to noisy neighbourhoods, endless domestic chores and constant disturbance. The lack of sufficient, conducive physical space at home was a major constraint for many students. Their houses were small. Due to the prevalent patriarchal restrictions on the girl's mobility, they were not permitted to go out frequently like their brothers, to receive better internet connectivity. The scope for concentrated learning in a quiet place with privacy was a luxury for a majority of the students. They shared mobile devices with their siblings and in many cases with parents. This was especially true for female students. A few students reported that there exists only one smartphone for everyone's use at home. If the father leaves for work at 9 am, no one could attend lectures after that, because the phone was not available. In homes where digital resources were scarce, girls were getting the short end of the stick. If a parent had to choose between giving the phone to a son or a daughter, it is the son who was given preference (Hindu, December 2020). In some cases, it was reported that as a consequence of the pandemic, girls were being pressured to get married rather than continue their education (Hindu/V. Madhurima 2020). There is a possibility that the dropout rate among female students has increased, though we do not have any concrete data at hand.

Around 65 per cent of the students reported that they miss vibrant campus life, in which they learn, bond, fight, negotiate, and share. The compulsion of learning online and the inability to leave home has particularly affected students from a lower economic stratum. Earlier for most of them, college or university campus was a space of relief from domestic chores, and domestic violence, and an opportunity to learn and realise their aspirations to be financially independent. Now that space is missing.

Quality of Education

It is too early to comment decisively on the impact of the pandemic on the overall quality of education. Findings from the online survey with teachers and students very clearly indicate that the quality of education is suffering to a great extent. In this context, three issues become very important, viz., issues related to the lack of physical presence, the safety of teachers and students while using online platforms, and the absence of pedagogical spaces for imbibing critical thinking.

First, classroom teaching, which ensures physical presence and interaction between teachers and students, is very critical according to almost 85 per cent of the teachers. The reactions of students, the body language of teacher and students, gestures, and intonations – all of these add to the quality of teaching when lectures are delivered in person. It is an integral part of the education system. In online education, this physical presence is missing and that has a detrimental impact on teaching as well as on learning and comprehension. Many students have reported an increase in depression and anxiety due to a lack of human contact. Retaining the attention of the students across all age groups is a challenge for all teachers. As V. Madurima (2020) suggests, to make online learning efficacious, we need to think of multimodal dispersal of learning material and maintenance of the balance between synchronous and asynchronous modes. Nayar (2020: 5) also mentions that 'with online education, multimodal literacy is poised for a boom. To ensure that the enhancement made possible by this form of literacy reaches more demographics, a radical rethinking of pedagogics seems inevitable'. I, too, strongly believe that the warmth, the fun, the dramatics, the whole act of teaching cannot be replaced completely by online methods alone – no matter how effective we try to make it. The learning process in classroom delivery is layered, multi-faceted, and multi-directional, and the lack of classroom teaching is going to have long-term consequences on the learning process.

Second, an important aspect is the safety of teachers and students while using online platforms. On the online platforms, teachers are not aware and cannot control who is listening to the lectures along with students. Many times it has been noticed that family members are also attending the classes – albeit often out of curiosity. We need to raise the question of ethics concerning the sanctity of the classroom, whether online or offline. This is especially relevant while teaching subjects like sociology, psychology, and gender studies and discussing social issues within families, sexuality, and several other sensitive issues. In the physical space of the class, while discussing domestic violence, abuse, and patriarchal experiences at home, students can speak openly in the safe environment of the classroom. Some of them have broken down and have shared their experiences since no family member was around, and they found it safe and secure to share the same in front of the small group of familiar faces. My experience as well as many colleagues' experiences tell us that offline classrooms can be made safe places for students, who otherwise are not able to share these experiences anywhere else. Now, in the new online scenario, one has to think twice before discussing such sensitive topics, since you do not know if a student's family member is also attending your class and whether it is a safe place for students to share such sensitive experiences about their family members.

The teachers are instructed to upload live videos of the class teachings on various online platforms. As the present classroom has porous boundaries, with friends and family of students potentially having access to the videos of teachers giving lectures, concerns about the privacy of the content and the risk of it being used inappropriately weigh on the minds of teachers. The cases of so-called Zoom bombing[7] are also on the rise across the globe. Teachers, as well as students, are susceptible to online sexual harassment since their video feeds are accessible to people outside the classrooms.

Third, while teaching social sciences and humanities, teachers give a lot of examples from and make connections with the current political scenario and discuss various political ideologies. References to contemporary socio-cultural setup is a very common scenario in social science classrooms. Taken out of context, examples and connections with current events may be interpreted erroneously and perceived as 'hurting sentiments' or, worse, used as evidence to complain about the teacher. Humanities and social science classrooms potentially offer a space for critical thinking and allow for a critique of the various structures of society. We run the risk of shutting down this space completely when classrooms are conducted in a porous, virtual classroom, where a permanent record of the lecture is maintained.

One of the important functions of the education system is to create citizens with critical thinking minds. Society needs well-informed citizens, who possess the ability to question the system and are instrumental in bringing about positive change. The ideals of justice, equality, equity, tolerance, and democracy need to be instilled in the growing minds and that is supposed to be the ideal function of the education system, particularly humanities and social sciences. When these ideals are compromised due to fear of getting quoted out of context, I strongly feel that the very purpose of education gets defeated. There is a strong chance of this happening if the liberty accorded by the safe and open classroom is taken away from the teachers and students.

Conclusion

Digital technologies have certainly enabled widespread access to some form of education for most students, even during an unprecedented pandemic. Nonetheless, the 'digital capital' replicates, reinforces, and reproduces inequalities within the society just as cultural capital does. While all of us are still grappling to understand how the new normal will emerge for the education system once the pandemic is behind us, one thing is becoming all too clear: digital-only classrooms are not desirable for various reasons. The quality and depth of education, especially for humanities and social sciences, imparted in a classroom-based education, cannot be replaced with online classrooms. Having access to a classroom in a controlled environment provides a segregated and safe discussion space, where there is potential for meaningful exchange of ideas during learning sessions. And this is critical for high-quality education. Education should not be reduced to reading out PowerPoint slides and avoiding 'controversial', yet important social issues due to the fear generated by the unknown, blank, faceless online spaces. Nayar (2020: 5), looking at the predictions of various reports about the increasing demand and supply of online teaching, warns us about the battles ahead: 'learner concentration, retention of motivation, behaviour – and attitude – development modes, appropriate content delivery, addressing opportunity gaps, and the age-old immersivity versus interactivity conundrum'. What we need to envisage is a blended system, which will combine online and offline modes of teaching–learning. At the same time, we need to ensure equal access to digital tools and make education engaging by introducing new pedagogical methods based on the availability of digital resources. We need to make education accessible to everyone so that no woman from the working class ever has to repent her decision to educate her children.

Notes

1 LMS is a generic learning management system. Moodle is one of the online education learning management systems, in which students can enrol themselves for the respective courses. They can access the lecture recordings, take notes for the subject, can submit assignments, and solve subject-related quizzes online.
2 In telephonic or in-person conversations during the strict lockdown and the following months, some of the students especially from regional language background and students from low socio-economic backgrounds expressed the fact that they were not able to pay fees or exam fees due to the financial crisis at home. Constant questions on these issues or comments on their lack of digital knowledge regarding Moodle or other interactive platforms such as Zoom and Google classroom during the online lectures was humiliating for them. Many students from my class learned to scan the pages and convert them into pdf very recently, during this pandemic. When teachers ask the so-called 'smart' students to help the underprivileged students, it is done in a way that humiliates the latter.
3 The concept of 'new now' is introduced by Professor Nayar in his book 'An Introduction to Cultural Studies', while explaining how consumer culture thrives on novelty which is created by the rhetoric of a new-now.
4 *Habitus* refers to the physical embodiment of cultural capital, to the deeply ingrained habits, skills, and dispositions that we possess due to our life experiences (routledgesoc.com)

5 Symbolic violence describes a type of non-physical violence manifested in the power differential between social groups. It is often unconsciously agreed upon by both parties and is manifested in the imposition of the norms of the group possessing greater social power on those of the subordinate group.

6 According to S. Claussen and J. Osborne (2012: 62) 'not all cultural capital is acquired in schools. Bourdieu and Passeron divide the ways of transferring cultural capital into three modes of "pedagogic action" – through diffuse education, through family education and through institutionalized education'. Informally, it is transmitted through diffuse education, which occurs through social interactions. Family education is viewed as the greatest source of any individual's embodied cultural capital and the final means of transmission is through institutionalised education – school (Claussen and Osborne 2012).

7 Zoom bombing or Zoom raiding refers to the unwanted, disruptive intrusion, into a video-conference call. In a typical Zoom bombing incident, a teleconferencing session is hijacked.

References

Anand, K. (2020). 'Why Education Must be an Essential Service: An Educator's Impassioned Plea', *Opinion-National*, 30 April [online]. Available at: https://www.scoonews.com/news/why-education-must-be-an-essential-service-an-educator-s-impassioned-plea-8975 [Accessed 9 May 2020].

Black, D., Bissessar, C. and Boolaky, M. (2019). 'Online Education as an Opportunity Equalizer: The Changing Canvas of Online Education', *Interchange*, 50: 423–443 [online]. Available at: https://doi.org/10.1007/s10780-019-09358-0 [Accessed 1 May 2021].

Bourdieu, P. (1990) *Reproduction in Education, Society and Culture*. London: Sage.

Claussen, S. and Osborne, J. (2012; 2013). 'Bourdieu's Notion of Cultural Capital and Its Implications for the Science Curriculum', *Science and Education*, 97(1): 58–79 [online]. Available at: https://doi.org/10.1002/sce.21040 [Accessed 1 May 2020].

Hindu. (2020). 'What Challenges do Online Classes Pose? An interview with V. Madurima and Gurumurthy Kasinath', *The Hindu*, 18 December [online]. Available at: https://www.thehindu.com/opinion/op-ed/what-challenges-do-online-classes-pose/article33358120.ece [Accessed 19 December 2020].

Nayar, P. (2020). 'The New Cultures of Learning – Pedagogy Online', *eSS Sunday Edit*, 28 December, pp. 1–5 [online]. Available at: http://www.esocialsciences.org/Articles/Show_Article.aspx?qs=9dkve6t4+5BDnt5o/XDm8feVIdyWtiw7fL1kTyOhvbWaWWGJzS7XVJtP6fjtS+FteYfHzRBJaBgd0L9kJAtFBA== [Accessed 1 May 2020].

Sarkar, S., Mohapatra, S., and Sundarakrishnan, J. (2017). 'Assessing Impact of Technology Based Digital Equalizer Programme on Improving Student Learning Outcomes', *Education and Information Technologies*, 22(1): 195–213 [online]. Available at: https://www.researchgate.net/publication/312196439_61_Subrata_Sarkar_Sanjay_Mohapatra_J_Sundarakrishnan_2017_Assessing_impact_of_technology_based_digital_equalizer_programme_on_improving_student_learning_outcomes_Education_and_Information_Technologies [Accessed 1 May 2020].

Sengupta, H. (2020). 'The Covid-19 Opportunity for Online Education', *Fortune India*, 2 April [online]. Available at: https://www.fortuneindia.com/polemicist/the-coronavirus-opportunity-for-online-education/104372 [Accessed 19 December 2020].

OF TRAUMA AND LOSS

27

GROUND ZERO AFTER GROUND ZERO

April 2020

Jacob M. Appel

My macabre joke with my colleagues – we are emergency room physicians in New York City – is that Covid-19 must kill only well-off white people because since the pandemic started, we no longer see any of them on the streets of Manhattan anymore. Of course, the tragic reality is rather the opposite. Preliminary data from across the United States suggests that coronavirus has hit hardest in lower-income African American and Latino communities. Non-whites in the United States are more likely to be employed as essential workers in fields like food delivery and home healthcare, increasing their exposure to illness. They are more likely to suffer at baseline from diseases exacerbated by economic disparity such as diabetes and hypertension, the same conditions that render one more vulnerable to death from Covid-19. They often live in tight quarters in inner cities, making social distancing both physically and psychologically challenging. Many are victims of limited healthcare literacy. After generations of second-class treatment in the medical system, large segments of these communities lack faith in the pronouncements of public health authorities. Who can blame them? And yet, looking out of the hospital windows, I see a number of dark-skinned workers, wearing flimsy surgical masks, attending to the tasks that keep the metropolis functioning. So where are the white folks? The good news is that they have not died off. The reality is nearly as dark: they have fled.

As the pandemic bore down upon New York City, an increasing number of my upper-middle-class Caucasian friends and acquaintances embarked on their own version of the Passover Exodus. From posh neighbourhoods like the Gramercy and Brooklyn Heights, they made their way to summer homes and seasonal rentals in the countryside – the Hamptons on Long Island, Cape Cod, the Catskill Mountains of Upstate New York. Or they ensconced themselves in the homes of relatives in the largely white, largely well-heeled suburbs of Westchester County and northern New Jersey. Or, for those who could not flee by car or jet, they sealed themselves inside their

DOI: 10.4324/9781003320524-36

upscale apartments, relying on the services of low-income essential workers to deliver their food, to keep their electricity and water and internet running, to police the streets to prevent looters and arsonists from wreaking havoc in their wake. Who can blame them either? If I were not working night shifts in the emergency room, I might have done the same. Social justice and equality are wonderful aspirations but not when a lethal virus threatens one's family.

I do not intend to sound cynical. But one cannot change the world unless one recognises the world as it is. And nothing does as effective a job of clarifying the reality of the society we have constructed than life-threatening calamities. I was within walking distance of Ground Zero on 9-11-2001 and witnessed United Airlines Flight 175, the so-called second plane, collide with the South Tower. For a brief moment, that terrorist attack of 9-11 generated solidarity, but it was a solidarity of fear – not of camaraderie of spirit not a unity of hope. The frontline workers that morning and in the days that followed were working-class New Yorkers: firefighters, cops, and construction crews. We cheered their bravery and determination. But when they fell sick as a result of their efforts, the goal of securing basic medical care for these heroes – ultimately achieved through the Zadroga Compensation Act – provoked a heated political battle. Today, at 7 o'clock every evening, New Yorkers shout and clap from their windows to cheer on the nurses who are risking their lives under the most wrought conditions to save their fellow human beings from Covid-19. I cannot help wondering, in six months or two years, when it comes time to negotiate labour contracts with these same nurses, whether the executives who profit off our hospitals will feel as generous.

Disasters tell us who we are. And who we are is not promising.

Covid-19 has led to challenging conversations regarding healthcare rationing. Some of these discussions have been frankly eye-opening, even for a professional bioethicist such as myself. Ever since the 1960s, when the allocation of scarce dialysis slots in Seattle on the basis of perceived 'social worth' led to a public backlash, one of the fundamental premises of American healthcare has been that rationing should not favour the rich or famous. Of course, controversies have arisen: most notably, accusations have been levelled that a number of celebrities from baseball star Mickey Mantle to actor Jim Nabors to tech guru Steve Jobs have received favouritism in the awarding of liver transplants. But on paper, at least, the allocation process is supposed to be blind to wealth or power. Yet in preparing for the distribution of ventilators, American hospital systems considered plans that favoured high-ranking political officials, such as Governor Ralph Northam of Virginia. The new message appeared to be, to channel George Orwell, that all people are equal but some are more equal than others. We are all in this together until we are not.

Amazingly, disasters tell us who we are *over and over again*: the horrors of racial and economic disparity laid bare by Hurricane Katrina; the civil unrest in Ferguson, Missouri; the riots in Los Angeles following the arrest and beating of Rodney King. And over and over again we do not listen. Covid-19 is frightening. As an emergency room physician, I do not mean to downplay the threat or horror of this shattering illness. But even more terrifying is that only history can tell the difference between a wake-up call and a final warning. And only a fool gambles upon the difference. This may prove our last opportunity to listen.

I do not mean to suggest that the world will come to an end. It won't. (The gallows humour I share with my colleagues includes the observation that "Covid-19 won't end the world, only our role in it.") To paraphrase Eliza Doolittle in *My Fair Lady*, there'll be spring every year without us. What might come to an end is the vast post-Enlightenment liberal project – the Pax Americana, the New World Order, call it what you will – that saw its apex in the first years of the twenty-first century. And I fear what replaces this flawed vision will not be an egalitarian utopia but rather a slide back down the far side of the mountain.

Several times an hour, in my hospital, a resuscitation code is called over the public address system, summoning the medical and/or anaesthesia teams to the bed of a critically ill coronavirus patient. Those of us in white coats understand that this announcement is tantamount to broadcasting an expiration. Never in my career have I encountered death so frequently, so intensely. Yet maybe one of the warnings of Covid-19 is that the security of healthy living is an exception – a historical aberration – not a rule. We are only a historical blink removed from the yellow fever epidemics that decimated New Orleans and the cholera epidemics that forced the partial evacuation of New York City, even closer to the mass deaths from diphtheria and polio that swept away generations of American children. In my grandparents' youth, before tetanus vaccines and the miracle of penicillin, even stepping on a rusty nail or a run-of-the-mill strep throat infection often proved fatal. As late as the 1960s, the accepted fate of American men was to keel over from heart disease in their sixties. Today, if one does not live beyond eighty in the West, one feels cheated. Yet tuberculosis still kills 1.5 million people worldwide each year; malaria strikes down another half million. For my New York neighbours, security from sudden death is very much a privilege of both history and geography.

On breaks from patient care, I used to duck across the street for a late-night cup of coffee or sit on the benches in the nearby park to enjoy a brief reprieve from urban chaos. Only now the chaos around the hospital is literal, rather than metaphoric, and I would not venture into the adjacent park without armed guards at my side. In the early 1980s, the neighbourhood surrounding my hospital was beset with homelessness, addiction, and crime – both petty and violent. Several 'law-and-order' mayors sanitised the streets by relocating city shelters to a distant island and incarcerating small-time offenders in droves. Gone, seemingly overnight, were the purveyors of graffiti, the 'squeegee' men who harassed motorists, the aimless youths who lurked on street corners conveying a sense of hopelessness and undefined menace. Suddenly, they have returned in full force. Or, more likely, they have been here all along, just not visible. Now the shops are all shuttered behind iron gates. Parking rules have become optional; traffic lights have melted into yield signs. My search for a late-night cup of coffee crosses paths with men 'tagging' storefronts and bus stops, with ever-expanding cardboard enclaves policed by the homeless themselves. So this is a warning too. We are all civil libertarians in moments of peace and security. But unless the rule of law serves the interests of all, those left out will see little benefit in upholding the rule of law. They will merely bid their time.

Yet maybe the most ominous part of the warning is that this is 'only' a pandemic. As one of my patients, who suffered from a mild case of Covid-19 said, it could be worse. I do not mean to mitigate either the emotional or economic toll of this tragedy. But the truth is that humanity, as a species, will move past this tragedy. But we might not have. Covid-19 could have been a disease with a much longer incubation period and a might higher fatality rate; it could have killed us by the billions, rather than the thousands. Or it might have been a solar storm like the Carrington Event of 1859, capable of melting the electric grid and starving humanity back to the Stone Age. Or it might have been a nuclear winter. All of these are lurking threats – and all preventable with meaningful preparation and collective action.

Covid-19 may be the universe's way of telling us to get our acts together, that humanity can only endure so many Trumps, Modis, Bolsonaros, Putins, Erdogans, Maduros, Orbans, and Dutertes before these malevolent dunces start becoming the norm, rather than the exception. Most of the world already knows this. But in New York City – or now in the Catskills and the Hamptons and on Cape Cod – my friends and neighbours, until recently, placed their trust in the inevitable, in the peace and prosperity as they experienced it, of secular rationality and liberal capitalism. Much as the Roman Emperors believed themselves invincible and the eminent Edwardians slumbered with confidence that the Pax Britannica would endure forever.

The Report of the 9-11 Commission in the United States attributed the success of the terrorist attacks of that day to a failure of imagination. Terrorists had previously blown up a federal building in Oklahoma City, attacked the Olympic Games in Atlanta, an even detonated explosives beneath the World Trade Center itself. In spite of all these warnings, the overwhelming evidence, Americans failed to imagine the inevitable. Covid-19 is a similar failure. But the pandemic has given us a chance to imagine – both the danger that lies ahead, but also the better world we might pursue to stave off the fire next time. Walking through my emergency room, seeing so much suffering, so much death, one cannot help but think that we have to stop fleeing and start imagining. And we need to start imagining as though the fate of the entire world depends upon it.

28

NARRATING THE MOMENT OF TRANSMISSION

Rosalie Purvis

Written in the summer of 2020 from a life at home in Worcester, MA, USA, sheltering from the coronavirus pandemic.

In the early days of Covid-19, a friend was convinced he had contracted the dreaded disease. While tests were still scarce and he could not confirm his self-diagnosis, his symptoms did seem to line up. He confided that he felt scared and also guilty towards his family for bringing the illness into his household. I tried to ease his conscience, telling him we are all living in the midst of a global pandemic, and contracting the disease was difficult to avoid. After all, the period leading into lockdown unfolded, inadvertently, in phases as we struggled to collectively and individually exit the daily activities upon which we build our lives. For a few days, unsure of how to proceed, we still conducted our usual errands, attended work, school, meetings, and social events. We could not abruptly cease all activities. In those days, we'd had no choice but to expose ourselves and one another to some risk.

'But that is the problem', my friend said,

> I mean yea … I had to go to work, stop by the pharmacy and buy groceries and all that, but I did something I did not have to do. Last minute I decided to make one last stop at the liquor store. And that is where I caught it. And now I've put my family at risk.

His voice sounded strained. From the notorious covid cough, I wondered, or from the weight of his regret?

'I should have never made that last stop'.

I pondered this for a moment and asked him how he knew he had contracted the virus specifically there in the liquor store.

He answered: 'Where else would I have caught it?'

I did not point this out to my friend, but at that moment, the virus was spreading rapidly in our region, so he could have caught it virtually anywhere. He could have caught it easily in his workplace, in line picking up his husband's prescription refill at the pharmacy, or while choosing a

DOI: 10.4324/9781003320524-37

cantaloupe in the produce aisle of his local supermarket. But I did not argue with him. Experience has already taught me that trying to alleviate irrational guilt is both futile and pointless.

Ten years ago, I co-led a writing and advocacy group for people living with Hepatitis in NYC. In the summer of 2015, I provided outreach and HIV testing to at-risk populations in the streets of NYC. I observed that when asked, people living with HIV or Hepatitis would pinpoint the moment they contracted the disease. Some stories that have stayed with me:

> One woman felt certain she had contracted HIV during a specific sex act her abusive partner had coerced her into agreeing to. At the time she had been struggling to make ends meet, and her partner had hinted that, if she didn't agree to indulge his high-risk sexual whims, he would not pay for her young children's back-to-school supplies.

Another man would point to one of his prison tattoos, his least favourite, the only one he regretted getting, a snake, pierced by a dagger. He would explain the moment of hopelessness the tattoo had symbolised, at the time. Now, as an older man, his despair had long dissipated. While he still looked upon his other tattoos with pride, nostalgia, even tenderness, the dying snake on his bicep only served as a painful reminder of those most bitter feelings. It was during the process of receiving this tattoo, he explained, that he had contracted hepatitis.

Another man told us he knew for certain he had contracted hepatitis as a young adult from sharing a razor with his old roommate, a close friend who had then later betrayed him by sleeping with his ex-girlfriend.

There are many more stories like this, and two things strike me about all of them. First of all, the narratives people constructed around their own moment of transmission often focus on one specific incident within the context of a lifetime of high-risk exposure. Alongside these specific stories, each of these individuals had described countless high-risk behaviours in which they had engaged throughout their lives. Nearly everyone in the group had injected drugs and, at some point, shared needles, engaged in unprotected penetrative sex with multiple, often unknown partners and received tattoos without proper sanitary precautions. Considering this multitude of risk factors, accurately identifying a single incident of transmission seems unlikely.

The second common link between the stories is that they tend to represent a traumatic moment of heightened emotion, anger, loss, or betrayal. When I first noticed this pattern, I thought back to the earlier decades of the AIDS crisis, where people tended to associate infection, not only with trauma but with virtue or lack thereof. This mindset did not limit itself to the religious right. I recall co-leading a safer sex workshop in the 1990s during which my fellow educator urged the young women in the room to 'still make a man wear a condom even if he says he's clean because, even if he seems really nice, he could be lying'. Aside from the glaring heteronormativity of the statement, her advice troubled me, as she likened sexually transmitted diseases with people who are 'not nice' or 'lying'. Highly educated friends in the United States would shock me, not only with their profound ignorance of the science and prevention of STD transmission but with their assumptions about who would or would not have STDs. 'Oh he/she doesn't have it' a young graduate student would say, waving a hand dismissively. If I asked whether they had discussed the sexual history and test results and, if not, how they knew for certain this person might not carry STDs. A smirk or scoff would follow along with an implication or direct statement that this person was 'nice' and/or 'trustworthy' and/or of the wrong look/type/class/background/culture/milieu to carry disease. Time and time again, however, these same friends would learn the hard way that no particular class background or personality type guaranteed immunity to HIV, gonorrhoea, herpes, or even genital warts and that, quite often, well-intentioned individuals did not even realise that they were carriers.

I recall one sexual encounter in particular, where a highly educated cisgender man, a scientist no less, tried to assure me we did not need to use a condom because he was 'clean'. I asked him how he knew this. He told me he was 'always very careful'. I told him that the fact that he had never once inquired after my status in this encounter was evidence to the contrary. Furthermore, the use of the term 'clean', as Americans seem to like to use as synonymous for STD-negative, in contrast to the word 'dirty' as synonymous with 'sexual', reveals disturbingly oppressive residual puritanism.

In Armistead Maupin's iconic *Tales of the City* series, one of the main characters, Brian, a heterosexual cisgender man, is confessing to his gay friend Michael that he fears he has put himself at risk for contracting HIV. This book takes place in the 1980s at the peak of the HIV crisis. As he awaits test results, Michael assures Brian that, just as he and many others have done, Brian will learn to cope with his results, either way.

'But there are innocents involved!' Brian says, referring to his wife and daughter.

'Are you saying my partner and I are not innocent?' Michael asks. This gives Brian pause enough to question his definition of 'innocence'.

Now, in spring 2020, NYC has become the epicentre of the coronavirus. As more and more of my friends, family, and colleagues have contracted the virus, I notice much of the same patterns around how people tend to succumb to judgments around moments of infection. Once again, people seem to attribute risk to people selectively, based on their own societal or personal biases of trust and trustworthiness.

A divorced mother told me she positively knew that her ex-husband's new girlfriend had 'brought Corona' into their family when she returned from Spain to spend the quarantine with him. She and her ex-husband have been co-quarantined, via their two children who continued to go back and forth as their custody arrangement specifies. Upon further reflection, it seemed the mother herself had put herself at equally high, if not higher risk of transmission, as she had continued her work in local New York City hospitals at the start of quarantine. But the husband's new girlfriend represented a new and emotionally charged element in her family, and thus she projected her uneasiness onto the pandemic or projected the pandemic onto her uneasiness.

In a similar vein, a colleague was convinced that he had caught Covid during a particularly frustrating meeting his team had been asked to attend in person, just before the lockdown. While he, himself, never developed any symptoms and never confirmed his suspicion with a test, his stepmother had grown ill after he delivered her groceries on the day of that work meeting. Even though her symptoms remained mild and ambiguous and she was also never tested, he remains convinced the virus was foisted upon her indirectly via that meeting. He still resents his supervisor for pressuring them all to attend.

These personal constructions of trust do not faze me much, as I understand how, in the face of so much that is unknown, we cling to whatever makes us feel safe. Unfortunately, however, the personal can quickly become political, leading to the stigmatisation of marginalised groups. We attribute risk to those whom we already distrust and the curtain is lifted on our biases and bigotry. When, in the early days of test shortages I, myself, came down with an, albeit mild, case of what my doctor now agrees was likely covid, a friend of mine, being shocked, asked me: 'Oh no! That is so crazy! Do you have any idea where you might have caught it?'

The question surprised me. After all, we are living through a global pandemic. As the word 'global' would suggest, I could have contracted the disease anywhere on the 'globe'. His tone, however, suggested that I had somehow subjected myself to nefarious elements. Intuitively, I chose not to correct him. After all, it occurred to me that he may have taken comfort in the narrative that, so long as one avoids such elements, one can completely avoid the pandemic.

All these narratives remain engrained, even as they remain impossible to prove. Even when the precise moment of risk and infection is indiscernible, people seem to fall into patterns of emotional, magical thinking to make sense of their condition. Observing these cultural thinking patterns makes me wonder: how can we investigate our narratives as windows into personal trauma? How can this investigation lead us to a deeper and more compassionate understanding of ourselves and one another?

As I considered this, I had to admit to myself that I have not been immune to this mode of thinking. While my particular narrative does not deal with an infectious disease, it nonetheless reveals how I experienced a condition of my own as a metaphor for trauma. Nearly three years ago, my spouse left me, taking with them their child, whom I had been co-parenting for several years and to whom I was deeply attached. While my partner may have been planning their leave in secret for some time, to me the departure seemed abrupt. During the last days of their stay, as they were packing to leave, I tried to conceal my fear and grief and put on a brave face for my beloved stepchild's sake. I may have also hoped, against mounting evidence, that if I supported my soon-to-be ex by helping them pack and move, and if I remained accommodating and loving, maybe this would temper their erratic behaviour and they might cease their threats to separate me from my stepchild.

One late night, my child crept into the kitchen where, through hours of insomnia, I had taken to silently weeping, so I could contain my tears by day. She wrapped her arms around me and whispered tearfully into my ear of her own sadness and fear of our impending separation. We held one another, and I struggled to find the right words for her when I lacked them for myself. This moment tore through the depths of my being, and I barely noticed when later that day, for the first time, my period returned only a week after my last. Gradually, during the departure and after, my stretches of bleeding increased and grew longer and heavier. At first, I did not have the wherewithal to go to the doctor, but when I did, she told me 'this happens sometimes' and there was no cause for concern. Most likely the extra bleeding was a result of 'stress', which I readily believed, as I was, after all, extraordinarily 'stressed'. Once in a while, I would mention the excess bleeding to doctors when I was seen for routine check-ups and other such reasons, but for months no practitioner conducted a single test, and my condition was generally chalked up, again, to the sweeping catch-all of 'stress'. On one occasion my doctor said the bleeding was a sign of 'too much exercise'. Another blamed it on my age and the assumption I had entered perimenopause.

All in all, with grief hungrily consuming all my mental and physical energy each day, I accepted these explanations. But, while I never told anyone, my bleeding did not truly surprise me as it felt part and parcel of my experience: a long, metaphorical miscarriage, in response to being separated from the only child I had ever parented, and to whom I had devoted the entirety of my maternal self. While she was not my biological child, in spite or perhaps because of this, I took the bleeding as my womb's rebellion. In my lowest point of inconsolable depression, the psychiatrist I saw called my condition – and I paraphrase – 'acute situational depression and PTSD from abrupt parental separation syndrome'. He described the symptoms and each one tracked; flashbacks, unwillingness, or what feels like sheer inability to get out of bed, intense fatigue, unexplained migrating pains, dizziness, difficulty catching my breath, and lung pressure. He did not mention it, but I mentally added 'bleeding from the maternal organs' to his list.

Finally, when my bleeding and pain began to hinder more days than not, a woman I had been dating urged me to see a new doctor and insist on an ultrasound. She herself worked in the field of women's health and wondered whether I might have fibroids. The ultrasound confirmed that I did, indeed have a small but un-fortuitously located and thus highly disruptive fibroid lodged within the lining of my uterus.

Even then, it took me some time to actively pursue a solution as the doctors I saw seemed to have ambiguous and wildly differing ideas of treatment ranging from dietary adjustments to hysterectomy. Eventually, however, I sought out a specialist who would offer to remove the benign growth in a relatively simple hysteroscopic procedure so, as she put it, I could 'get on with my life'.

These words resonated more deeply than intended. I had not considered that, without my stepchild, I would ever find the wherewithal to truly 'get on with my life'. The doctor knew nothing of my personal history and she was certainly not referring to it now, but, somehow I believed her promise on multiple levels. Perhaps this is why, during the procedure, I felt gratitude far more laden than I had expected, and I wept in recovery, emotionally thanking each doctor, assistant, and nurse charged with my care. They took this in stride. Many people behave oddly after surgery. Little did they know I was thanking them for helping to ease what had felt like my haemorrhaging grief.

Indeed, I began to 'get on with my life' more fully. The surgery had been simple and required virtually no recovery. I did, however, spend months rebuilding the blood I had lost in the months leading up to the procedure, during which time I had bled nonstop, often a dizzying amount. Now that the bleeding had ended, tests confirmed my dire shortage of stored iron, the abnormality of that blood loss sank in. I might add, it also confirmed that I was, in fact, not perimenopausal.

A friend asked me whether I was angry.

'Angry? About what?' I asked.

'Are you angry that the doctors failed to correctly diagnose you for so long?'

I thought about it. Indeed, my situation seems to serve as an example of the ubiquitous dismissal of women's health concerns, and would, thus, merit anger. Yet somehow I was not able to access this justifiable anger on command. Strangely, however, a wave of unprocessed fury surged back into my system from nearly ten years prior. During our marriage, my spouse had been struggling with illness. In those early days, we saw many doctors and specialists, none of whom could provide a resolute explanation for my spouse's alarming cluster of symptoms. Even once a presumptive diagnosis was reached, treatment plans varied from expert to expert and remained generally elusive. While I never expressed it, I took note of the fact that each time I left a doctor's office feeling first intense fear for my beloved's survival, which quickly morphed into silent rage, irrationally directed at each well-meaning doctor we had just seen. Anger does not appear to be among my default settings and when I do experience it, it puzzles me. I spoke of this anger to only one person, a colleague, a professor of religious studies.

'Oh', he said, 'That is Thich Nhat Hahn's screaming baby'.

He proceeded to explain that Thich Nhat Hahn often likens anger to a crying baby that must be comforted. If we cannot soothe our crying baby, and the baby continues to scream and squirm in our arms, we may become exhausted and, out of despair, try to hand the baby to someone else to hold.

I think of this each time I see people becoming incensed over personal handling of the pandemic. When we do venture out, we are irritable. We cannot seem to soothe Thich Nhat Hahn's baby. Distressed by his persistent crying, we seek to pass it along and are quick to point to the wrongdoings of others. See how that person is washing their hands the wrong way or failing to disinfect the counter or doorknob before or after touching it. Look, over there someone has failed to wear a mask at the right time or in the correct way. Or, conversely, someone becomes furious at being forced to wear a mask in a setting where there may not be a risk of transmission. Someone misses a sign in the grocery store and walks the wrong way into head-on foot traffic and risks facing off with another shopper. Anger ensues and permeates our lives. Thich Nhat Hahn's baby screams relentlessly. Pandemic rage exposes the worst of us. Well-off white-collar professionals with the luxury to quarantine indefinitely yelling at an underpaid delivery worker for pausing to remove her mask and catch a breath on a ten-hour shift. The maskless curse at the masked, calling them sheep. The masked curse the maskless calling them 'covidiots'.

Two masked neighbours agree to meet for the occasional 'self-care walk' outside. During their physically distanced stroll, they notice the family down the street is holding a suspiciously crowded backyard cookout. 'Are they really quarantined with that many people?' asks the one neighbour, as she furrows her brow. Somehow the brow reads even angrier without the support of the mouth, which remains hidden beneath the mask and the other neighbour, who had just agreed to allow her own nephews to play in her yard the other day, feels offended, and points to studies that show outdoors poses little to no risk. The neighbours disagree. They argue. They argue in vicious, anxious circles, for, across the globe, guidelines on how to manage the pandemic largely remain, much like my spouse's diagnosis and treatment plan, varied from expert to expert and generally elusive.

In its own way, medicine can feel a lot like an act of faith, a religion even. Is it any wonder we often conflate or intertwine the two? As we pass around Thich Nhat Hahn's relentlessly screaming baby, we try to make sense of our mysterious world and, like our ancient and perhaps less ancient ancestors, we mythologise that which we cannot fully comprehend, filling in the unknown spaces with speculation and imagination. In public and/or private, we mythologise 'the virus'. Much of science remains interpretive or relatively invisible to us and our emotions offer shape to what we cannot see and vice versa. When science seems inaccessible, we seek metaphors to guide us. At the start of the pandemic, some suggested we imagine the virus as an invisible glitter that needs to be scrubbed vigorously off our hands and the surfaces it populates. Later, as research findings shifted, we were told to imagine the virus-like cigarette smoke and use masks, airflow, and physical distance to limit its reach and our exposure. The virus, we are told, has a life of its own. The virus is a social disease, and at the same time, social diseases are also viruses. The virus is 'the universe telling us to take a break'. The virus is our punishment for abusing our planet so egregiously. The virus is a threat to our freedom and we must not let it win. The virus exposes our inequities. Or the virus is an equaliser. The virus is an enemy. We are at war with the virus. The virus is at war with us.

At the moment, we are piecing together evolving collective interpretations of Covid-19 that range from the poetic to the prosaic, from the public to the personal, and from the secular to the spiritual. As I absorb our early, often clumsy renderings in the current crisis, I wonder how this pandemic will find its way into our long-term artistic consciousness. Tony Kushner's iconic play *Angels in America*, encompasses the complexity of the AIDS crisis through searingly provocative magic realism.

Accuracy is paramount in every detail of a work of history. Here's my rule: Ask yourself, 'Did this thing happen?' If the answer is yes, then it's historical. Then ask, 'Did this thing happen precisely this way?' If the answer is yes, then it's history; if the answer is no, not precisely this way, then it's historical drama.

There is no innate harm in seeking metaphorical meaning in that which quite literally plagues us, so long as we do not destructively turn on ourselves and on one another in the process. In fact, the thing I realised from gathering stories from people living with stigmatised diseases is how anxious people were to tell their stories and how deeply relieved and fulfilled they would feel afterwards. It was often through telling their narratives, especially with someone present to listen and bear witness that they came to new revelations of action and healing. As we tell our stories, we craft, construct, speculate, editorialise, edit, fill in gaps, and even poeticise. Because of this, we might indeed question the accuracy of these narratives. Yet, I ask myself; to what extent does attachment to accuracy serve us here? After all, there is fact in fiction and fiction in fact. Perhaps our own personal 'historical dramas' can tell us things a doctor's report cannot. While I have facilitated others to tell their stories of illness, this chapter is the first time I sought to narrate my own. The narrative of physical pain had intertwined itself with the most painful part of my life story. Did I develop a fibroid due to being separated from my stepchild as my narrative would suggest? From a medical perspective, probably not. But physical pain seems to prefer to cohabitate with emotional pain and perhaps my system spun the yarns of grief and illness together for that reason. Perhaps the one pain taught me something about the other. Along these lines, might the image of a stabbed snake facilitate processing of a life-altering diagnosis or the other way around? Can we view all of our narratives through this lens? The current pandemic will eventually touch each of our individual lives in one way or another. Our narratives can offer us windows into our own as well as our collective experience. In this time of inevitable transition, let us listen.

CREATIVE RE-IMAGININGS

29

SHAKESPEARE AND KAFKA

Telling Stories in Times of Uncertainty
June 2020

Jim Ife

[This chapter was written in June 2020, when the extent of the Covid-19 pandemic was still uncertain, and no vaccine was in sight]

Shakespeare

We live at a time of crisis, transition, and uncertainty. There are many ideas about what the future might hold – some optimistically foretelling a transition to a more just and sustainable world, some foretelling a 'return to normal' (and all the associated problems), or to a 'new normal' (as if that is even possible), some foretelling an increase in inequality, surveillance, and oppression, and some – seemingly an increasing number – foretelling the collapse of Western civilisation. At this time, the stories we tell each other about our predicament become particularly important, as these stories will shape our immediate responses and our future actions. Our stories tell us what is possible, and what is not. At such a moment, it is interesting to speculate on how the greatest storyteller in the English language, William Shakespeare, might have characterised our present predicament.

History. Many stories of our current predicament are told as history. Shakespeare's histories, such as Richard II, Henry V, and Richard III, are enthralling and insightful stories of personalities, clashes, personal tensions, power, bravery, envy, betrayal, ambition, and so on, with hardly any reference to the turbulence of late 14th-and-15th-century England when the events took place, the decline of feudalism, or the lived experience of the bulk of the population at that time. Like Shakespeare's histories, many of our current stories concentrate on the actions and the interplay of individual actors, reducing history to human personalities and human dramas. We tell stories of the actions, the conflicts, the inadequacies and the triumphs of presidents, prime ministers, oil company executives, epidemiologists, activists, journalists, generals, scientists, investors, entrepreneurs, police, celebrities, whistle-blowers,

DOI: 10.4324/9781003320524-39

and so on. This is 'personalised' history removed from structural forces, removed from cultural context, removed from ecological reality, and removed from the lived experience of most of the human race. It is 'comfortable' history, which does not ask too many confronting questions about the need for structural change. There are, of course, exceptions, as there are also stories that seek to ask the radical questions, though these stories are not strongly present in mainstream media, or social media; you can find them if you look for them, but they are not the dominant narratives of our time. This is history of a certain kind: history as a totality of micro-level human dramas. It results in elections fought based on personalities, scandals, and reputations, rather than policies, and it also results in an inability to understand and address major issues such as capitalism and climate change. Here feminism, with its insistence on connecting the personal and the political, suggests important ways forward, and it is this connection between personal stories and structural changes that have to be emphasised if we are telling stories of our current predicament as history.

Another problem with stories of history is that they concentrate on what has happened only in the past, rather than what could happen in the future. The assumption is that by understanding the historical story, by telling ourselves what has led us to our present predicament, we will know what actions to take in the future to move beyond our present crises and predicaments. This, however, is a questionable assumption. Unfortunately, as has been frequently pointed out, one of the lessons of history is our inability to learn the lessons of history. Understanding the past may be important, but it does not seem to stop humans from repeating the mistakes of that past. At a broader scope than Shakespearian historical drama, human history since the Neolithic Revolution, with the exception of First Nations cultures, is a story not of discrete dramas but of *continuing* conflict, oppression, exploitation, patriarchy, greed, war, and the rise and collapse of civilisations, with human hubris as a constant background.

Telling the stories of our current predicament as history may help us understand how we got here, but it does not tell us much about the future and about what we should do. Indeed, the Shakespearian stories of history can give us a false sense of agency. By reducing history to personal and interpersonal conflict and drama, we can readily assume that our individual actions are, or can be, dramatically important. It leads to the mantra 'you (as an individual) can change the world', by concentrating on those rare occasions when an individual person, usually male – Nelson Mandela, Hitler, Jesus, Julius Caesar, Genghis Khan, Buddha – has profoundly influenced history by the force of their personality and actions. These are rare exceptions, and telling such stories can give people an exaggerated sense of their own agency and lead to inevitable disillusionment. It also emphasises individual rather than collective agency, so does not challenge dominant individualism. It is true that, from an ecological perspective, all human actions change the world, but in subtle, undramatic ways that nevertheless have 'ripple effects' within complex ecological systems. This is a potentially more realistic and more empowering story for those alarmed at the state of the world.

Comedy. The contemporary world certainly lends itself to stories of comedy. Many world leaders seem like cartoon characters, and there are plenty of fools and buffoons. There is ample room for satire, and comedians are spoilt for material. We can craft clever satirical comedies from current events, whether international or local, as can be seen in social media, mainstream media, cartoons, street theatre, placards at demonstrations and stand-up comedy. Laughing at the awfulness of current events can give a sense of relief and escape, and can be good for our mental health. Comedy can also provide a sharp critique. But while comedy is both healthy and appropriate, there are dangers in allowing comedic stories to dominate. One message of comedy is it suggests that things are not to be taken too seriously, yet the problems we are facing are extremely serious. It is easy to laugh at the buffoons leading the nations of the world, thereby deflecting attention from the harm they are doing and the need for serious and urgent action. Comedies are played out for our amusement and entertainment; we play the role of the detached audience, whose role is to laugh at the jokes, but we are not implicated as actors with agency. Shakespeare's comedies, like most other comedies, have happy endings: *Twelfth Night*, *As You Like It*, and *A Midsummer Night's Dream* all end with happy weddings as the intricacies of the plot are resolved. Telling stories of our present predicament as comedy allows us to believe that somehow everything will work out well in the end, and to downplay the seriousness of our present predicament. Of course, comedy is culturally and socially constructed, and modern forms of comedy do not simply reflect the comedic traditions of Shakespeare's experience. Black comedy is perhaps the more relevant form of comedy for our times, as it blurs the boundary between comedy and tragedy.

Romance. A few of Shakespeare's later plays, which do not fall readily within the history/comedy/tragedy typology, have been classified as romances; perhaps the best known are *The Winter's Tale* and *The Tempest*. Like the comedies, the romances tend to have happy endings resolving the complexities of the plot, although without so much reliance on comedy. Again, we can see stories of our current predicament taking the form of a romance. These are the narratives of the triumph of humanity against the challenges of climate change and other potential ecological crises. Usually, these narratives rely on the ability of technology to solve our problems: human ingenuity, research, and the entrepreneurial spirit, like the magic of Prospero, are seen as having the boundless capacity to extract us from whatever mess we find ourselves in. This is well illustrated with the Covid-19 pandemic, where there is an assumption that before too long a vaccine will be developed which will solve the problem, with a happy ending assured. There is a similar faith in scientific or technological 'solutions' to problems of energy supply, carbon capture, food shortages, over-fishing of the oceans, and so on. Watching a romance, we know that somehow everything will end well for the principal characters, and telling our stories as romances can result in a similar naïve optimism. The possibility that there may not be a magical/technological fix for our problems or a happy ending, is too confronting; it challenges our myths of human supremacy and human infallibility. The Western Enlightenment worldview, of continuous human 'progress' towards a better future, has led to this optimism in the human ability to manipulate the world to our own ends. Such optimism is not well-founded in these times.

Tragedy. Telling the stories of our present predicament as tragedies is not easy, yet in the circumstances, it is perhaps the most realistic. As we watch performances of Shakespeare's great tragedies – *Hamlet, King Lear, Othello, Macbeth, Romeo and Juliet* – we sense the ominous inevitability of defeat, destruction, and death. The major characters are often brave and noble but with a fatal flaw that eventually drags them down. Events overtake the characters, who in the end become powerless to prevent their own fate. There is not the happy ending of the comedies or the romances, with the promise of happiness into the future. Nor is there the uncertain future of the histories. Rather, there is decline and fall. These are the stories for the present because we are witnessing the decline and collapse of Western civilisation, a civilisation that has been imposed on the rest of the world and held up as the ideal, through colonisation and globalisation. Western civilisation, like Shakespearean tragic heroes, has its fatal flaws: its unsustainable obsession with growth, its belief in perpetual linear progress, its valuing of the individual rather than the collective, its taking rather than giving, its Western hubris, its patriarchy, its whiteness, and its anthropocentrism. These fatal flaws will bring it down, just as surely as Macbeth, Othello, Lear, and Hamlet met their fates.

This is a hard reality to accept. The dominant narratives of progress require us to believe that things are getting better and better, and that somehow human progress, ingenuity, and technology will solve all our problems. Indeed, the very narrative of 'problems' to be solved leads us to accept the legitimacy of the existing order, and to assume that we can use the strengths of the existing order to 'solve' problems and move 'forward'. But what if there are no adequate solutions within the existing paradigm? What if there is no effective vaccine for Covid-19? What if 'carbon capture and storage' is simply not feasible? What if the technologies we have developed are doing us more harm (physically, socially, emotionally, cognitively) than good? Several commentators have pointed out the simple unsustainability of the existing social, economic, political, and ecological order, and this is becoming increasingly obvious. Others such as Jem Bendall[1] and Paul Kingsnorth[2] claim that the evidence is now overwhelming that civilisational collapse is now inevitable. It has become fashionable to describe almost any 'crisis' as 'existential', but we must face the fact that Western civilisation – increasingly globalised – is now facing a genuinely existential crisis.

Thinking of our present predicament in terms of tragedy may seem like accepting 'defeat', and giving up. In the face of the great tragedy we now see enacted, there doesn't seem to be much that anyone can do about it; that is the nature of tragedy. But there are ways in which telling our story as tragedy can be surprisingly liberating. First, it allows us to take an overview. It is easy to be overwhelmed by the multiplicity of 'problems' with which we are confronted. We may think we are making some progress with one problem (such as climate change), only to be brought up sharp by the overwhelming threats of the others (Covid-19, biodiversity, toxic pollution, and so on). But if we understand all these as part of the larger tragic story of the collapse of Western Society we can at least understand these problems systemically, rather than putting all our energy into 'solving' specific 'problems' which are really just the symptoms of system collapse. This is not to say such efforts are unimportant, but rather to see them in an overall context. And doing so enables us to start telling alternative stories, to imagine other futures, to recognise that things can and do move on after a tragedy. We may not, indeed cannot, know what form this future will take, but we can at least ask questions that are not asked when we are in problem-solving mode. In other words, it makes it easier for us to question the dominant paradigm, and to dare to think outside it.

In this way, perversely, tragedy helps us to cope and to move beyond existential despair. By taking an overview, at a paradigmatic level, we can conceptualise our predicament and think about what to do about it – even if the answers are far from obvious. Watching a Shakespearean tragedy leaves the viewer not totally disillusioned or disempowered, but rather asking some fundamental questions about the human condition. If confronting our world as a world of tragedy can help us to do that, it is surely worth doing. It suggests a different strategy from one of trying to deny the awfulness of our present predicament because we do not want to induce fear or despair. Rather, fear and despair are more likely to be induced if we look at 'problems' in isolation, rather than at the systemic whole.

One of the characteristics of much comment on social, economic, and ecological 'problems' is the perceived imperative to 'say something hopeful', to give some cause for optimism. This imperative is partly driven by a wish not to leave people with a sense of despair and lack of agency, and partly because the narrative of Western Modernity – that we are on a path of linear progress – makes it necessary to show a 'way forward'. To accept that there is no hope, at least within the dominant paradigm, is almost unthinkable. Yet that is precisely what we need to do, to stop inventing false causes for optimism. But we must also understand that to accept that Western civilisation is in a state of terminal decline is not simply a message of total gloom but can also be an invitation to tell different stories, to ask different questions, and to imagine other possibilities. It can help to put the old unsustainable paradigm to bed and to start thinking about what that means for humanity and the non-human world.

There are no simple answers, no obvious ways forward, no ten-point plans, that will work. To seek them is to remain within the dominant paradigm.

We need therefore to stop trying to find them. But as Kingsnorth points out, we can tell stories.[3] We can recognise that Western Modernity is just one story, and we can seek others, from Indigenous traditions, from mythology, from art, from a liberated imagination, from literature, and from other forms of cultural expression. We can reject the idea of coming up with a grand plan, a program for change, and recognise that if change is to happen it will emerge from below, from many attempts to reaffirm our humanity and our embeddedness in the non-human world, and we can tell stories to that effect.

Kafka

Kafka, perhaps more than any other, is the writer for our times. His characters are lost, alienated, and disoriented in a world, where they are made to feel powerless by a stifling bureaucracy of rules that keep changing and by authorities that are anonymous and unreachable. There can be no future, and no certainty, as they are trapped in a world that they can neither understand nor control. In contemplating this world, a well-known quote from Kafka serves as a potent descriptor of our times:

> We human beings ought to stand before one another as reverently,
> as reflectively, as lovingly, as we would before the entrance to hell [4]

The future is bleak, frightening, and dire. We are indeed standing before the entrance to hell: a hothouse and degraded planet, species extinction, mass starvation, pandemics, authoritarian regimes, wars, genocide, total surveillance, nuclear threat, enforced 'compliance', and the exercise of raw power in the interest of greed. We have to face this; to do anything less is to deny the awful truth of our predicament. That is extremely difficult, as we all want to believe in a future that is somehow more positive, or with at least a glimmer of hope. But it is only by facing our 'hell', by staring into the abyss, without compromise, that a glimmer of something else might be visible.

Kafka suggests we 'stand before one another'. We do not face the future alone, but with others. But we must not just stand together but *stand before* one another. This implies an openness to each other as flawed humans, a willingness to judge and be judged by each other, a preparedness to share our vulnerabilities, our weaknesses and our fears. We must learn to undo the separation of our public and private selves. To the extent that each of us is complicit in the crises we face, we must be prepared to understand and acknowledge that before our brothers and sisters. Only then will we be able to stand together in genuine solidarity.

Then there are Kafka's three adverbs: *reverently*, *reflectively*, and *lovingly*. First, the need for *reverence*. It sounds so much like the word 'relevance'. Yet in these times we will probably hear the word 'relevance' at least 100 times more often than the word 'reverence' – a telling indictment of the values of our culture. The two words convey two contrasting attitudes towards the world around us. 'Relevance' suggests an instrumentalism, that we value things that are materially useful to us, and that readily fit in with our world-view and help us unquestioningly create a place for ourselves in that world. Reverence, on the other hand, implies awe, wonder, and respect for the world around us. It is our acknowledgement of a world that is bigger, richer, deeper, and more varied than we can possibly understand. It assumes a more humble humanity that is not 'in charge' but rather that is enmeshed in a far more wondrous universe, that is worthy of respect. It is an outlook that refuses to see the natural world as 'resources' but rather sees it as sacred. And this applies not only to the natural world, but to other humans, and to all non-human life forms. If we are to stand together reverently, we must seek to rediscover the sacred, not in the perverted form of most insti-tutionalised religions, but in a much more animistic or pantheistic way, and to recognise how we have not just destroyed, but have desecrated our world. Indigenous cultures understand this in ways that 'modern western' cultures do not. The secularisation of society and the institutionalisation of religion have denied and perverted our sense of the sacredness of the world. This humble and ecological stance at the entrance to hell acknowledges our part in the desecration of the Earth.

Kafka's next adverb is *reflectively*. We need not just to react but to reflect, and this is not easy in an era where anti-intellectualism has strong currency, where simplistic answers are the norm, and where the many demands on us, the rate of change and the '24-hour media cycle' leave little time or space for reflection. The current assault on humanities teaching in universities,[5] sadly supported by so many in the name of 'relevance', is a symptom of the superficiality and the anti-intellectualism of modern life. Critical thought, reflection, and analysis have come to be seen as luxuries for the few, rather than necessities for the many, and this needs to change if we are to help craft alternative futures. If we are to face the future, we must do so reflectively, recognising and valuing our uncertainty, our perplexity, our partial under-standing, our confusion, and realising that making sense of the world, and our place in it, is an ongoing struggle and is always tentative. Our humanity requires continuing questioning, analysis, dialogue, and a recognition that a search for meaning is the essence of being human but also that we can never reach the end of that journey.

Finally, Kafka mentions *love*. In Modernity, love has been exiled to the private sphere. It has no place in political debate or public policy and is mar-ginalised in the professions, even the 'helping professions', where it should surely dominate. Love is one of the strongest and most important human emotions. Its exclusion from the public sphere, from anything beyond inti-mate personal relationships, is one of the tragedies of the Modern Western (and increasingly global) world. As we face the awfulness and the uncer-tainty of the future, humanity must learn to love again. To love not just our intimate partners, but to love each other, to love our communities, to love other humans wherever and whoever they may be, to love both the Earth and the earth, and to love other living beings. This is not something Western Modernity has understood, and we need to learn to love again. Fromm, in his 1956 classic *The Art of Loving*, suggested that the components of love are care, respect, responsibility, and knowledge, each of which must be learned and fostered. This understanding of love incorporates Kafka's reverence and reflectiveness and suggests that, in these awful and perplexing times, thinking about, nurturing, and enacting love is a good place to start. In telling new stories, stories of love may be the most important.

Notes

1 https://www.lifeworth.com/deepadaptation.pdf
2 https://emergencemagazine.org/story/the-myth-of-progress/?fbclid=IwAR2A0f51 UzdaxYa9mN6nSDGjCkHN6uG7sLTzrtNkyE59s2N34HW26p8SpwI
3 https://emergencemagazine.org/story/the-myth-of-progress/?fbclid=IwAR2A0f51 UzdaxYa9mN6nSDGjCkHN6uG7sLTzrtNkyE59s2N34HW26p8SpwI
4 https://www.goodreads.com/quotes/397635-we-are-as-forlorn-as-children-lost-in-the-woods
5 https://www.theguardian.com/australia-news/2020/jun/19/australian-university-fees-arts-stem-science-maths-nursing-teaching-humanities

30

SOCIALISM, LANGUAGE, AND VALUES FOR POST-CORONA WORLD

April 2020

Stuart Rees

New words and phrases, lockdown, self-isolation, and flattening the curve have been coined to explain ways to cope with Covid-19. Language to promote the traits of a post-corona society is also needed.

It will come from words in common usage, and from the visions of artists, musicians and poets who helped their nations to overcome oppression as life-threatening as Covid-19.

A Reluctance to Change

Keywords to express ideals of a common humanity include sufficiency, enough, inclusiveness, justice, equality, universal, green, sharing, feminist, and socialist. Compound ideas can be added: global commons, peace with justice, not-for-profit, public sector, social justice, human rights, humane governance, non-violence, nuclear disarmament, overseas aid, gift relationships and, for worldwide application, altruism over egoism.

Such language can influence public understanding but in spite of Covid-19 motivating people to share resources and help the vulnerable, support persists for a repeat of the past.

In Sydney, a well-heeled superannuant told me, 'Only prophets of doom think that the economic system can't be revived'. He supported Mrs. Thatcher's view about neoliberalism, 'There is no alternative', and Prime Minister Morrison refers to 'snap back', 'We have to get back to what it was like before'.

In Sydney, a friend met a well-educated neighbour who expressed his conspiracy theory, 'This pandemic is a media beat-up'. My friend responded, 'No, it's dangerous, don't you hear the warnings from the ABC?' He reacted, 'The ABC is left-wing, you can't believe what they say'.

DOI: 10.4324/9781003320524-40

In Melbourne, a colleague reported his exchange with a high-profile businessman with a prescription for ways to revive the economy. 'It depends on how many elderly people are wiped out, thereby releasing valuable real estate into the market. Profit from deceased's sales will go into the pockets of children who will spend wildly and so regenerate the economy'.

These comments suggest reluctance to speak of a less destructive society and economy. If a careful, highly professional organisation like the ABC can be dismissed as leftist, what chance of highlighting values to craft a more humanitarian future.

Demystifying Socialism

Cherishing a vocabulary for humanity also requires that the eternal bogey of right-wing politics and media – socialism – be demystified. With neither reflection nor definition, that word is used as a political and cultural scapegoat to describe what people are against, not what they are for.

In Sydney in August 2019, the Conservative Political Action Conference (CPAC) met 'to protect Australia's future'. Participants included former Prime Minister Tony Abbot, representatives from Fox News and the US National Rifle Association. Conference contributors spoke of achieving freedom for 'real people' by protecting the country from socialism.

In similar vein, in the campaign during the 2019 Federal election, Dan Tehan, Minister of Education ridiculed labor proposals for free child care for families earning less than $79,000 a year. This proposal, he said, was 'a fast track to a socialist if not a communist economy'.

A Professor of International Economics at Oregon State told me that in early April he spoke to postgraduate students about societies which invested in public sector health and education. After his lecture, which ended with emphasis on citizens not being financially penalised for being sick, a couple of students emailed him, 'Are you a socialist?'

He explained that in this US university, even at a time of coronavirus lockdowns, and when Senator Bernie Sanders had been derided for his proposals for universal healthcare, it was wise to sidestep the students' question. He advised them, 'Try not to label people, just listen to the message and decide what's right for society and act accordingly'.

Stereotyping promotes baseless fears. Socialism does include principles concerning ownership of the means of production and exchange, but 'ownership' appears in diverse forms. These range from wide public ownership as in the Australian government's virtual nationalisation of private hospitals, to local cooperatives, or to collective initiatives concerned with equity, as in grassroots efforts to contact the lonely and deliver food.

The significant economic historian R H Tawney, usually remembered for warning against private affluence and public squalor, showed that socialism was characterised by dispersion of power and participation by citizens. This, he said, amounted to a recognition of people's interdependence and their enthusiasm for fellowship, which should be good for all citizens.

So, ignore the stereotypes peddled by conservative US commentators, by right-wing evangelists. Avoid the derision of human rights by neo-liberal worshippers. Demystify socialism. Embrace the values. Forget the fears. Get over it.

Not-Quite-Ready Attitudes

For decades citizens have been bombarded with the language of neo-liberal economics, which John Quiggin concludes has been treated as 'common sense'. In consequence, voters perceive security through militarism, and they assume the benefits of lower taxes, privatisation, the protection of borders, flag waving for sovereignty and a mysterious brew called market-oriented reform.

Even in apparently enlightened circles, there's caution to talk about radical change, for fear that to do so would encourage suspicion that a different society might need socialistic policies. It's as though commentators on current affairs apply their ideological brakes. 'We are not ready', as in repetition of clichés about 'returning to normal', 'regaining equilibrium', and hopes for a sort of Moses-led recovery by 'getting to the other side'.

Those clichés suggest confusion about socialism and unwillingness to reject policies which foster inequality and reward affluence. In spite of investments in backup for workers' wages, for free child care and support for diverse businesses, there remains a reluctance to insist that if these policies are beneficial, they could be permanent.

Chastity belt restraints evident in not-quite-ready attitudes, suggest reluctance to envisage a socialist-led economy, which nurtures social justice, fosters equality, improves education and health outcomes, respects human rights, and ends cruelty as a hub of domestic and foreign policies.

Throughout history, this 'not-quite-ready' dictum has been used to oppose significant reforms. Wilberforce and his supporters heard that ending slavery would be premature. Suffragettes were told that women would be too emotional to vote. Until a referendum in 1967, Australia was not ready to treat Indigenous people as citizens.

The corona pandemic has uncovered an economic system which has not valued essential workers and has justified massive, some would say obscene, inequalities in pay. The female head of a Spanish hospital's infectious diseases department was grilled by the press as to why it would take so long to create a vaccine against Covid-19. She replied, 'You give a footballer one million euros per month and biological researchers one thousand eight hundred euros. If you are looking for a vaccination now, go to Cristiano Ronaldo or Lionel Messi, they will find you a cure'.

Language of Musicians and Poets

When politicians are agonising about an economy, though they seem to have overlooked the consequences of climate change, it may seem esoteric

257

to speak about the influence of music and poetry. Yet those art forms illustrate inspiring responses to previous life-threatening crises, persecution, pandemics, and wars.

Beethoven said of his Peace Symphony that he wanted it to be a victory for all humanity. The words in the last movement came from the German poet Schiller's work, 'Ode to Joy'. Schiller wrote that he wanted his words to be 'a kiss for the whole earth'.

In 1899, to evoke the struggles of the Finnish people against Russian control and censorship, the composer Sibelius wrote Finlandia, a musical plea for freedom.

In 1937, at the height of Stalinist tyranny, and in a carefully disguised protest, Shostakovich wrote his Fifth Symphony. At the first performance in Leningrad, the audience wept.

In 19th-century England, Percy Bysshe Shelley insisted that poets were the unacknowledged legislators of the world. During the industrial revolution, as though he was following Shelley's advice, William Wordsworth wrote in 'Humanity', 'What a fair world were ours for verse to paint, if power could live at ease with self-restraint'. He was protesting cruelties in factory labour.

In the United States in the 1960s, during the civil rights movement and the anti-Vietnam war protests, Pete Seeger sang 'If I had a hammer'. He finished by singing that he had a hammer, a bell and a song to sing. It was a hammer of justice, a bell of freedom, a song of love 'between my brothers and sisters, all over this land.

In Britain, Roger Waters, singer-songwriter for Pink Floyd, uses his music to seek justice for refugees, for Palestinians, and for journalist whistleblower Julian Assange. His song 'Each Small Candle' typifies his advocacy that respect for universal human rights is the alternative to 'the blind indifference of a merciless, unfeeling world.

Contemporary poets paint visions to influence a post-corona world. A few weeks ago, Kitty O'Meara wrote that in the absence of people living in ignorant, dangerous, mindless, and heartless ways, the earth began to heal. She summarised that when the danger passed, people joined together, grieved losses, made new choices, dreamed new images, 'created new ways to live and heal the earth fully, as they had been healed

Language to promote the interest of a common humanity envisages societies based on respect for human rights, for internationalism, and on policies for planetary survival. Such vocabulary crafts a future based not entirely on shopping but on sharing and self-sufficiency, on realising that greater equality can contribute to health and happiness and even to a robust economy.

(First published on 17 April 2020 in *Pearls and Irritations* https://johnmenadue.com/stuart-rees-socialism-language-and-values-for-post-corona-worlds/)

31

THE COVID-19 PANDEMIC AND ITS IMPACTS

A Dialogue on Intersectional Vulnerabilities and Resistances[1]
May–June 2020

Francesca Esposito, Gaia Giuliani, Emerson Pessoa, and Vera Silva

Introduction

In the past few months, we have been experiencing unprecedented levels of turmoil and unpredictability due to the outbreak of Covid-19 around the globe. During this time, the slogan 'we are all together in tackling a common enemy' became a recurring theme in mainstream media and political discourses. However, while it is true that the virus affects people regardless of their gender, race, sexuality, and class, as shown by its rapid spread, it is also evident that pre-existing structural disparities significantly influence the risk of being exposed to and infected with Covid. Moreover, now that the 'emergency' phase is passing in many states, we are beginning to ask what will come next. Many of us are concerned with the relief efforts governments are going to introduce and how they will build on pre-existing inequalities, while also deeply entrenching them (as Kimberlé Crenshaw [2020] argued in a recent livestream talk). Some of us are also trying to imagine how we can move on from this pandemic, or rather 'syndemic'[2] as interestingly argued by some scholars (Irons 2020), without going back to a pre-Covid scenario or getting into an even worse one, instead building an alternative and more just world. At this point, we believe radical ideas are needed more than ever.

To address these questions and respond to the call launched by the editors of this volume, in the period between May and July 2020 we decided to engage in an exercise of critical reflection about Covid-19 and its impacts and collective imagination of a post-Covid era. Each of us contributed to this process through their positioned gaze and situated experiences and emotions, as well as with insights gained from the contexts and solidarity networks they have been engaging with. These contexts are interconnected: Portugal,

DOI: 10.4324/9781003320524-41

where we all met and where Vera Silva and Gaia Giuliani still live and work; the United Kingdom, where Francesca Esposito currently lives; Brazil, where Emerson Pessoa returned after completing his PhD in Lisbon; and Italy, where Esposito and Giuliani were born and raised. These very different contexts challenge any universalistic take on our analysis yet offer a clear picture of the unevenness of the pandemic's impact. This unevenness is here explored also through the various perspectives that arise from our different fields of expertise and activism: Francesca on intersectional feminisms, border abolitionism, and migrant justice struggles in the UK, Italy, and Portugal; Gaia on critical whiteness studies, and anti-racist feminist analyses of transnational postcolonial (visual) archives of monstrosity; Emerson on sex workers' rights, migrant justice and LGBTQIA+ people's struggles in Brazil and Portugal; Vera on feminist anthropology, feminist ethnography in women prisons in Portugal, gender, carcerality and abolition feminism.

Our chapter is based on a transcription of our discussion, as a form of a polyphonic dialogue between places, contexts, times, embodied experiences, and emotions. The choice of this format is rooted in the belief that transformative changes and alternative worldviews can only emerge through bottom-up processes of collective radical imagination and enactment of these same changes and alternatives.

The Intersectional Impacts of Covid-19

GAIA: In a recent six-handed study (Giuliani et al. 2020) with a performer and a photographer – a sort of small home-based collective – we reflected on ideas and feelings related to the biopolitics of confinement imposed by European (and global) governments. We used two kinds of plastic film, one for wrapping food and the other for covering furniture, to physically represent, by exhibiting our plastified bodies, a set of emotions: solitude and obsession caused by the presence and absence of the Other and by domestic space as an intensifier of fears, moral panic, and social distancing. The set was organised in an apartment at Rua Rafael de Andrade 19 in Lisbon where Gaia Giuliani and the photographer Ida Fiele (aka Fidelia Avanzato) lived. After a long quarantine alone, they prepared the set together with the HIV+ activist and performer Paolo Gorgoni, who was also emerging from a long self-isolation. The scene and selection of materials were the results of a close dialogue between the three, based on years of artistic and intellectual collaboration and a strong friendship. The set was the fruit of improvisation, starting with a shared storyboard structured in indoor scenes that depicted sensations and moods, as well as actual bodily conditions. The inside of a house/prison in the time of Covid-19 is thematised here as a place/shelter and at the same time a precursory place of dangerous absences that ensnare desires, reduce affects, and cause obsessions to run rampant. It is a place of reflection – for us, it was a laboratory for anything and everything, but also and most of all it was a lab of estrangement and solitude, different than the media vulgarity and the biopolitics of containment that described closing oneself in one's home as residing serenely in the safest and reassuring place.

I wanted to start my chapter by mentioning this recent exploration because it forced me to think about the very peculiar kind of confinement we have experienced en masse during this period and the ontological differences it has with imprisonment. These differences are the core of our discussion here because they define the line that separates those who still have the privilege of 'temporary confinement without criminalisation' (i.e. confinement meant to 'preserve' the life of the confinee) and the many others who, for different reasons, do not have the conditions to experience this: people with no home to be confined in, people whose home is not a safe place, people who live in overcrowded houses, people who are compelled to go to unsafe workplaces, people who are locked up in prisons and detention centres. All these specific conditions are marked by lines that define race, gender, sexuality, and class privilege. In this context, the body – the marked body of hegemonic as well as unprivileged people – defines access to a 'temporary confinement without criminalisation' that is only made possible by a certain amount of cultural, racial, gender and economic capital. Our chapter to the call can therefore be seen as stemming from these premises.

As discussed in the conclusion to the monograph *Monsters, Catastrophes, and the Anthropocene*, a Postcolonial Critique, published in 2021, the impact of this pandemic is unimaginably widespread, since it has to do with our most intimate feelings (of vulnerability and fear) towards social and moral panic and includes a normativisation of ideas of illness and social illness that acts on the social fabric of societies and communities. It will influence the way people reflect on their own bodies, individual and social relationships, their effects, and society as a whole. In this sense, the pandemic is a semiotic event, whose bio – and necropolitical mechanisms are changing imaginaries and ideas of the self and others, paving the way for new forms of neo-liberal restructuring and authoritarian control over individuals and societies.

EMERSON: I agree with Gaia that it is important to adopt an intersectional analytical perspective and look at issues of privilege and vulnerability. After all, in a world marked by class inequalities, colonialism, racism, and cis-heteronormativity, who are the people that have access to technologies, body care, well-being, health, and art? Looking at the current economic, social, and cultural context in my country, Brazil, I cannot help thinking of my students from the Amazon region. They are mainly working students, who cannot access distance learning because they lack quality internet. In addition, Brazil is facing a serious political and pandemic crisis that started in large cities but is currently attacking people in different states in very unequal ways, both in the cities and

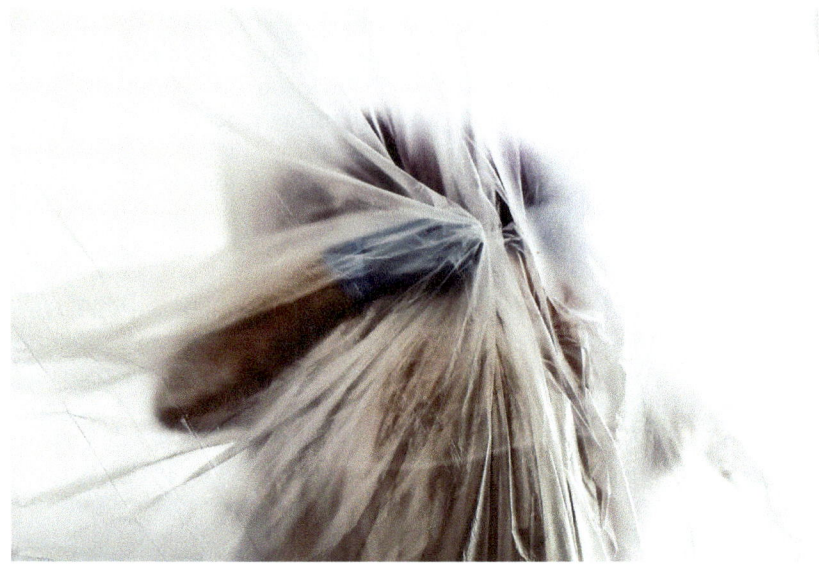

Artwork 31.1 Photo by Fidelia Avanzato. Gaia Giuliani and Paolo Gorgoni in "Pandemic: a six-handed study".

the countryside and including Indigenous and Quilombola communities. To give an example, the northern region of Brazil, where I currently live has the highest mortality rates in the country per 100,000 inhabitants and twice the national rate. This reflects the precariousness and vulnerability of the local population and healthcare system. I have been experiencing a lot of anxiety in the last couple of months, as I have witnessed the state's neglect of the most vulnerable and marginalised groups and the lack of uniformity between policies implemented by the federal government on the one hand, and those implemented by states and municipalities on the other. However, I have also witnessed numerous initiatives implemented by civil society groups to momentarily address the problems of individuals and communities living in precarious and vulnerable situations, such as the actions of the sex workers and Indigenous peoples' movements. Nevertheless, I often feel powerless in the face of the social and political tragedies that my country is experiencing daily.

VERA: I agree with Gaia that we are experiencing a semiotic event, although this is either partly or fully built on previous sediments. The strategies and responses to the pandemic put in place by governments and corporations show how our neo-liberal societies are organised, materialising in different ways in diverse geographical and political contexts.

Following Angela Davis (BCRW 2020), the experience of incarceration has nothing to do with what we are going through now, although there are possible parallels. For instance, in some countries, such as Portugal, we can observe similarities between crime control and the measures adopted to prevent and tackle Covid-19. In addition to quarantine and social distancing, some of the measures that have been introduced include monitoring, control, persecution, and punishment. Accordingly, the arbitrary power of the security forces has been reinforced and, predictably, police repression has mainly targeted marginalised groups and communities already affected by poverty and social exclusion. Significantly, these groups and communities are also the ones most vulnerable to the pandemic, as they have fewer resources to tackle it. Overall, contention measures have had multiple effects on people's lives and, in some cases, we can make connections with the experiences of people who are incarcerated, criminalised, or on welfare (Fraser and Gordon 1992), that is those subjected to the controlling and monitoring mechanisms of the carceral-assistential complex (Wacquant 2008).

In reflecting on my lockdown experience as well as the experiences shared by friends, relatives, and colleagues, I can identify some similarities with the accounts of the women and transgenders I used to meet in prisons. What emerges as common in both cases is a sense of isolation, powerlessness, despair, mental confusion, lack of concentration, insomnia, and anxiety. Despite these similarities, the effects of lockdown and imprisonment are still significantly different. Notably, in prisons, the lockdown was extremely harsh, as prisoners were locked in cells for an average of 22 hours a day and denied any visits from relatives and friends. At the same time, prisoners have been facing a higher risk of contagion due to poor health and hygiene conditions and overcrowding. The particular example of the prison context well illustrates how lockdown experiences have varied from one context to another, as well as from person to person, as Gaia and Emerson observed, with the White middle and upper-class experience having been established as normative.

In general, I also think that our lives are increasingly being controlled through biopolitics and technological devices, and this is only getting worse as time passes. During this period, I have been thinking about communities' tendencies towards social control. In particular, I reflected on how the idea of acting as a 'public health agent'[3], marketed by public health authorities, has ultimately led to policing attitudes in the general public, rather than a communal and solidarity-based vision of health, protection, and care. By declaring a 'state of emergency' Portugal government responded to the Covid-19 outbreak with force, instilling fear, moral panic, and punitivism. As a consequence, health protection and care have, for many people, translated into acts of self-policing and policing of others or, alternatively, into the transgression of rules. This favours the creation of scapegoats to justify the spread of the virus, blaming individuals and hiding the real causes for this public health calamity that derive from the lack of resources and public health policies, among other structural issues arising from the neo-liberal governance. Unfortunately, a truly community and solidarity-informed understanding of health, protection, and care have largely been lacking.

FRANCESCA: At the beginning, this situation was quite unsettling for me, as I felt a sense of uncertainty and disorientation, both externally and internally. As soon as I started to realise what was actually going on, I also felt a sense of helplessness, the helplessness that Emerson was talking about. I felt helpless and also confused, without knowing exactly what responses to give, how to react to this event. So my first impulse was to look for immediate actions, such as participating in solidarity networks to support those most affected by Covid-19 in our communities or launching public campaigns (e.g. for the release of people in immigration detention centres and prisons; VV.AA 2020). I initially went in this direction, but at some point, I also started to question my actions – or reactions – and the extent to which they were having a transformative impact. Also, one of the things that wearied me the most in this period was the information overload we have been exposed to. At first, like everyone else, I tried to follow all the news, reading articles about what was happening in different countries and monitoring the 'epidemic curve', but then I felt that the information circulating in the mainstream media was completely saturated, that is, it did not provide me with any critical tool to deal with what was going on – in the world and within myself too. And all of a sudden I decided to start reading books that had nothing to do with Covid, for example, diaries written by imprisoned people. The experience of imprisonment, as Gaia and Vera said, is completely different from what we have been living through, but I think this literature has enormous value. It offers us critical analytical tools and, above all, it teaches us unique resistance strategies – originally used in much more violent circumstances.

From the very beginning of the Covid-19 outbreak the narrative that 'this is a shared crisis for us to overcome' has circulated on social media and permeated public discourses, but this is a false narrative as we are not 'all in this together': we are not all exposed in the same way and we do not all have access to the same resources to deal with this health emergency. What has been happening recently has reflected, highlighted, and amplified all the inequalities that already existed, which have now become striking. This pandemic did not come from nowhere, as there were known trends and contributing factors as well as measures that could have been put in place long ago to prevent it. More importantly, the pandemic did not come to revolutionise our neo-liberal capitalist societies and show how we are all deeply interconnected. Instead, it highlighted the longstanding inequalities and many differences in how people are made vulnerable, in different times and contexts. So, I agree with what Emerson said: any reflection on this situation needs to put intersectionality at the centre of the discussion and take privilege, power, oppression, positionality, and subjectivity into account.

For instance, since the beginning of the health emergency, count-less measures have been implemented, but while some of them have been celebrated as advances for those who are most marginalised and at risk, the truth is that they have only reached certain people and excluded others, thus reinforcing and reconfiguring the blurred line between 'desirable' and 'undesirable' subjects. Some people have been released from prison, while others have not. In many countries, asylum seekers confined in detention centres were released, but the same did not happen to those who had any kind of criminal record, who were abandoned in these sites (see, for instance, Esposito et al. 2020). As for borders, while the majority of countries have closed their borders to curb the spread of Covid-19 and many people have been prevented from travelling and reuniting with their loved ones, many governments have also encouraged the entry of certain groups, such as healthcare professionals and seasonal workers to be employed in the agro-industrial sector (individuals deemed 'desirable' in the pandemic times) (Sekalala and Rawson 2020). In other words, I think that during this period we have been witnessing a proliferation of boundaries and hierarchies – the proliferation of borders mentioned by Mezzadra and Neilson (2013) – and further entrenchment of the blurred line between who is 'desirable' and 'deserves' (to be liberated, to be protected, to live) and who is 'undesirable' and 'undeserving'. This divide operates across lines of colour, race, gender, class, gener-ations, and nationality among others, and is illustrative of the inter-secting power relations at stake in our Western societies and how these latter are moulded and transformed according to the hegem-onic needs of the moment.

VERA: I agree with Francesca and I think that the exploitative relationship with nature – and the disconnection that has been imposed on us through-out modern, Western and colonial history – is also another intersection that should be addressed in our analysis. During the lockdown, I started two vegetable gardens and this process has helped me a lot to deal with the pandemic. It has also made me think about the importance of per-maculture and the need to build a sustainable way of life that reconnects with nature. Significantly, our relationship with nature is intertwined with the notion of subject, the relationship with our bodies and the pro-cesses of othering. I think that we are disconnected from ourselves and from the world that surrounds and nurtures us.

I am still exploring and learning about the concept of intersection-ality, but I am aware of the importance of understanding the various power complexes and intersections. I think intersectionality is not only about identifying the 'many exclusions' and the 'different excluded groups', as there is a risk of essentialising them, but is also (and above all) about understanding how power operates. Power is not unidirec-tional, which makes it difficult to dismantle. The main challenge is therefore to develop an awareness of the racist, patriarchal, and capitalist nature of power, without legitimising and reproducing it. To do so, we need to critically reflect on our positionality while we engage either in direct action or theoretical analysis.

EMERSON: I fully agree with Vera's argument about the heightening of the control mechanisms that were already operating on our bodies and subjectivities before the virus. There has been a great debate about Agamben's reflections on Covid-19, published in the *Boitempo Dossier*[4]. Thinking about it, I find it very interesting to reflect on the theoretical radicalism of some philosophers, researchers and academics. In particular, I believe that we cannot be tempted to rely on ready-made theories to understand the current context within the pandemic. As a pragmatic researcher, I frequently adopt Foucault's (1986) perspective on control mechanisms, and I agree with Agamben (2020) when he argues that the pandemic has been used to legitimise a state of exception, but we cannot dismiss all the scientific evidence about the pandemic and the importance of the lockdown to stem the spread of the virus. Still thinking about Agamben's chapter and the criticism it attracted, Frateschi (2020) concludes her article with the following challenge: 'Go back to the city, philosopher'. I believe that at this moment we do need to leave our privileged 'academic bubbles' and go back to our communities to understand people's different realities and avoid 'theoretical masturbation'. The reality is indeed much more complex than our theories. We have to think about this to avoid theoretical extremism and denial of the existing scientific knowledge on Covid-19, as Agamben does when he argues: 'Are you willing to allow the pandemic to legitimise a state of exception?' I agree that many governments have been using the pandemic to take backwards steps in terms of public policies – the Brazilian government is one of them. However, we cannot deny the importance of the state in dealing with the pandemic. In the case of Brazil, public hospitals are primarily responsible for the care of sick people. I believe that this reality will change people's representations of public health and its importance.

The information overload that Francesca mentioned is another issue that has intensified my feeling of helplessness. The dozens of *lives* of teachers, researchers, NGO members, and artistic collectives made me think that in the context of a pandemic everyone wants to become a digital influencer. In the online debates I was invited to, I always asked myself what would be the purpose of the material/information produced. Who would actually be able to access and consume it? To what extent is our 'organic processor' capable of retaining all the information produced during the pandemic? And I am not only thinking about information for the general public but also information produced by the network of intellectuals and researchers that I follow. That is why I decided to start filtering the information I consumed daily.

GAIA: Besides referring to the impact of the official information on Covid and its broader media and social media dimensions, I also believe it is important for us to discuss how it forges a very biased idea of the catastrophe. If we feel like we are being bombarded, and actually we are, the kind of information dropped on us every day describes the catastrophe as something new and global, not because it is unparalleled (in fact, it came in the wake of many other zoonotic pandemics that have spread in the last 20 years) but because it hit the so-called Global North first. After China, Europe has been the target of the pandemic for all the well-known reasons related to global capitalism. In European media such as Italian and Portuguese online television channels and the BBC, which I watched during the lockdown, the pandemic was portrayed as something which was occurring only in the West. While Al Jazeera makes it clear that the impact outside Europe and the West is generating a series of different kinds of unchecked catastrophes and will continue to do so, given that the pandemic has exacerbated all the inequalities produced by global neo-liberal extractivist capitalism, the media and governments in Italy and Portugal only focus on their 'imagined communities' and bombard us with anything that generates moral panic against situations and people seen as carriers of the virus. Together with other public discourses, this information contributes towards building up the idea of a safer space, namely the West, Europe, 'our' homeland, 'our' home, based on the distinction between what I have defined as 'places *of* disaster' and 'places *for* disaster' (Giuliani 2017), to identify the current understanding of the civilised 'here' – the West (where disasters are not systemic) – and the uncivilised 'out there' – the formerly colonised world (where disasters are endemic and are also generated to maintain the privilege of the 'here'). As is evident, this distinction is structured by colonial logics and ontologies. According to this distinction – which is epistemic as well as epistemological – what happens beyond the line that separates the two worlds is less important, forgettable, inconsequential for the 'here', and the populations of the 'out there' – as Judith Butler (2009), Talal Asad (2007), and Achille Mbembe (2003) have argued – are expendable for the good of global capitalism that still guarantees us (White Europeans) wealth, protection and safety. Therefore, 'we' do not know anything about the impact of the pandemic on the population of the Global South and those on the margins of our societies. Nor do we know about the Indigenous forms of resistance and resilience in the face of the environmental effects of neo-liberal capitalism (such as pandemics, floods, air and water pollution, and climate change), and the struggles waged against them in the internal social margins of Western societies. The line separating 'places *of* disaster' and 'places *for* disasters' is thus not merely a line separating the Global North from the Global South, but a set of multiple intersecting and contextually shaped race, gender, class and territorial lines, deeply affected by border regimes and neo-liberal restructuring across nations and continents. Moreover, in alternately obfuscating and shedding light on phenomena and the differential impacts of Covid in the world, this kind of information creates the semiotic space for a reshaping of the Western idea of 'subject', described as constrained between state control and catastrophe, and based on a de-politicisation and de-responsibilisation of capitalism and its public and private agents. Capitalism, by the way, is never mentioned by Agamben (2003), who describes the new biopolitical regimes as if people were only faced with a state superpower, similar to the one described by Carl Schmitt (2007), rather than with warfare and control capitalism trading big data and pharmaceuticals. State bio- and necropolitics are the results of a very complex set of capitalist restructurings that benefit multinational corporations extracting data and environmental resources, whose activities are at the root of the current pandemic. Biopolitical and control technology – from drones to vaccines, leading to extreme restrictions on privacy and control of mobility – is what the world's population will be increasingly and differentially facing, generating forms of resistance that we need to look at to limit the authoritarian outcome of this extractivist capitalism. Counteracting the information regime that overwhelms us means being able to reject a simplistic and universalistic vision of the world in which we are, and will be, living, a vision that does not reflect power relations. It allows us to grasp the contradictions of a discourse which, in levelling out the impact of the pandemic – 'we are all in the same situation' – constructs a conformist and authoritarian narrative that sees in the unchecked actions of the state, directed towards its national community – and of the West, directed towards the rest of the world – the very possibility of 'our' salvation. We need to look back to the genealogy of forms of resistance from the margins – local and global – whose experience of catastrophe since the dawn of modernity and colonialism could help us understand how to fight this pandemic – I mean how to fight both its material causes and biopolitical outcomes – and draw up a political project for the future.

Responses to Covid-19: Reacting, Resisting, Transforming

EMERSON: I perceive a sense of hopelessness among people and organisations here in Brazil. Gaia emphasised that we need to look back to the genealogy of forms of resistance from the margins. I feel quite dystopian right now. I cannot think that we – the isolated population, non-governmental organisations, resistance groups – have the power to reverse everything that is happening. The impression I have of Brazil is that people were already experiencing many difficulties due to the political, economic, and social crisis, and this situation has been exacerbated by the pandemic. This has created these feelings of frustration and help-lessness. We feel as if our hands are tied in the face of all the urgent matters and needs looming over us. I think particularly of the Brazilian left, which in the current situation is attempting to build and present a political project for Brazil. In my view, at the moment we do not have a political party and/or public figure that I regard as a possible represent-ative of the people. This situation has greatly affected those around me and is aggravated by the information overload and the numerous prob-lems/urgencies that have recently emerged.

FRANCESCA: It is true that at the moment there are so many urgent matters that it is difficult to navigate and address them all. I think that the sense of helplessness we all feel partly stems from this: from experiencing difficulty in responding to the many issues which have emerged – and are still emerging – in this period which, as we said, are linked to pre-existing problems in terms of inequalities and differential access to resources and rights. We have witnessed the development of numerous community-based initiatives, as Emerson mentioned before, but some of them relied on very assistentialist and individualised notions of 'help' and 'care', thus reproducing problematic state-sponsored practices. On the other hand, some grassroots initiatives and community-based soli-darity networks have provided meaningful platforms for the exchange of mutual forms of support on an emotional, economic, and material level, especially among those who are most marginalised. In Portugal, we have the example of the Anti-Racist Campaign for Immediate Support – Lisbon or the Anti-Racist Campaign for Immediate Support – Coimbra which, together with local community organisations, have been provid-ing solidarity networks for Black, Roma, and migrant communities as well as for families in very vulnerable situations – all groups that have been hit badly by the pandemic (Gomes Duarte and Lima 2020). These campaigns/networks are more or less purposefully reconfiguring the meaning of basic notions such as 'care', 'love', 'family' and their related practices in a more solidarity-based and communal (and therefore polit-ical) way. In doing so, they are challenging the state's individualistic neo-liberal modus operandi. Refugee organisations in Portugal have been working to support asylum-seeking people, providing them with personal protective equipment and other essential resources that state authorities did not supply. If these practices are maintained beyond this emergency period and accompanied by critical reflection on the under-lying values and ideas (e.g. love, care, solidarity), I do believe they can have a transformative impact and contribute to the creation of alterna-tive and meaningful ways of living in our communities.

I also think that important forms of resistance have emerged dur-ing this period, informed by radical political visions and demands, such as the struggles of people in prisons and detention centres. In Spain, the struggles of the migrants detained in the CIEs (*Centros de Internamiento de Extranjeros*), supported by external activists, have forced the government to close all detention centres in mainland Spain and the islands (although in the North African enclaves of Ceuta and Melilla this has not happened yet, and the situation has worsened (Gabrielli 2020)). This was an unprecedented victory as it was the first time these centres in Spain had been emptied since they were created (Global Detention Project 2020). We know that this may not be a permanent change, given that it is actually linked to the Covid-19 emergency, and questions remain about what will happen to the facilities and to formerly detained people in the near future, but even so it is extremely important, even in terms of our collective imaginary. It shows that we can live without these horrific institutions. It demonstrates that it is not too difficult to end migrant detention and let people live free in our communities: it is a concrete, not a utopian scenario. For ordinary people, this may cause a 'shift' in terms of imaginary, possible realities, although the same is unlikely to happen with policy-makers, as we know the political-economic interests at stake in the detention industry and in the border industrial complex more broadly. Overall, what I want to say is that amid this tragic situation there is some transformative potential and some forms of resistance are taking place which can significantly change our present and, above all, our future.

VERA: In Portugal, almost 2,000 people were released from prison during the lockdown. However, this was a very small number compared to the total prison population, which amounts to 13,000 people. At the beginning of the pandemic, I was hoping that the general public could develop a kind of empathy with those incarcerated in prisons. Unfortunately, this was not the case, as there was great opposition from the right-wing parties and a large part of civil society to any measure to release people from prisons during the pandemic, evidence which highlights the widespread popular punitivism and the dominant patriarchal culture of punishment.

Concerning grassroots actions and practices during this period, I was also involved in a solidarity network created in my neighbourhood. I think these initiatives are important as they show that we are still supportive and compassionate to each other, even in such difficult times. However, I agree that we must be very careful not to slide into the reproduction of assistential models. Helping a person by providing food or addressing their immediate basic needs is important, but it is not enough. The political and capitalist structures can even profit from these actions, which ultimately replace the state in terms of responsibility to provide social welfare. Moreover, when these practices defy the hierarchical and discriminatory capitalist order on which our societies are based, they are repressed by means of force or depletion of their resources. If, on the one hand, this pandemic is unveiling the operations of power, allowing us to see the cracks and failures in the state and the political and economic systems in which we live, it is also making clear the need to reflect and mobilise our strategies of resistance.

EMERSON: Yes, the risk is falling into community assistentialism. For example, the university is collecting food for vulnerable students, many of whom are without money and/or work. But what resolution are we taking in the macro sense? It is rather like giving aspirin to those who have cancer. We are not solving the problem. There were many solidarity campaigns here that involved making masks for the Indigenous population, but in the grand scheme of things, these initiatives mean very little. The situation of the Indigenous population in Brazil is one of poverty and genocide, and the current government has intensified policies for the death and destruction of Indigenous reserves. Environmental issues are considered an obstacle to the country's development. In a government meeting leaked by the media, the current Minister for the Environment, Renato Salles, went so far as to affirm that the pandemic was an 'opportunity' to change the rules related to environmental protection and agriculture without being questioned by the mainstream media and judicial system. In other words, we are facing constant attacks on human and non-human populations in the country. Everything is very bleak.

FRANCESCA: I agree with Vera and Emerson, and I think that as long as we are 'reacting' to a situation that is imposed on us and which places many constraints on our actions and transformative possibilities, it is very exhausting and we do not change much, especially if we focus on individual needs. Although I recognise the importance of these efforts, I believe the challenge is to address the structural bases of the problems and be able to identify and transform the roots of individual and collective suffering, rather than just the 'symptoms'. But this is a much more complex operation. And I think that in this period we witnessed both types of responses, that is, people 'reacting' to the pandemic and its violence, and people trying to address the problems that have arisen while also pushing to transform the system as a whole. In this second category, I include, for example, the struggles to abolish the prison and immigration industrial complexes and guarantee a document for all (regardless of their personal and immigration background).

VERA: I believe that one of the reasons why we fall into assistential practices is because we consider ourselves external to some problems. This is what feminist abolitionists in the United States taught us. These political perspectives and practices emerged from the movements of Black and Indigenous women who have long been advocating transformative justice and community accountability as means to deal with structural and interpersonal violence (Kim 2018). I think that, as researchers and activists, we urgently need to reflect on and transform the way we position ourselves as subjects and in relation to others, as well as how we theorise and act.

There is a need in Western societies to rebuild community practices, empathy and *vincularity* (Segato 2018), which have been eroded by a capitalist way of life – and the pandemic crisis has made this need more evident and urgent. Vulnerabilised groups – such as women, Black and Indigenous communities, transgender people, refugees, prisoners and their families, among others – are the ones who, throughout history, have been resisting and developing community bonding and bridging as well as political practices for mutual care.

Looking at prisons and the repressive measures of the state enables us to understand how they ultimately work to disrupt affective, social, and political ties between people and communities. These ties are fundamental to allowing communities to organise themselves politically and achieve economic sustainability, direct democracy, transformative justice, and a life in harmony with the natural world and the planet.

Re-imagining Our Present for a Political Project for the Future

In White, Eurocentric colonial thinking, the distinction between 'places *of* disaster' and 'places *for* disasters', defined by a series of lines – based on race, gender, sexuality, and religion but also generations (and in the case of Covid, this is an important intersectional marker) – separates ontologies of places, people, and forms of more than human life according to an extractivist and exploitative rationale. Now, the world 'out there', the world of ongoing apocalypse, has managed to expose the weakness of an unequal system based on privatisation and dispensability. The dispensability of racialised subjects, the poor and older adults, which appeared to have been held in check by a system of governmentality based on the welfare state and biopolitical control, is revealing itself to be violent, underpinned by arguments that claim to be universal. The fear is that Western geography, the history behind the division into the world (*of* disaster) 'here' and the world (*for* disaster) 'out there' that characterises the West as master and conceals its internal contradictions and violence, is disappearing, bringing colonial violence into the safe space of the postcolonial metropole.

This vision is, once again, Euro/Western-centric and racist because it hides both the complexity of planetary relationships between phenomena which Karen Barad (2007, 2008) describes as 'intra-active' and Rita Segato (2018) as 'vincularity' and the 'interdependence of beings' according to Stacey Alaimo (2010) or our 'radical dependency' in the words of Ruth Gilmore (2020) and also because it denies the systemic violence of the Anthropocene. The media narrows down the vision, focusing only on what is happening in the here and now, in a utopian West that must be saved, in Atreyu's Fantasia in the anthropocentric version of the never-ending story that leaves out all the contradictions. In short, the idea that our 'here and now' is the 'society that must be saved' from barbarian invasion and brutality, including Covid, is reconstructed. The brutality of Sars-CoV-2 is represented as a force from outside the Anthropocene and the Anthropocene is described as the best world possible for all (Giuliani et al. 2020).

Self-care – as Audre Lorde stated – and care for the Earth are what we need to escape from the patriarchal reasoning of the Capitalocene, and the rationale of slavery and racist and colonial oppression which obliterate the subjectivity and autonomy of oppressed people, as well as the oppressive mindset of accelerated capitalism, which obliges us to work like maniacs even during a pandemic, destroying us physically, mentally and spiritually, and exposing the Earth to a suicidal level of exploitation. This set of inter-dependent rationales establishes the degree of vulnerability to exploitation and death for people (as anti-racist movements like Black Lives Matter are reminding us these days) and the environment, and the different levels of responsibility for this vulnerability. Neo-liberalism makes us believe that we can love and care for ourselves without others or, alternatively, that we can satisfy our needs for love and care in a family or a romantic relationship alone. These beliefs are two sides of the same coin, both deeply shaped by individualised notions of possession and control. Hence, it is crucial to crit-ically re-think and re-shape notions and practices of care and love within our own communities, while also discovering ways to reproduce love and care equally among people.

The self-care which Inna Michaeli (2017), Sara Ahmed (2014), and Gaia Giuliani (2021) refer to, following Audre Lorde (1988), is not a 'neo-liberal trap' based on consumerism and privatisation but an ongoing – individual and communal – war, a political stance, an act of assuming responsibility. It is what racialised and Indigenous, feminist, transgender and queer communi-ties practice: 'self-care' – argues Ahmed – is 'not about self-indulgence, but self-preservation …. This kind of self-care is not about one's own happiness. It is about finding ways to exist in a world that is diminishing' (Ahmed 2014).

An intersectional and anti-capitalist critique of care and self-care is, therefore, necessary for both a critical understanding of our world and an 'epistemology in action' against inequalities: an intersectional perspective indeed allows us to grasp how structural inequalities and contemporary technologies of social control affect different people in a different way, as well as how they shape and operate in our relationships of self-care and care for others. At the same time, intersectionality allows us to apprehend the 'precariousness of life' mentioned by Judith Butler (2009), that is, the evidence that the persistence of life, and one's survival, is intrinsically related to and dependent on existing social and political conditions, but also to the 'social network of hands' (Butler 2009: 14) that we establish with others in the current global context.

Finally, intersectionality is a necessary political tool to build alliances and make our 'actions in solidarity' respectful of the different positionalities and political agendas, since without an intersectional approach even the more radical action of care and self-care can turn colonial and patriarchal. Conceived in these terms, self-care can include self-protection for Indigenous peoples and racialised and gendered minorities faced with the violence of the Anthropocene and its related disasters and pandemics. In the case of Brazil, for instance, care and love have offered hope in these dark times. Despite all the attacks that the most vulnerabilised groups are facing at the moment, there have also been initiatives by associations, collectives and individuals from civil society seeking better living conditions and rights for all. The Observatory on Prostitution at the Federal University of Rio de Janeiro (UFRJ), for example, recently reported on campaigns by Brazilian sex workers movements and associations in different cities throughout the country aimed at helping to tackle the pandemic and/or establishing public policies for sex workers (Simões *et al.* 2020). The Articulação dos Povos Indígenas do Brasil has also launched campaigns for resources and/or to counter the effects of the pandemic in Indigenous communities.

These bottom-up solidarity networks, like others we mentioned in our dialogue (i.e., the Campanha Antirracista de Apoio Imediato – Lisboa (2020) and the Campanha Antirracista de Apoio Imediato – Coimbra (2020), Boleto +1 (2020), are transformative experiences that have far-reaching potential. If they are continued beyond the Covid-19 emergency and transformed into long-term socio-political infrastructures for our communities, these experiences can help us forge a different world, a world based on care, responsibility, and reciprocity among humans and with the more-than-human world of nature, as Elisabeth Povinelli (2016) stresses. Only in this way can self-care, self-love, care, and earth-care form the pillar of the new world that our project envisions. This project, it is worthwhile to re-emphasise, has intersectional feminist visions at its core.

Notes

1 This chapter was conceived and written on an equal basis by all the authors, who are listed in alphabetical order.
2 The term 'syndemic' was first developed by Singer and Snipes (1992), Singer (1994) in her critical work on the AIDS epidemic in the United States to call attention to the synergistic nature of the health and social problems facing the poor and underserved. In particular, Singer situated the ADIS disease in terms of the broader configuration of health and social conditions that structured the epidemic. An extensive literature has been produced over the years on syndemics, and recently this notion has been used by some scholars, such as Rebecca Irons (2020), to describe the Covid-19 emergency and call for a more nuanced approach to tackle it.
3 https://covid19.min-saude.pt/wp-content/uploads/2020/05/MEDIDAS-GERAIS.pdf
4 https://blogdaboitempo.com.br/dossies-tematicos/dossie-coronavirus/

References

Agamben, G. (2003). *Stato di Eccezione. Homo sacer II*. Turin: Bollati Boringhieri.

Agamben, G. (2020). *Reflexões sobre a peste: ensaios em tempos de pandemia*. São Paulo: Boitempo editorial.

Ahmed, S. (2014). 'Selfcare as Warfare'. *Feminist Killjoy* [online]. Available at: https://feministkilljoys.com/2014/08/25/selfcare-as-warfare/ [Accessed 11 March 2020].

Alaimo, S. (2010). *Bodily Natures: Science, Environment, and the Material Self*. Bloomington: Indiana University Press.

Asad, T. (2007). *On Suicide Bombing*. New York: Columbia University Press.

Barad, K. (2007). *Meeting the Universe Halfway: Quantum Physics and the Entanglement of Matter and Meaning*. Durham: Duke University Press [online]. Available at: http://doi.org/10.1215/9780822388128 [Accessed 10 March 2020].

Barad, K. (2008). 'Posthumanist performativity: toward an understanding of how matter comes to matter'. In: Alaimo, S. and Hekman, S. (eds.) *Material Feminisms*. Indianapolis: Indiana University Press, pp. 120–156.

Barnard Center for Research on Women – BCRW. (2020). Abolition Feminism: Celebrating 20 Years of INCITE! [Video file] [online]. Available at: https://www.facebook.com/BCRW.Feminism/videos/367419774199654/?t=2 [Accessed 25 June 2020].

Boleto + 1. (2020). Available at: https://www.facebook.com/boletomaisum [Accessed 25 June 2020].

Butler, J. (2009). *Frames of War: When Is Life Grievable?* New York: Verso.

Esposito, F. Caja, E., and Mattiello, G. (2020). 'No one is looking at us anymore': *Migrant Detention and Covid-19 in Italy* [online]. Available at: https://www.law.ox.ac.uk/sites/files/oxlaw/no_one_is_looking_at_us_anymore_1.pdf [Accessed 21 June 2020].

Campanha Antirracista de Apoio Imediato – Lisboa. Available at: https://www.facebook.com/pages/category/Community-Organization/Covid-19-Campanha-Antirracista-de-Apoio-Imediato-Lisboa-100984081570759/ [Accessed 25 June 2020].

Campanha Antirracista de Apoio Imediato – Coimbra. Available at: https://www.facebook.com/events/212458623313044/permalink/218900026002237/?ref=3&ref_newsfeed_story_type=regular&action_history=[%7B%22surface%22%3A%22newsfeed%22%2C%22mechanism%22%3A%22feed_story%22%2C%22extra_data%22%3A[]%7D [Accessed 25 June 2020].

Crenshaw, K. (2020). *Intersectionality Matters: A Conversation with Kimberlé Crenshaw* [Video file] [online]. Available at: https://www.youtube.com/watch?v=otload6iBhA [Accessed 25 June 2020].

Covid 19 e os povos indígenas. (2020). Available at: https://covid19.socioambiental.org/?gclid=Cj0KCQjwiYL3BRDVARIsAF9E4GeejJMcOaFd_woiA0AZBwmqLLEjeGL4rBqBLIWnRIO88A3KtfUA7jwaApNsEALw_wcB [Accessed 25 June 2020].

Foucault, M. (1986). *Microfísica do Poder*. 6ª edição. Rio de Janeiro, RJ: Graal.

Fraser, N. and Gordon, L. (1992). "Contract versus charity: Why is there no social citizenship in the United States?", *Socialist Review* 22(3), pp. 45–68.

Frateschi, Y. (2020). *Agamben sendo Agamben: o filósofo e a invenção da pandemia*. [Blog] [online]. Available at: https://blogdaboitempo.com.br/2020/05/12/agamben-sendo-agamben-o-filosofo-e-a-invencao-da-pandemia/ [Accessed 30 May 2020].

Gabrielli, L. (2020). *Migrazioni sottosopra. L'impatto del Covid-19 sui movimenti di persone alle frontiere tra Spagna e Marocco* [online]. Available at: https://www.fieri.it/2020/06/04/migrazioni-sottosopra-limpatto-del-covid-19-sui-movimenti-di-persone-alle-frontiere-tra-spagna-e-marocco/ [Accessed 30 May 2020].

Gilmore, R. (2020). *Geographies of Racial Capitalism with Ruth Wilson Gilmore – An Antipode Foundation Film.* [Video file] [online]. Available at: https://www.youtube.com/watch?v=2CS627aKrJI [Accessed 25 June 2020].

Giuliani, G., Gorgoni, P., and Avanzato, F. (2020). *Pandemico: Sex-hands Study, From the European South* (forthcoming).

Giuliani, G. (2021). *Monsters, Catastrophes and the Anthropocene. A Postcolonial Critique.* London: Routledge, forthcoming.

Giuliani, G. (2017). "Afterword: Life adrift in a postcolonial world." In: Baldwin, A. and Bettini, G. (eds.) *Life Adrift: Climate Change, Migration, Critique.* London and New York: Rowman & Littlefield International, pp. 227–242.

Global Detention Project. (2020). *Country Report: Immigration Detention in Spain: A Rapid Response to Covid-19.* [online]. Available at: https://www.globaldetentionproject.org/immigration-detention-in-spain-a-rapid-response-to-covid-19 [Accessed 30 May 2020].

Gomes Duarte, L., and Lima, R. (2020). "On intersectional solidarity in Portugal". In: Sitrin, M. and Sembrar, C. (eds.) *Pandemic Solidarity: Mutual Aid during the Covid-19 Crisis.* Pluto Press, pp. 123–137.

Iron, R. (2020). "Pandemic … or *syndemic*? Re-framing COVID-19 disease burden and 'underlying health conditions'", *Social Anthropology*, 28(2), pp. 286–287.

Kim, M. E. (2018). "From carceral feminism to transformative justice: Women-of-color feminism and alternatives to incarceration". *Journal of Ethnic & Cultural Diversity in Social Work*, 27(3), pp. 219–233. doi: 10.1080/15313204.2018.1474827 [Accessed 26 May 2020].

Lorde, A. (1988). *A Burst of Light and Other Essays.* New York: Ixia Press (this edition 2017).

Mbembe, A. (2003). "Necropolitics". *Public Culture*, 15(1), pp. 11–40.

Mezzadra, S. and Neilson, B. (2013). *Border as Method, or, the Multiplication of Labor.* Durham: Duke University Press.

Michaeli, I. (2017). "Self-Care: An Act of Political Warfare or a Neoliberal Trap?" *Development* 60, pp. 50–56. https://doi.org/10.1057/s41301-017-0131-8 [Accessed 2 April 2020].

Povinelli, E. (2016). *Geontologies. A Requiem to Late Liberalism.* Durham and London: Duke University Press.

Segato, R. (2018). *Contra-pedagogías de la crueldad.* Ciudad Autónoma de Buenos Aires: Prometeo Libros.

Sekalala, S. and Rawson, B. (2020). *Navigating the Paradoxes of Selective COVID-19 Border Closure* [online]. Available at: https://www.law.ox.ac.uk/research-subject-groups/centre-criminology/centreborder-criminologies/blog/2020/07/navigating [Accessed 30 May 2020].

Schmitt, C. (1962). *Theory of the Partisan: Intermediate Commentary on the Concept of the Political.* New York: Telos Press Publishing (this edition 2007).

Simões, S. S., Murray L., Toledo, P., Blanchette, T. G., and Silva, A. P. (2020). *A prostituta, o vírus e a cidade* [online]. Available at: http://ippur.ufrj.br/index.php/pt-br/noticias/outros-eventos/672-a-prostituta-o-virus-a-cidade [Accessed 30 June 2020].

Singer, M. and Snipes, C. (1992). "Generations of suffering: Experiences of a treatment program for substance abuse during pregnancy". *Journal of Health Care for the Poor and Underserved*, 3(1), pp. 222–234.

Singer, M. (1994). "AIDS and the health crisis of the U.S. urban poor: The perspective of critical medical anthropology". *Social Science & Medicine*, 39(7), pp. 931–948. https://doi.org/10.1016/0277-9536(94)90205-4 [Accessed 5 May 2020].

VV.AA. (2020). Carta aberta. Covid-19 e os Centros de Detenção em Portugal: 41 associações e mais de 100 cidadãos pedem libertação dos migrantes [online]. Available at: https://expresso.pt/opiniao/2020-04-09-Carta-aberta.-Covid-19-e-os-Centros-de-Detencao-em-Portugal-41-associacoes-e-mais-de-100-cidadaos-pedem-libertacao-dos-migrantes [Accessed 20 May 2020].

Wacquant, L. (2008). The place of prison in the new government of poverty. In: Frampton, M., Lopez, I., and Simon, J. (eds.), *After the War on Crime: Race, Democracy and the New Reconstruction*. New York: New York University Press, pp. 23–37.

32

BEYOND CRISIS

Building Child-Friendly Cities as Bird-Friendly Spaces
December 2020

Chandni Basu

Stray birds of summer come to my window to sing and fly away.
– Rabindranath Tagore, Stray Birds (1916)[1]

Bulbuli, Benebou, Boshonto Bouri, Tia…(Bulbul, Oriole, Barbet, Parrot…) the list is pretty endless. These feathered creatures visiting neighbourhoods all over the city from their green ghettos seem to outwit the otherwise pensive mood of the viral attack rocking the earth in many ways than one over the last months. Only the visiting birds in the city neighbourhoods along with the bats flying in and out of their nests on the date palm tree, after dusk, in front of my home possibly are the happiest with the spread of the virus all around. Their visit from the nearby *Rabindra Sarovar*,[2] the lake area, has created an atmosphere of happiness in our neighbourhood. My elderly mother's lockdown moment anxieties eased a bit watching the birds sing while dancing around with the hoppers and butterflies. Surely she missed her 11-year-old grandchild while enjoying these moments with the bird visitors in her South Kolkata[3] apartment.

This chapter has three sections. The first section delves into the impact of the 2020 lockdown on the environment. It is followed by a reflection on the imagination of a child-friendly city, and finally, the third section discusses the concept of a green childhood.

Lockdown and the Environment

The lockdown phase (March–June 2020) in India has been an environment conservator's relief till now. It saw Olive Ridley Turtles laying eggs in peace at the coast in Rushikulya[4], Flamingo visits in Mumbai or the visible Himalayan range standing gorgeously in front of Jalandhar.[5] Lokhandwala and Gautam (2020)[6] observe the positive impact on the environment, which came along with the lockdown, "worldwide spread of COVID-19 in

DOI: 10.4324/9781003320524-42

a quite short time has brought a dramatic decrease in industrial activities, road traffic, and tourism. Restricted human interaction with nature during this crisis time has appeared as a blessing for nature and environment." They note the improvement in the air quality in India along with improvement in river quality in a number of rivers, including the Ganga, Cauvery, Sutlej, and Yamuna, due to lesser industrial activity during the lockdown period. Further, they note, "undoubtedly COVID-19 has brought a fearful devastating scourge for human beings but it has emerged as a blessing for the natural environment providing it a 'recovery time'" (Lokhandwala and Gautam 2020). Arora et al. (2020)[7] mention, "[D]uring the period of lockdown across the world, the sight of the blue sky created a sense of optimism among the people towards a clean and better environment." Animals and birds were observed in spaces that were previously occupied by humans. Deer, peacocks, monkeys, elephants, birds, dolphins, etc., were seen in greater numbers near human-occupied spaces and settlements. During the lockdown, experts noted the breeding of birds in spaces that were otherwise human occupied. As migratory birds visited lakes and water bodies in greater numbers, the reduction of traffic noise in the cities made birds' chirping and songs more audible (ibid).

At my Kolkata home, the freshness in the air was matched with the glistening coconut leaves and the songs of the *Doyel* (Magpie Robin) to wake us up for the day in the neighbourhood. The lockdown phase has given many of us privileged ones a scope to pause and reflect even while encountering bouts of frustrated attacks from intimate others.[8] I suddenly take account of my room, which has kept transforming itself over the last 30 years from the children's play zone into the adult workspace now. In a kaleidoscopic moment, my love for children and birds blended. The Childhood Researcher in me laid down her post lockdown agenda: child-friendly cities as bird-friendly spaces. Such an agenda lies at the crossing of childhood research, urban planning, and the green movement. Imagining urban spaces for the twenty-first century in post-Covid times, therefore, ought to bring together pending agendas. It is not only time to reimagine childhoods but also to put childhoods along with nature at the centre stage of metropolitan existence in this century.

Child-Friendly Cities

Until now there have been calls to make city spaces bird-friendly by urban planners. Timothy Beatley at the Department of Urban and Environmental Planning, University of Virginia, says, "hearing birds is one of the joys of life and for me triggers intense memories of childhood" (2015). He refers to research and practice, one where children responded positively to bird songs played to them during vaccination at the Liverpool hospital. His commentary highlights watching and listening to birds as an important element of urban stress reduction. Notably, Timothy Beatley[9] (2020) is an advocate of intertwining built and natural environments. In recent times, calls for Ecourbanism or Biophilia[10] have led to initiatives like Child-Responsive Urban Planning (UNICEF 2018). In India, the National Institute of Urban Affairs, New Delhi, in partnership with the Bernard van Leer Foundation, has set its goal towards Child Friendly Smart Cities. Bhubaneswar has been declared a child-friendly city in India. It includes a sensory park for children with special needs.

Identity of a child-friendly city remains in its bird-friendliness. The lockdown experience urges us to imagine child-friendly cities as bird-friendly spaces. The green city initiative by now includes ten cities in India and waits to be expanded to the metropolitan cities. Environmental degradation and ill health are on the rise in cities the world over and are particularly damaging to children. An emerging global child-friendly cities movement is focused on children's rights and participation (Gill 2017: 5). By 2030, it is expected that 70 per cent of the world population will inhabit urban areas and among these, children are projected to be the majority of the population (ibid). This puts urban planning and designing in front of a challenge. Designing for urban childhoods makes it imperative to put children's needs, experiences, and views at the centre stage in order to respond to the challenges of urban existence. In other words, it could be said that a city's sustenance, success, and health depends on its child-friendliness.

Within the field of urban planning, child-friendliness is an emerging concept. It argues that a city's wellness could be measured by the quality of its child-friendliness. Hence, a child-friendly city indicates the quality of living in the city not only for children but for all its inhabitants irrespective of age. Tim Gill defines child-friendliness in urban planning as "a coherent and systematic approach to planning and designing cities that improves children's development, health and access to opportunities, moving well beyond simply providing playgrounds" (Gill 2017: 7). Further, it recognises "the fundamental importance, not just of independence and play, but of the built environment as a whole in helping to shape a child's development and prospects, and hence their adult lives." Child-friendliness of a city could be measured by "the amount of time children spend playing outdoors, their ability to get around independently, and their level of contact with nature are strong indicators of how a city is performing, and not just for children but for all city dwellers" (ibid).

A child-friendly city is a new concept. The first global Child Friendly Cities Summit was held in October 2019 in Cologne, Germany on the occasion of the 30th anniversary of the United Nations Convention on the Rights of the Child, 1989.[11] At this event, the Cologne Mayor's Declaration for Child Friendly Cities was signed by more than 100 city mayors and regional leaders from different parts of the world. It is built on a manifesto called 'Our cities. Our lives. Our future.' where 120,000 young people from more than 160 countries contributed towards creating safer, more inclusive, healthier, and greener cities. Notably, the Child Friendly Cities

Initiative was launched in 1996 by UNICEF. In the child-friendly cities' handbook, a child-friendly city is defined as "a city, town, community or any system of local governance which recognises the voices, needs and priorities of children as an integral part of public policies, programmes and decisions" (UNICEF 2018: 10). In this sense, a child-friendly city is a city that is fit for all.

The major challenges to urban childhoods comprise the following: traffic and pollution; high-rise living and urban sprawl; crime, social fears and risk aversion; isolation and intolerance; and inadequate and unequal access to the city (Gill 2017: 8). The concepts of 'everyday freedom' and 'children's infrastructure' become important here. It urges us to see the city from a child's perspective while enhancing children's experience of the city. In other words, a city that prioritises children's free movements in different spaces along with building children's connections to green and healthy environments could be considered to follow child-friendly practices.

Green Childhood

The lockdown phase (2020) has been one of reminiscences too. Watching the circling cranes in an early morning sky as the coconut leaves rustle surely brought back memories of visits to my grandparent's garden house as a child. Laying forth the agenda of a child-friendly city resonates with youth movements in recent times like 'Fridays for Future', which started in Bad Segeberg, Germany, in December 2018. The demands by young people for a cleaner earth also conceived green childhood for the twenty-first century. Such protests for a greener earth by young people synergise with imaginations of childhoods from the early decades of the twentieth century. Rabindranath Tagore remains a pioneer in this direction. As the first Nobel Laureate beyond the North Atlantic hemisphere, Tagore's vision of childhood had a romantic flavour, much beyond the already critiqued Romantic primitivism. His poems for children or stories involving child characters sketch his romantic vision of childhood in its postcolonial essence. A biophilic green childhood for the twenty-first century therefore could tune its resonance from such romantic visions. Tagore's vision of childhood, which was biophilic in essence led him to model the nature-based education centre in Shantiniketan[12] (the abode of peace) near the Santhal villages of Birbhum – the land of red soil away from the British capital of Calcutta. In *Tapaban* ('The Forest' 1910), he emphasised a child's spiritual relation with nature. According to him, true education is the realisation of the universe by spirit, volition, and mind. This ushers in spiritual universalism as the ultimate truth of life (Podder 2018: 101).

The positive influence of green exposure on children's well-being has been accounted for in recent scientific studies. Childhood research further puts forth the need to dismantle the standardised notion of normative modern childhood predominant in mainstream society. A move towards green childhood in this sense not only will ensure children's well-being but will also lay forth the ideals of a romantic imagination of childhood, as the litterateur Rabindranath Tagore envisaged. Significantly, Tagore advocated assimilation of the nature, world, and the human in his literary pieces (Podder 2018: 99). Child-friendly cities as bird-friendly spaces remain the call of the hour and the way forward in the twenty-first century. It enriches the imagination of postcolonial childhoods in contemporary times, which endeavours to reorganise normative childhood from its colonial influences. The romantic vision of childhood bringing young people and nature together, along with a model of nature-based education as a foundation of green/postcolonial childhoods remains an essential component of ecourbanism-biophilia.

Tagore's idea of romantic childhood resonates in the concept of the 'Waldkindergärten'[13] in contemporary times in Germany. These are preschool centres for children between three and six years of age. It socialises children through open-air activities with natural materials, thus educating them to lead a responsible life close to nature. Encouraging children irrespective of their social profiles towards more green engagement along with the practice of gratitude in their everyday life will establish the norms and foundation of a more harmonious coexistence and interaction among all living species, especially within urban spaces. Such a foundation will uphold the deeper interconnectedness of the earth and the world, as the overarching common social reality influencing policy and educational decisions impacting urban children's lives in different societies. More open spaces within the city limits, with an increased green cover, water bodies along with better mobility access for young people will ensure their interactions with birds along with butterflies, hoppers, and others. In a tropical climatic zone as in parts of South Asia, child-friendly cities as bird-friendly spaces could go a long way towards maintaining the variety of flora and fauna in urban spaces.

Conclusion

At a time when urban spaces are ever-increasing in terms of their geographical limits and population density, especially in postcolonial societies[14], the call for a child-friendly city as a bird-friendly space remains the need of the hour. This is significant in postcolonial cities, given the rise in pollution levels due to increased traffic and industrial activities. Envisaging the model of a green childhood in a child-friendly city, hence, is important with its multifarious positive impacts like lowering of pollution levels by increasing the green cover of the city to invite more bird visitors and of making the city space safer for its young inhabitants.[15] It, therefore, remains an ethical vision of making urban habitation more inclusive of different forms of life with the spirit to create child-responsive cities and communities.

Notes

1 Rabindranath Tagore (1861–1941) was a polymath born in Bengal. He received the Nobel Prize for literature in 1913 for his collection *Gitanjali*. https://www. ibiblio.org/eldritch/rt/stray.htm [Accessed 29 January 2021].

2 The Rabindra Sarovar lake area in the southern part of Kolkata was envisaged in the 1920s. It is an artificial lake and has water bodies spread over 73 acres. The rest (over 100 acres) is covered by trees ranging up to 50 species. It is home to birds and is also visited by migratory birds.

3 Kolkata (Calcutta) is a metropolitan city in eastern India with a population of 4,496,694. It is the capital of the state of West Bengal sharing a land border with Bangladesh. Its urban/metropolitan population is 14,035,959, according to the Census Report, 2011, Government of India. It is known as the cultural capital of India. South Kolkata is a newer part of the city that mostly came up in post-independent (1947) India. https://www.census2011.co.in/census/city/215-kolkata.html [Accessed 29 January 2021].

4 Rushikulya is a beach in the state of Odisha, next to the Bay of Bengal.

5 Jalandhar is a city in the state of Punjab.

6 For details see, Lokhandwala and Gautam (2020), https://www.ncbi.nlm.nih. gov/pmc/articles/PMC7299871/ [Accessed 29 January 2021].

7 See, https://www.ncbi.nlm.nih.gov/pmc/articles/PMC7323667/ [Accessed 2 February 2021].

8 The lockdown phase (2020) saw a surge in domestic violence towards women in India. See 'Lockdown and rise in domestic violence: How to tackle situation if locked with an abuser', The Indian Express, https://indianexpress.com/article/lifestyle/life-style/lockdown-rise-of-domestic-violence-how-to-tackle-situation-if-locked-with-abuser-national-commission-for-women-6406268/ [Accessed 29 January 2021].

9 For more understanding, see Beatley (2020).

10 The term was coined by Dr. Edward O. Wilson. It refers to the innate tendency among humans to bond with nature and other species. For further understanding, see Edward O. Wilson (1984) Biophilia, Harvard University Press.

11 See, https://childfriendlycities.org/mayors-commit-to-action-for-children-at-the-child-friendly-cities-summit/ [Accessed 30 January 2021].

12 Tagore founded Shantiniketan near Bolpur, West Bengal, in 1901. Here children are taught under the trees, in the open air. In post-independent times, it became a central university named Viswa Bharati.

13 See, https://smartergerman.com/blog/waldkindergarten-forest-kindergarten/ [Accessed 1 February 2021].

14 For further understanding on postcolonial cities, see King (2009).

15 The *Sabooj Sathi* scheme by the West Bengal government since 2015 has earned the WSIS winner award in 2020. Under the scheme, bicycles are distributed among students in high schools within the public education system. It encourages retention of students within the formal education system by motivating both girls and boys to continue their education. The scheme envisages coverage to 40 lakh students in different districts of West Bengal. For details see, https://indianexpress.com/article/cities/kolkata/had-contested-with-800-projects-after-kanyashree-bengal-govt-bags-wsis-award-for-its-sabuj-sathi-scheme-6589951/ [Accessed 2 February 2021]; https://wbsaboojsathi.gov.in/v2/ [Accessed 2 February 2021].

References

Arora, S., Bhaukhandi, K. D., and Mishra, P. K. (2020). 'Coronavirus lockdown helped the environment to bounce back'. *Science of the Total Environment*, 1–25.

Beatley, T. (2020). *The Bird Friendly City: Creating Safe Urban Habitats*, Washington, DC: Island Press.

Gill, T. (2017). *Cities Alive: Designing for Urban Childhoods*, London: ARUP.

King, A. D. (2009). *Postcolonial Cities*, Binghamton: Elsevier.

Lokhandwala, S., and Gautam, P. (2020). 'Indirect impact of COVID-19 on environment: A brief study in Indian context', *Environmental Research*, 1–25.

Podder, K. (2018). 'Tagore's view on liberty of childhood: A closed study on Gitanjali', *International Journal of Research and Analytical Reviews*, 5(3), 99–101.

Tagore, R. (1916). *Stray Birds*, New York: The Macmillan Company.

UNICEF. (2018). *Child Friendly Cities and Communities Handbook*, United Nation's Childrens Fund.

INDEX

Pages in *italics* refer to figures.